Y0-CBB-195

Physical Medicine and Rehabilitation

Rehabilitation of Fractures

Guest Editor:

Arun J. Mehta, MB, FRCPC

Associate Clinical Professor
Division of Rehabilitation Medicine
Department of Medicine
University of California, Los Angeles, School of Medicine
Los Angeles, California
        and
Physical Medicine and Rehabilitation Service
Veterans Affairs Medical Center
Sepulveda, California

Volume 9/Number 1   February 1995
HANLEY & BELFUS, INC.   Philadelphia

STATE OF THE ART REVIEWS

Publisher: **HANLEY & BELFUS, INC.**
210 South 13th Street
Philadelphia, PA 19107
(215) 546-7293
(215) 790-9330 (Fax)

PHYSICAL MEDICINE AND REHABILITATION: State of the Art Reviews is included in *BioSciences Information Service, Current Contents, ISI/BIOMED,* and *Cumulative Index to Nursing & Allied Health Literature.*

PHYSICAL MEDICINE AND REHABILITATION: State of the Art Reviews   ISSN 0888-7357
Volume 9, Number 1   ISBN 1-56053-183-5

PHYSICAL MEDICINE AND REHABILITATION: State of the Art Reviews is published triannually (three times per year) by Hanley & Belfus, Inc., 210 South 13th Street, Philadelphia, Pennsylvania 19107.

POSTMASTER: Send address changes to PHYSICAL MEDICINE AND REHABILITATION: State of the Art Reviews, Hanley & Belfus, Inc., 210 South 13th Street, Philadelphia, PA 19107.

The 1995 subscription price is $72.00 per year U.S., $82.00 outside U.S. (add $30.00 for air mail). Single copies $34.00 U.S., $37.00 outside U.S. (add $10.00 for single copy air mail).

Physical Medicine and Rehabilitation: State of the Art Reviews
Vol. 9, No. 1, February 1995

REHABILITATION OF FRACTURES
Arun J. Mehta, MB, FRCPC, Editor

CONTENTS

CONTRIBUTORS

Rajnikant K. Bakhda, MD
Assistant Clinical Professor, Department of Radiology, University of California, Los Angeles; Staff Radiologist, West L.A. Veterans Affairs Medical Center, Los Angeles, California

Sidney J. Blair, MD, FACS
Professor Emeritus, Department of Orthopedic Surgery, Loyola University Medical Center, Maywood, Illinois

Cynthia C. Catindig, RN
Staff Nurse, Orthopedic/Rehabilitation Ward, Veterans Affairs Medical Center, Sepulveda, California

Anna Marie Cheney, RN, BS, MS
Medical/Surgical Clinical Nurse Specialist, Veterans Affairs Medical Center, Sepulveda, California

David X. Cifu, MD
Assistant Professor, Department of Physical Medicine and Rehabilitation, Medical College of Virginia, Richmond, Virginia

Marlyn Delim, RN
Veterans Affairs Medical Center, Sepulveda, California

Caridad B. Divina, RNC, MSN
Community Health Nurse Coordinator, Nursing Service, Veterans Affairs Medical Center, Sepulveda, California

Thao Thi Thu Duong, MD
Assistant Professor, Department of Rehabilitation Medicine, University of Colorado Health Sciences Center; Director, Rehabilitation Services, Denver General Hospital, Denver, Colorado

Barbara Andre Flynn, RN
Veterans Affairs Medical Center, Sepulveda, California

Steve R. Geiringer, MD
Associate Professor, Department of Physical Medicine and Rehabilitation, Wayne State University; Medical Director, Outpatient Services and Electrodiagnostic Services, The Rehabilitation Institute of Michigan, Detroit, Michigan

Gerard Glancy, MD
Department of Orthopaedics, The Children's Hospital, Denver, Colorado

V. Nanda Kumar, MD
Clinical Professor, Department of Rehabilitation Medicine, University of Kansas Medical Center, Kansas City, Kansas

Sulabha Masih, MD
Assistant Clinical Professor, Department of Radiology, University of California, Los Angeles; Staff Radiologist, West L.A. Veterans Affairs Medical Center, Los Angeles, California

Edward G. McFarland, MD
Director, Section of Sports Medicine and Shoulder Surgery; Assistant Professor, Department of Orthopaedic Surgery, The Johns Hopkins University School of Medicine; Consulting Team Physician, The Baltimore Orioles, Baltimore, Maryland

Kenneth J. McLeod, PhD
Associate Professor, Department of Orthopaedics, State University of New York, Stony Brook, New York

Arun J. Mehta, MB, FRCPC
Associate Clinical Professor, Division of Rehabilitation Medicine, Department of Medicine, University of California, Los Angeles, School of Medicine, Los Angeles; Physical Medicine and Rehabilitation Service, Veterans Affairs Medical Center, Sepulveda, California

Scott Naftulin, DO
Physical Medicine and Rehabilitation Services, Coordinated Health Systems, Bethlehem, Pennsylvania

Steven Niergarth, DO
Department of Orthopedic Surgery, Michigan State University, College of Osteopathic Medicine, East Lansing, Michigan

Abna A. Ogle, MD
Assistant Professor, Department of Rehabilitation Medicine; Medical Director, Rehabilitation Unit, University of Kansas Medical Center, Kansas City, Kansas

Bryan J. O'Young, MD
Department of Rehabilitation Medicine, The Johns Hopkins University School of Medicine, Baltimore, Maryland

Mersamma Philip, MD
Assistant Professor, Department of Physical Medicine and Rehabilitation, Northwestern University Medical School, Chicago, Illinois

Puliyodil A. Philip, MD
Assistant Professor, Department of Physical Medicine and Rehabilitation, Northwestern University Medical School; Associate Director, Brain Injury Program, Rehabilitation Institute of Chicago, Chicago, Illinois

Clinton T. Rubin, PhD
Professor of Orthopedics, Musculo-Skeletal Research Laboratory, State University of New York, Stony Brook, New York

Pamela E. Santellano, RN
Nurse Manager, Veterans Affairs Medical Center, Sepulveda, California

Mehrsheed Sinaki, MD, MS
Consultant, Department of Physical Medicine and Rehabilitation, Mayo Clinic and Mayo Foundation; Professor of Physical Medicine and Rehabilitation, Mayo Medical School, Rochester, Minnesota

Jeffrey W. Spychalski, MD
Department of Orthopaedics, University of California, Los Angeles, Medical Center, Los Angeles, California

Lynne M. Stempien, MD
Assistant Medical Director, Rehabilitation Center, The Children's Hospital, Denver, Colorado

Marilyn R. Strong, RN
Veterans Affairs Medical Center, Sepulveda, California

Jay V. Subbarao, MD, MS
Clinical Professor, Department of Orthopedic Surgery, Physical Medicine and Rehabilitation Section, Loyola University Medical Center, Hines Comprehensive Rehabilitative Services, Maywood Illinois

Bert J. Thomas, MD
Associate Professor of Orthopaedic Surgery, Department of Orthopaedics, University of California, Los Angeles, Medical Center, Los Angeles, California

Edward S. Traisman, MD
Assistant Clinical Professor, Departments of Pediatrics and Physical Medicine and Rehabilitation, Northwestern University Medical School, Chicago, Illinois

Mark A. Young, MD
Assistant Professor, Department of Physical Medicine and Rehabilitation, The Johns Hopkins University School of Medicine, Baltimore, Maryland

Robert S. Zucker, MD, MPH
Clinical Assistant Professor, Department of Physical Medicine and Rehabilitation, The Ohio State University; Chief, Physical Medicine and Rehabilitation Service, Veterans Affairs Outpatient Clinic, Columbus, Ohio

PUBLISHED ISSUES 1987–1992
(available from the publisher)

1993 ISSUES

Long-Term Consequences of Stroke
Robert W. Teasell, MD, Editor
London, Ontario, Canada

Management for Rehabilitation Medicine II
F. Patrick Maloney, MD, and Richard P. Gray, MD, Editors
Little Rock, Arkansas

Neurologic and Orthopaedic Sequelae of Traumatic Brain Injury
Lance R. Stone, DO, Editor
Downey, California

HIV-Related Disability: Assessment and Management
Michael W. O'Dell, MD, Editor
Cincinnati, Ohio

1994 ISSUES

Prosthetics
Alberto Esquenazi, MD, Editor
Philadelphia, Pennsylvania

Cancer Rehabilitation
Fae H. Garden, MD, and Martin Grabois, MD, Editors
Houston, Texas

Spasticity
Richard T. Katz, MD, Editor
St. Louis, Missouri

1995 ISSUES

Rehabilitation of Fractures
Arun J. Mehta, MB, FRCPC, Editor
Sepulveda, California

Sexuality and Disability
Trilok N. Monga, MD, Editor
Houston, Texas

The Autonomic Nervous System
Robert W. Teasell, MD, Editor
London, Ontario, Canada

Subscriptions for full year and single issues available from the publisher—
Hanley & Belfus, Inc., 210 South 13th Street, Philadelphia, PA 19107.
Telephone (215) 546-7293; (800) 962-1892. Fax (215) 790-9330.

PREFACE

The most important goal in the treatment of any injury is to regain the maximum level of function in physical, psychological, social, vocational, and avocational spheres of life. To achieve this goal, all health professionals should make every effort to prevent complications and treat functional deficits that result from injury. This makes rehabilitation the most important phase in the treatment of fractures. The fracture may heal in perfect alignment, but if adjacent joints are stiff or muscles are weak, the patient will not be able to use the extremity in an optimal fashion. Some patients with fractures have other medical problems that may need attention. It is important to take into account all the factors that may interfere with the maximum level of function and not restrict our attention only to the fracture or the involved extremity.

Physiatrists should be involved in the rehabilitation of patients with fractures from the very beginning to prevent complications such as stiffness of joints and atrophy of muscles and to look into psychosocial, vocational, and avocational concerns of the patient. General principles of rehabilitation need to be applied to this group of patients. The physiatrist involved in the rehabilitation of patients with fractures should be familiar with mechanisms of skeletal injury, general principles of fracture treatment, radiologic features of stages of healing, complications of fractures, and recent developments in the field of orthopedics. This knowledge will help in communicating with orthopedic surgeons and planning treatment strategies. An interdisciplinary treatment approach has become an accepted concept in which few health professionals are trained and/or willing to put into practice because it is very time-consuming. A successful team approach requires frequent communication with the team members, knowledge of their strengths and weaknesses, and a special mental attitude of considering the patient as an individual with more than a broken bone. A physiatrist brings in this special knowledge and training for a successful outcome.

Skeletal injuries are very common, and their treatment consumes a significant percentage of the total health care dollars. Most fractures, even those that do not require admission to a hospital, affect activities of daily living, and additional assistance at home may be required. Intervention by rehabilitation professionals can improve outcome, return patients to gainful employment, prevent unnecessary admission to a nursing home, and ultimately save money by reducing dependence on health care providers or family members. However, there is great need for research studies to show how rehabilitation interventions help improve functional outcome and reduce costs to society.

I have been very fortunate to have an excellent faculty to contribute chapters on various aspects of the rehabilitation of fractures. I am very grateful to all of the authors for their time and effort. This volume should be especially useful to residents in training and physiatrists who have recently finished their training.

Arun J. Mehta, MB, FRCPC
Guest Editor

ARUN J. MEHTA, MB, FRCPC

AN INTRODUCTION

From the Physical Medicine &
  Rehabilitation Service
Veterans Administration Medical
  Center
Sepulveda, California

Reprint requests to:
Arun J. Mehta, MB, FRCPC
Physical Medicine & Rehabilitation
  Service (117)
Veterans Affairs Medical Center
16111 Plummer Street
Sepulveda, CA 91343

Rehabilitation is the most important phase in the treatment of fractures.[1] Most of the patients require rehabilitation to regain function after an injury that results in a fracture even if it does not require reduction or immobilization. The fracture may heal in perfect alignment, but if the adjacent joints are stiff or muscles are weak the patient will not be able to use the extremity in an optimal fashion. Some patients with fractures have other medical, psychological, social, vocational, or avocational problems that may interfere with optimal functioning and may need attention. It is important to take into account all the factors that interfere with maximum level of function and not just pay attention to the fracture or the involved extremity.

Physiatrists should be involved in the rehabilitation of fracture patients from the initial stages to prevent complications such as stiffness of joints and atrophy of muscles and to look into psychosocial, vocational, and avocational concerns of the patient. General principles of rehabilitation need to be applied to this group of patients to achieve the maximum level of function. Physiatrists involved in the rehabilitation of patients with fracture should be familiar with mechanisms of skeletal injury, general principles of fracture treatment, radiologic features of stages of healing and complications of fractures, and recent developments in the field of orthopedics. This knowledge will help in communicating with orthopedic surgeons and planning treatment strategies.

EPIDEMIOLOGY

Skeletal injuries are very common, and their treatment takes up a significant part of the total health care dollars in the United States. In 1990, 1,017,000 cases of fractures were reported in the U.S.[6] In Norway Sahlin reported an incidence of 22.8 fractures per 1,000 population per year. In general, some of the most common fractures, in decreasing order of frequency, are distal forearm, rib, foot, carpal or metacarpal bone, hip, and finger. Fractures of the forearm, rib, and hip are the most common among the elderly. After the age of 50, the incidence of these fractures increases considerably, doubling for every five years' increase in age.[8] In the United Kingdom the incidence of fracture of the femoral neck increased by 10% per year from 1971 to 1977 even though the elderly population increased by only 2%.[23] The rate of occurrence of hip fractures in the U.S. is highest in women of European descent and lowest in men of African descent.[10] The overall age-adjusted rate for hip fractures in women of different racial backgrounds in California was examined by Silverman and Madison.[19] The overall rate was much lower in Hispanic, black, and Asian American women than in white females. Visits to the emergency room for fractures are also very common in children.

Nearly a third of all patients with fractures require admission to a hospital for treatment. Half of all the hospital days necessary for the treatment of all fractures are required by fractures of the proximal femur. Reduction of fractures (excluding the skull, nose, and jaw) was the third most common surgical procedure performed in 1989 on males of all ages (342,000) after cardiac catheterization and prostatectomy.[6] For fractures the average length of hospital stay in the U.S. was 8.3 days in 1990.

High-energy accidents such as motor vehicle accidents lead to multisystem trauma. They occur in about 2–5% of all fractures, but because of the complexity of these injuries, an inordinate amount of resources are required to treat them. Specially trained trauma surgeons and highly skilled nursing and other professionals are essential for a good outcome. The average age of the patients in this category is 34.[9] These patients are in the prime of their life, and concentrated effort should be made to rehabilitate them to the best of their ability. However, because of the expense of running a trauma center, training staff, and preventing burnout and early turnaround of staff, some trauma centers in the U.S. are being closed.

PATHOLOGY

Most fractures occur as a result of injury—a fall, motor vehicle accident, or some other form of violence. When a person falls, a bone further away from the site of impact may be broken. This is described as indirect violence. Fracture due to direct violence occurs when forearm bones are broken in a fight after the patient has tried to protect himself from being hit by a stick by bringing the forearm in front of his head. A fracture through a metastasis in a bone is called a pathologic fracture. Sometimes a fracture develops in a normal bone due to repeated stress over a period of time—e.g., fracture of a metatarsal in an Army recruit during basic training. The skin over the fracture is usually intact. In open, or compound, fractures there is communication with the outside, and these fractures require special treatment to prevent infection.

Elderly people can fall while walking and break a bone. The fracture occurs because of deterioration in the bone mass due to osteoporosis. Poor balance, orthostatic hypotension, and deteriorating vision are some common reasons for a fall. Parkinson's disease, cerebrovascular accidents, and generalized weakness can also lead to loss of balance. It is difficult for elderly people to clear the ground by lifting their feet up while walking. They can trip and fall easily when they encounter a loose piece of rug.

Fracture Healing

The rate of fracture healing varies with age and is much faster in young children. There is less chance of stiffness of joints and greater possibility of correction of deformity by remodeling. Children require less formal rehabilitation than the elderly for these reasons. The time it takes for the soft tissues and bone to heal needs to be considered when planning rehabilitation therapies. Delayed union, nonunion, or instability of a joint may result if vigorous exercises or weightbearing are started prematurely.[2]

The process of healing is different in cortical and cancellous bones. Healing also is affected by the distance between the bone fragments and movement at the fracture site. Many blood vessels are torn at the time of the injury. Bleeding from these vessels forms a hematoma at the fracture site. The periosteum is lifted off the bone, and ends of the bone become necrotic. Muscles and ligaments also suffer the effects of this injury. The cells lining the periosteum and endosteum start dividing, and most of them mature into osteoblasts. Some of them become chondroblasts and form cartilage tissue. The osteoblasts form an intercellular matrix of collagen fibers in which calcium hydroxyappatite is deposited. This tissue is called the callus. The callus matures into bone with a mature lamellar structure. The excessive bone gets resorbed over a period of many months. In children this remodeling process may even correct deformity to a certain extent. The process of healing in cancellous bone is more efficient, and fractures of bones with a large proportion of cancellous bone, such as an intertrochanteric fracture of femur, heal most of the time. There is always some soft tissue injury with any fracture. Unlike bone, ligaments and muscles heal by formation of fibrous tissue that has different mechanical properties than the original tissue. The scar tissue does not perform as well as the uninjured tissue.

ORTHOPEDIC MANAGEMENT

The initial management of fractures is beyond the scope of this book. The clinical diagnosis of a fracture is confirmed by x-rays. The clinician then determines whether the fracture fragments need to be manipulated and reduced to bring them back to as normal an alignment as possible. This can be done without an open operation (closed reduction), by open reduction, or by continuous traction. The fracture fragments need to be immobilized until there is bony union. Free movement at the fracture site is very painful initially and may lead to malunion or nonunion of the fracture if allowed to continue during the healing process. Movement of fragments is usually prevented by a plaster cast. While the patient is in a cast, the clinician should encourage the patient to perform range of motion exercises for the joints that are not immobilized. It may be possible for the patient to do some isometric exercises for the muscles enclosed in the cast. Skin ulceration and nerve injury are common complications, and every effort should be made to prevent them or, if they do develop, diagnose them early. Ischemic necrosis of muscles enclosed within the cast is a very serious complication that requires emergency treatment.

Fixation devices are sometimes used and are put inside the medullary cavity or over the cortex of the bone (internal fixation) to maintain fracture reduction. Fractures that are likely to be displaced after reduction or are not likely to unite without a rigid internal fixation (such as fractures of the femoral neck) are treated this way. These patients may not show much callus on x-rays. The internal fixation devices are not strong enough to withstand weightbearing stress before the fracture is healed. However, internal fixation may reduce the length of stay in the hospital and allow range of motion exercises for the adjacent joints and nonweightbearing activities sooner. This may be a distinct advantage for elderly patients because it may allow them to avoid some complications of prolonged bedrest. Internal fixation devices are a foreign body, and infection at the operation site can be a disaster that should be prevented at all cost. Fracture bracing is another method of allowing range of motion exercises and walking early.

GENERAL PRINCIPLES OF REHABILITATION

Evaluation

The usual history and physical examination gives the clinician an idea of the medical problems faced by the patient. Evaluation of a patient before embarking on a program of rehabilitation includes many aspects that are not covered in routine history and physical, such as functional level before the injury, psychological reaction of the patient to the injury, occupation, social support the patient is likely to get after discharge, and others. The rehabilitation professional should know the common signs and symptoms of fractures and soft tissue injuries. It is possible that some of these injuries might have been missed during the first visit to emergency room[15] or after a major accidental injury. A fresh set of x-rays and clinical reevaluation may throw more light on the patient's problems. Osteogenesis imperfecta or child abuse should be ruled out in children with a history of multiple fractures. Osteoporosis is a very common cause of fractures in white menopausal women. Any treatable cause of osteoporosis should be investigated to prevent fractures in the future. Neurovascular injury at the site of the fracture or as a complication of the treatment requires a neurologic examination and palpation of distal pulsations. These injuries may be confirmed by Doppler, electromyography, or nerve conduction studies.

It is important to evaluate how the patient will be able to function at home after a fracture. The Barthel Index is a functional assessment instrument with a numerical scoring system that is used to evaluate 10 activities of daily living. This index was used in one study for patients who were older than 70 and had minor fractures that did not require admission to a hospital. This group of 105 patients, with an average age of 77, showed a significant drop in the Barthel Index after a fracture of the wrist, humerus, or ankle. The drop in score was even more after fractures around the knee and tibia.[17] Determination of functional deficits helps in planning physical and occupational therapy, the need for equipment, help at home, and other needs.

The Team Approach

Evaluation of the patient is carried out by all the members of the team who will be treating the patient. Interdisciplinary team meetings are an integral part of the rehabilitation process. Information from all team members is exchanged during these meetings, and treatment strategies are planned. All the team members are familiar with the special knowledge and expertise other members are able to offer and have respect for each other. Good communication is the cornerstone for successful working of a team, and this is usually achieved by team meetings at regular intervals. Information regarding the patient's medical diagnoses, complications, results of evaluations by all the health professionals, changes in the patient's condition, therapies tried, and the results of all treatments are discussed at these meetings. Accurate and detailed records of the team meetings are useful. Activities of all of the members are coordinated to achieve optimal results for the patient. After a team meeting, all participants should feel that they have achieved something positive. Meetings should start on time and finish within a reasonable amount of time. All team members should have an opportunity to express their views freely, and the team leader should be able to resolve all differences and conflicts amicably. The role of the leader as a facilitator is very important for smooth running of the team. The team needs to be focused on the goals. Personal egos may come in the way of good working relationships and create conflicts between team members. It is essential to develop trust among all professionals.

The team can include professionals who are involved in taking care of the patient. The nurse keeps track of vital signs and how the patient functions on the ward. There should be carry-over from the therapy area to the ward. Patients who are able to put on their shirts in occupational therapy should not expect the nursing staff to do it for them on the ward. Nurses play a very important role in the prevention of decubiti.

The physical therapist works on improving balance, transfer training from bed to chair or standing, and gait training with different aids. Specific exercises are performed to increase range of movements of joints and to increase strength and endurance. Other modalities include local heat, ultrasound, shortwave diathermy, traction, and transcutaneous electrical stimulation.

The occupational therapist evaluates the patient's ability to perform activities of daily living. The need for special equipment to perform some of these activities more easily also is determined by the occupational therapist. The therapist usually provides therapy for hand and upper extremity problems.

Patients may experience fear, anxiety, and depression after an injury. Patients who sustained a fall may be very reluctant to get up and walk. Patients living alone are especially concerned about going home without any social support or help for routine chores such as cleaning and shopping. Anxiety may lead to depression, lethargy, and poor performance in therapy departments. Services of a psychologist or psychiatrist may be required for some patients who are depressed or are difficult to manage because of their behavior. After major trauma, patients may go through a period of denial, depression, or anger toward staff and family. Appropriate advice on how to handle these situations may be necessary.

A medical social worker looks into dynamics of the patient's family to see who may be able to help the patient during the hospitalization and after discharge. The financial situation is adversely affected when patients are not able to return to their job for a prolonged period. Discharge planning can be facilitated by a social worker. It is difficult for patients who live alone to manage at home immediately after discharge from the hospital without any help from relatives or friends. These patients need to be placed in a nursing home or board and care facility where tasks such as preparing meals and washing laundry are done for them. Modification of the workplace environment is an alternative that should be considered. Permanent inability of patients to perform their previous job is a good reason for vocational counseling and training.

After a fracture, most patients are started on narcotics to control pain. These medications need to be slowly discontinued as the severity of pain subsides. The physiatrist should go over all of the medications and discontinue those that are not necessary or change the dose as necessary. More addictive drugs can be substituted by less addictive or nonaddictive medications. Drug dependence develops more easily in people who have a history of alcohol and drug abuse.

The Treatment Plan

The rehabilitation treatment plan is developed in consultation with the orthopedic surgeon. Every orthopedic surgeon, like any other professional, has his or her own method of dealing with different fractures. The orthopedic surgeon may have a specific reason for using a particular method of treating a fracture, and it will be in the interest of good patient care for everyone involved to know why that particular method was selected, its advantages and disadvantages, complications that might occur, any therapy modalities to be avoided, and the outcome that can be expected. The staff should be aware of the general protocol for that type of fracture or method of fixation. Misunderstandings can be avoided by frequent personal communication with the surgeon.

Younger patients require shorter periods of immobilization, do not usually have other medical problems, and, unlike the elderly, do not need very formal rehabilitation programs. Unstable fractures such as comminuted or spiral fractures require closer follow-up to watch for redisplacement of fragments. The rehabilitation management will also depend on whether the fracture required manipulation and closed reduction or open reduction and internal fixation (ORIF). If the surgeon was able to achieve a very strong fixation by a device, the therapy program can be more vigorous.

The treatment program is changed as the fracture heals and the bone can withstand more stress. The x-rays may show increasing callus formation, and the fracture line becomes less distinct. X-rays also help in the diagnosis of complications such as avascular necrosis or nonunion. Appearance of changes suggestive of avascular necrosis in the head of the femur will delay weightbearing on the affected side.

The treatment plan depends on the list of problems of the patient and any of the problems or complications that can be foreseen and avoided (Table 1). This list

TABLE 1.   The Problem List

Number	Problem	Plan	Responsible Professional	Date Initiated	Date of Completion	Comments
I	Pain	Analgesic	MD			
II	Swelling	Elevate hand	RN			
III	ADLs	Teach one-handed activities	OT			
IV	Stiffness	Active ROM exercises	PT or OT			
V	Carpal tunnel syndrome	Prevent swelling	RN, OT			
VI	Degenerative joint disease	Accurate reduction of fragments	MD			
VII	Fasting blood sugar	Control within 95–160 mg/dL	MD			
VIII	Foot drop	Ankle-foot orthosis	MD, orthotist			
IX	Diminished sensation in fingers	Prevent injuries, patient education	OT, RN			

Each problem on the problem list can be given a number, and progress of the patient may be recorded in the format suggested above. A patient with a Colles' fracture and diabetes mellitus may have some of the problems mentioned above.

is not the same as the list of medical diagnoses. For example, a patient with a Colles' fracture may have pain during early stages, swelling of fingers distal to the cast, and inability to make a fist, hold things in the hand, or use the hand functionally. The treatment plan will include analgesics, elevation of the hand while in bed, use of a sling while sitting or standing, active range of motion exercises for fingers, and occupational therapy to teach activities of daily living. The shoulder and elbow joints on the affected side also need to be mobilized. Prevention of complications of the fracture and its treatment need to be considered in the initial treatment plan. In this case, it may include edema of fingers, atrophy of the forearm and hand muscles, and shoulder pain and stiffness while the patient is in a cast. After the cast is removed, carpal tunnel syndrome and degenerative arthritis of the radiocarpal joint may occur. In lower extremity fractures in elderly patients, decubitus ulcers, pneumonia, and urinary tract infection are common complications. The treatment plan will change when the cast comes off to include range of motion exercises for the wrist. Exercises to increase strength are added later. If the patient is osteoporotic, an appropriate workup should be ordered. Another method of writing goals and the treatment plan is shown in Table 2. The goals may be set to avoid future complications or correct existing problems.[14]

Elderly patients who are confined to bed for a long time because of fractures of the lower extremity develop flexion contractures at the hip and knee and plantar flexion contractures at the foot and ankle. Muscles that commonly become tight are the gastrocnemius, rectus femoris, hamstring, and pectoralis major muscles. A tight rectus femoris will prevent full flexion of the knee, whereas hamstring tightness will lead to flexion contracture of the knee.

The presence of other medical problems needs to be considered before formulating a treatment program. Patients with dementia are not able to follow instructions for walking nonweightbearing or remember what was learned the previous day. This may slow their progress. The capacity to learn new things and

TABLE 2.   Goals of Treatment

Goals	Treatment
Relief of pain	Analgesics Immobilization of fracture
Bony union in ideal position	Accurate reduction Maintenance of reduction
Maintain normal range of motion of joints	Immobilize minimum number of joints ROM exercises to joints that are not immobilized
Prevent muscle atrophy and weakness	Isometric and resistive exercises
Restoration of function	Ambulation Activities of daily living Vocational and avocational training
Prevention of complications Deep vein thrombosis	Active foot and ankle exercise Elastic stocking
Pneumonia	Deep breathing exercises
Decubitus ulcers	Avoid pressure on bony prominences

Adapted from Mehta AJ, Nastasi AN: Rehabilitation of fractures in the elderly. Clin Geriatr Med 9:717–730, 1993; with permission.

the ability to follow instructions should be considered in the decision for the type of surgical procedure. In patients with dementia, arthroplasty of the hip may be a better alternative than pinning for fracture of the neck of femur so that the patient is able to start walking the next day. Diabetic peripheral neuropathy may lead to bilateral foot-drop and difficulty in walking. Prescription of an ankle-foot orthosis can make a difference between safe and unsafe ambulation. Some elderly patients with stroke and hemiplegia may also be in similar situations. Children with osteogenesis imperfecta can fracture their bones very easily. Physical and occupational therapists treating these children have to be especially careful to avoid new fractures. Patients with ankylosing spondylitis are especially vulnerable to fractures of the spine.[22] They are also more likely to develop neurologic complications as a result of these fractures. Educating patients may reduce the rate of these serious complications.

Prevention of fractures should be considered in all patients. Important areas to be covered in preventive rehabilitation include avoiding trauma to children with osteogenesis imperfecta and avoiding falls among the osteoporotic elderly. A prospective population study in southern California showed the protective effect of dietary calcium in Caucasian women.[7] The age-adjusted risk factor for hip fracture was inversely related to calcium in the diet. Increasing the peak bone mass and slowing its deterioration by adequate calcium intake and not smoking may reduce the incidence of fractures secondary to osteoporosis.[11] Walking one mile three times a week as a form of exercise helped to reduce the risk of fracture in a study of 3,110 elderly men and women with an average age of 73 years.[20]

Alcohol, antihypertensives, tricyclic antidepressants, and phenothiazines have been implicated in falls.[13] Careful attention should be paid to the medications each patient is taking to eliminate those that may not be safe. Home evaluation for risk factors for falling such as loose pieces of rug or furniture on the floor should be carried out to prevent falls after discharge home. A patient with foot drop should be provided an ankle-foot orthosis. Equipment needs for special problems faced by individual patients can also be assessed at the time of home visit. Vision can be improved by proper prescription of glasses or a cataract operation. All medications prescribed are evaluated to determine if any of them may contribute to orthostatic hypotension or dizziness.

OUTCOME

The outcome of some fractures can be very serious. The mortality rate after a hip fracture is reported at 20–40% within 6 months of injury.[18] On the other hand, when multidisciplinary rehabilitation is provided under the guidance of an interested and knowledgeable physician, there can be significant reduction in the number of placements to nursing homes and improvement in activities of daily living.[12] Mortality after cemented arthroplasy for intracapsular fracture of the femoral neck was studied by Eiskjaer and Ostgard[3] in 240 patients. They found that cardiac disease, residence in a nursing home, chronic pulmonary disease, serum creatinine level more than 1.7 mg/100 mL, pneumonia, and previous myocardial infarction were some of the important factors in fatal outcome.

The effect of a prospective payment system (PPS) on patients with fracture of the neck of the femur was studied by Fitzgerald et al.[4,5] They showed that the length of stay in the acute care hospital decreased by nearly 40% after implementation of a prospective payment system even though patients' age, race, type of fracture, and type of operation remained similar. Decreased lengths of hospital stays were achieved at the cost of an increased number of transfers to nursing homes, which increased from 38% before implementation of PPS to 60% after. The authors also found that a much larger proportion of patients remained in the nursing home for 1 year (from 9% before PPS to 33% after). In other words, the benefit achieved by a shorter length of stay in the acute care setting was offset by larger numbers of patients requiring more help from health professionals at a greater expense to the society in general. The average Medicare payment for a month's stay in a nursing home was $2,141 in 1985. Intensive rehabilitation management immediately postoperatively in an acute hospital may be able to reduce the number of people placed in a nursing home after a hip fracture and thus save a tremendous amount of money. These studies show the importance of rehabilitation in improving outcomes and ultimately saving money by reducing dependence on health providers or family members.

There is still a great need for studies to show how rehabilitation interventions help improve outcome. Authors of a study of 31 patients with intraarticular fractures suggested that early mobilization was beneficial in preventing degenerative changes in the joint at a later date.[21] Ideally one would like to see the results of a controlled trial to prove or disprove this point. In practice, however, it is difficult to deny patients treatments that may be beneficial and to follow these patients for a long time. Use of continuous passive motion in treatment of certain fractures is another area that requires further study (chapter 5). Involvement of professionals trained in rehabilitation medicine in the management of fractures should improve the outcome, the patient's quality of life, and may even reduce the total burden on society.

REFERENCES

1. Adams JC: Outline of Fractures. 9th ed. New York, Churchill Livingstone, 1987.
2. Cornell CN, Lane JM: Newest factors in fracture healing. Clin Orthop 277:297–311, 1992.
3. Eiskjaer S, Ostgard SC: Risk factors influencing mortality after bipolar hemiarthroplasty in the treatment of fracture of the femoral neck. Clin Orthop 270:295–300, 1991.
4. Fitzgerald JF, Fagan LF, Tierney WM, Dittus RS: Changing patterns of hip fracture care before and after implementation of the prospective payment system. JAMA 258:218–221, 1987.
5. Fitzgerald JF, Moore BS, Dittus RS: The care of elderly patients with hip fracture. N Engl J Med 319:1392–1397, 1988.
6. Health United States 1990: US Dept of Health and Human Services, National Center for Health Statistics, Hyattsville, MD, 1991.
7. Holbrook TL, Barrett-Connar E, Wingard DL: Dietary calcium and risk of hip fracture: 14 year prospective population study. Lancet 2:1046–1049, 1988.
8. Jette AM, Harris BA, Cleary PD, Campion EW: Functional recovery after hip fracture. Arch Phys Med Rehabil 68:735–740, 1987.
9. Jurkovich GJ: The role of trauma surgeon in the management of orthopedic trauma. In Hansen ST, Swiontkowski MF (eds): Orthopedic Trauma Protocols. New York, Raven, 1993, pp 9–16.
10. Kellie SE, Brody JA: Sex-specific and race-specific hip fractures rates. Am J Public Health 80:326–328, 1990.
11. Kelsey JL: Risk factors for osteoporosis and associated fractures. Public Health Reports—Hyattsville. 104(suppl):14–20, September-October 1989.
12. Kennie DC, Reid J, Richardson IR, et al: Effectiveness of geriatric rehabilitative care after fractures of the proximal femur in elderly women: A randomised clinical trial. BMJ 297:1083–1086, 1988.
13. MacDonald JB: The role of drugs in falls in the elderly. Clin Geriatr Med 1:621–636, 1985.
14. Mehta AJ, Nastasi AN: Rehabilitation of fractures in the elderly. Clin Geriatr Med 9:717–730, 1993.
15. Moore MN: Orthopedic pitfalls in emergency medicine. South Med J 81:371–378, 1988.
16. Mossey JM, Multran E, Knott K, et al: Determinants of recovery 12 months after hip fracture: The importance of psychosocial factors. Am J Public Health 79:279–286, 1989.

17. Nankhonya JM: Social and functional impact of minor fractures in elderly people. BMJ 303:1514–1515, 1991.

18. Rodriguez JB, Sattin RW, Waxweiler RJ: Incidence of hip fractures, United States, 1970–83. Am J Prev Med 5:175–181, 1989.

19. Silverman SL, Madison RE: Decreased incidence of hip fracture in Hispanics, Asians, and Blacks: California hospital discharge data. Am J Public Health 78:1482–1483, 1988.

20. Sorock GS, Bush TL, Golden AL, et al: Physical activity and fracture risk in a free-living elderly cohort. J Gerontol 43:134–139, 1988.

21. Volpin G, Dowd GS, Stein H, Bentley G: Degenerative arthritis after intraarticular fractures of the knee. J Bone Joint Surg 72B:634–638, 1990.

22. Wade W, Saltzstein R, Maiman D: Spinal fractures complicating ankylosing spondylitis. Arch Phys Med Rehabil 70:398–401, 1989.

23. Wallace WA: The increasing incidence of fractures of the proximal femur: An orthopedic epidemic. Lancet 1:1413–1414, 1983.

24. Wood DJ, Ions GK, Quinby JM, Stevens J: Factors which influence mortality after subcapital hip fracture. J Bone Joint Surg 74B:199–202, 1992.

V. NANDA KUMAR, MD

FRACTURE BRACING

From the Heartland Health System
St. Joseph, Missouri
and
Department of Rehabilitation
Medicine
University of Kansas Medical
Center
Kansas City, Kansas

Reprint requests to:
V. Nanda Kumar, MD
701 Faraon Street
St. Joseph, MO 64501

Early application of a fracture brace after acute symptoms have subsided encourages function. Increased stress is placed on the limb before inherent stability is regained with soft tissue or bony healing.[14] This stage is called stage 1 of fracture healing or stage of instability. Motion at the fracture site encourages cartilage and fibrous tissue formation in the early callus, which is soft and cannot be seen in radiography. This is stage 2 of fracture healing or the soft callus stage. This soft callus can provide rigidity and strength to the bone because of the large moment of inertia. Motion at the fracture site as a result of early functional activity has been documented by various techniques. Such motion has not proved detrimental to fracture healing as long as the surrounding biologic environment is stimulated by functional activity.[9] The enhancement of blood supply and flow of nutrients into the area may contribute to the healing process even in the presence of high levels of tissue strain associated with motion at fracture site.[1,5] When controlled by soft tissue compression with casts and fracture braces, this motion can be maintained to within a few millimeters under functional loading conditions. The soft tissue compression provides enough stiffness to the limb and provides mechanical support to maintain the level of tissue strain within limits allowable for healing of tissue during functional activity.[8]

Soft tissues confined in a cylinder that provides compression have a mechanical advantage in three-point resistance to angulation of the confined bone fragments. Rotational and length stability, however, is significantly poorer than angulatory stability. By the time the callus has reached stage 2 of fracture healing, the soft tissue in the callus provides sufficient inherent stability to resist rotation and pistoning of the fragments. The soft tissues form in the periphery of the callus around the fracture site and provide early blood supply to the fracture site. Thus, calcification begins in the periphery. The callus changes from its "rubbery" state to a hard callus (stage 3 of fracture healing), and radiographs show only minor changes. At this stage of fracture healing, the structural strength of the callus can be equal to or even greater than that of the adjacent bone because of the mechanical advantage provided by the size of the periosteal callus.

As the functional recovery progresses, the fracture line consolidates (stage 4 of fracture healing) and demonstrates calcification of an endochondral nature, which obliterates the original fracture line on radiographs. During this stage, however, only a minor alteration of mechanical properties of the callus is evident.

The final stage of fracture healing (stage 5) may last for many years. During this stage, the callus structure remodels to reconstitute the normal diaphyseal bone and its medullary canal.

FRACTURE BRACING IN THE UPPER LIMB

Humeral Shaft Fractures

Historically, the most common methods of nonoperative treatment have included the use of coaptation splints, hanging casts, and Velpeau bandages.[2,12] However, many problems have been associated with these methods, including adhesive capsulitis of the shoulder, elbow stiffness after removal of the device, transient inferior shoulder subluxation caused by disuse atrophy, and lengthy periods of rehabilitation following immobilization.

Design Considerations.   The humerus is an inherently unstable limb segment, with only one bone surrounded by a thick layer of soft tissue and often a thick layer of adipose tissue. Fracture bracing is designed to take advantage of the early instability in the arm by achieving elbow extension as early as possible. Bracing provides gravity alignment of the arm and early functional activity, with natural alignment of the fragments. The humerus fracture brace provides adjustability by means of anterior and posterior interlocking shields that are molded to the shape of the arm and maintained together with Velcro straps.

Contraindications.   Contraindications include massive soft tissue or bony loss in the extremity, unreliable or uncooperative patients, and inability to obtain or maintain acceptable alignment.

Treatment Protocol.   Treatment consists of alignment of the fracture, application of a prefabricated device over the cast padding, and application of a sling on the initial day of injury. One week after injury, the cast padding is removed and a double layer of cotton stockinette is applied to the extremity. The brace is reapplied, and a radiograph is obtained to check for satisfactory alignment. The patient is instructed to begin pendulum exercises of the shoulder, passive flexion of the upper extremity, and active function of the hand, wrist, and elbow within the brace. The patient is reevaluated after 2, 4, and 6 weeks and, each time, clinical and radiographic evidence of healing is noted. When evidence of healing is confirmed, brace use is discontinued.

Complications.   In a large study of 208 humeral fractures treated with bracing,[14] the following complications were noted: nonunion, 2%; skin maceration, 1%; refracture, 1%; transient inferior shoulder subluxation, 4%; and excessive angulation (more than 25°), 1%.

Ulnar Shaft Fractures

Isolated fractures of the ulnar shaft are typically caused by a direct blow to the forearm, thus acquiring the name "night stick" fracture. Less commonly, these fractures may be caused by an indirect mechanism such as a fall on the extremity.

Design Considerations. If the radioulnar joints are not disrupted, isolated ulnar fractures are inherently stable because the strong interosseous membrane tethers the fragments of the ulna to the intact radius. Thus, soft tissue compression directed into the interosseous space tends to separate the radius from the ulna and places tension on the interosseous membrane to enhance the angular stability of the ulnar. To achieve the necessary tension, the brace should have interlocking shells with a molded interosseous groove anteriorly and posteriorly.[16]

Contraindications. Contraindications are Motaggia fracture-dislocations, intraarticular fractures, and severe fracture angulation of more than 10°.

Treatment Protocol. Initially, a closed reduction is indicated if fracture angulation is 10° or more. If angulation is less, no specific reduction is necessary. A long-arm cast is applied with the forearm in neutral position and elbow at 90° flexion. Radiographs are taken at the end of 2 weeks and, if alignment is satisfactory, the cast is removed and a prefabricated fracture brace is applied. In the brace, the patient is allowed active range of motion of the hand, elbow, and shoulder. The fracture position is ascertained at the end of 3 weeks after the fracture, and further follow-up is carrried out every 3 weeks until clinical union is confirmed, at which time the brace comes off. Also at the end of 3 weeks, the brace can be removed for brief periods of hygiene purposes. Further rehabilitation follow-up is necessary until full functional recovery is achieved.

Colles' Fractures

In 1975, Sarmiento et al.[7] reported on the use of fracture bracing in supination for fractures of the distal radius. The reasons for treatment in supination include inactivation of the brachioradialis muscle, reduction of dorsal ulnar dislocations, and improved leverage on the radial collateral ligament. Also, the parallel position of forearm bones facilitates evaluation of reduction and effective immobilization; rehabilitation is facilitated; the loss of pronation is compensated for by shoulder abduction;[6] scapholunate dislocation is earlier and more easily recognized, and late complications can be prevented; and the flexor muscle mechanical advantage maintains volar compression and minimizes extensor deforming forces.

Design Considerations. The ideal brace is composed of a dorsal and volar component. The dorsal component maintains the wrist in ulnar deviation and prevents extension by blocking it at 30° of volar flexsion. Full wrist flexion is allowed within the brace, but extension and radial deviation are blocked. The forearm is in supination. A volar shell compresses the volar surface to control rotation and maintain a snug fit. There is a supracondylar elbow extension that prevents rotation and also helps with suspension by preventing slippage of the brace distally. Velcro straps are used to maintain the fit. The braces are constructed of low-density polyethylene and have vent holes to allow for comfort.[13]

Treatment Protocol. On the day of the injury, the Colles' fracture is treated with manipulation and closed reduction under general anesthesia or axillary block. A long-arm cast is applied in supination with the wrist in 30° flexion and maximum ulnar deviation. Fracture alignment is reevaluated by radiograph at the end of 1 and 2 weeks. After 2 weeks, if the alignment is well maintained, the cast is removed and the Colles' prefabricated fracture brace is applied over a double cotton stockinette.

The patient is instructed to use the hand, wrist, and elbow. If the alignment is well maintained after 3 weeks, the brace can be removed for short periods for hygienic purposes only. After 6 weeks, the fracture brace is removed and radiographs are obtained, function is evaluated and encouraged and further follow-up is done as needed.

Complications. The most common complications associated with use of a brace in Colles' fractures are loss of reduction, reflex sympathetic dystrophy (RSD), severe edema, and median nerve palsy.

FRACTURE BRACING IN THE LOWER LIMB

Femoral Shaft Fractures

The treatment of choice for most femoral shaft fractures is intramedullary nailing, because of its low morbidity, high union rate, and the physiologic advantages to the multiply injured patient.[3] However, when surgical treatment is not feasible or practical, skeletal traction remains an important method of management of femoral shaft fractures.[17] After 4–6 weeks of skeletal traction, cast bracing has been suggested to allow activity and return to ambulation and weightbearing with good results.[4] The disadvantages of cast braces are that wound access and proper hygiene are limited and the chance of developing angulatory deformity is high.

A plastic fracture brace has several advantages.[10,18] The brace can be easily removed and the wound accessed, and good hygiene can be maintained. The thigh section of the brace can be adjusted easily for swelling or atrophy. Patient acceptance is high, and durability of the brace is good.

Design Considerations. In view of the large amount of soft tissue in the proximal thigh, it is quite difficult to control varus angulation with a fracture brace. In the distal half of the femur, the soft tissue is not as bulky and the fracture is inherently more stable and more controllable with a fracture brace.

Double upright knee joints provide added mediolateral stability. These joints are coupled to the leg by a component similar to the tibial fracture brace. A foot piece is essential for maintaining suspension of the brace. Since mediolateral instability is the most common problem in the femur, the closure of the proximal sleeve is mediolateral, with medial and lateral interlocking shells.

Active range of motion of the knee should be achieved as soon as possible in order to activate the muscles surrounding the fracture site and thus maintain function during early phases of fracture repair. Because of the possibility of developing angulatory deformity, late stage 2 or stage 3 fracture healing should be achieved before using the fracture brace and weightbearing.

Contraindications. Femoral fracture bracing should not be used with insufficient fracture stability, with most fractures located in the proximal third, with displaced intraarticular fractures, in patients with obese thighs, in patients with neurovascular impairment, or in patients who will not cooperate with the protocol.

Protocol. After 4–6 weeks of skeletal traction, radiographs are taken and evidence of early callus established. The tibial pin is removed, the fracture brace applied, and partial weightbearing ambulation initiated. A weightbearing radiograph of the femur in the brace is obtained to confirm that the fracture site is stable. The patient is scheduled for follow-up in 2 weeks. If the fracture alignment is maintained at the follow-up visit, progressive weightbearing is encouraged and the patient is seen at monthly intervals until clinical union has been achieved. Rehabilitation should be continued until joint motion and muscle strength are maximized.

Tibial Shaft Fractures

Sarmiento and others have done extensive work using bracing techniques for tibial fractures with excellent results.[11,15]

Design Considerations. The limb segment of which the tibia is a part is inherently stable. It consists of the tibia and fibula, which are connected by an interosseous membrane surrounded by very muscular soft tissue, and is well suited to soft tissue control with fracture braces. The role of the fracture brace is to control angulation. Rotational and length stability must be achieved prior to bracing. In a study using instrumented fracture braces,[9] it was demonstrated that approximately 80% of the loads are borne in the proximal half of the fracture brace. Although it is impractical to mold an interosseous groove in the leg as in the forearm, the natural triangular shape of the leg can be molded by the proximal portion of the sleeve of the tibial brace. To maintain this soft tissue molding in the proximal half of the brace during circumferential adjustment of the device, an interlocking shell design was developed that maintains its triangular cross-section with circumferential adjustments. A simple heel cup is sufficient to suspend the brace. The preferred material for the brace is low-density polyethylene because of its flexibility.

Indications. Indications for bracing in the treatment of tibial shaft fractures are closed diaphyseal fractures, open tibial fracture with an intact fibula, and an undisplaced intercondylar fracture of tibia.

Contraindications. These include uncooperative patients, the presence of neurologic or vascular impairment, inadequate fracture stability, unstable segmental fractures, and extremities with massive soft tissue or bone loss.

Protocol. After adequate reduction of the fracture is attained, a well-padded cast is initially applied and the patient is given a cast boot. Partial weightbearing is begun, and patients are encouraged to advance to full weightbearing as soon as possible. Alignment is checked radiographically. Follow-up is arranged in 1–2 weeks.

If the fracture is stable after 3 weeks, the long-leg cast is replaced by a short-leg functional cast. X-rays are done to confirm alignment. Five weeks following reduction, the short-leg cast is removed and a prefabricated tibial fracture brace is applied. X-rays are done to confirm alignment, and full weightbearing is continued in the device. Patients are seen at monthly intervals and radiographs are done. Once the union is confirmed clinically and radiographically, the brace is removed.

Results. Zych et al. report a study[17,18] of 753 patients with 773 tibial fractures; 180 patients had inadequate follow-up, and 92 patients were excluded from the study because they required treatment in addition to fracture bracing and could not follow standard protocol. Thus, 481 patients with 501 fractures were included. The average time to union for closed injuries was 15.5 weeks; the average time to union for open fractures was 23 weeks.

Complications. Minimal complications are noted in Zych's study, and they include angulatory deformities, limb shortening, skin maceration, and nonunion.

CONCLUSIONS

The special indications for fracture bracing continue to be developed and refined as clinical experience grows. Using braces for various indications has reduced patient morbidity. Patients with braces function better than those with casts. The combination of flexible internal fixation and fracture bracing holds great promise for many applications.

REFERENCES

1. Kruse RL, Kelly PJ: Acceleration of fracture healing distal to a venous tourniquet. J Bone Joint Surg 56A:730–738, 1976.
2. La Ferte AD, Nutter PD: The treatment of fractures of the humerus by means of hanging plaster cast—"Hanging cast." Ann Surg 114:919–924, 1941.
3. Miller CW, Anderson L, Grossman J, et al: Comparison of three treatments for fractures of the diaphysis of the femur. Surg Gynecol Obstet 146:572–576, 1978.
4. Mooney V, Nickel VL, Harvey JP, et al: Cast brace treatment for fractures of the distal part of the femur. J Bone Joint Surg 52A:1563–1568, 1970.
5. Perren SM: Physical and biological aspects of fracture healing with special reference to internal fixation. Clin Orthop 138:175–181, 1979.
6. Raisbeck CC, Ungeisma JA: Paradoxical reduction of Colles' fracture. J Bone Joint Surg 49A:1246–1258, 1967.
7. Sarmiento A, Prett GW, Berry NC, et al: Colles' fracture: Functional bracing in supination. J Bone Joint Surg 57A:311–320, 1975.
8. Sarmiento A, Latta LL: Principles of fracture healing. Instr Course Lect 1:1–20, 1984.
9. Sarmiento A, Latta LL: Closed Functional Treatment of Fractures. New York, Springer-Verlag, 1981.
10. Sarmiento A: Functional bracing of tibial and femoral shaft fractures. Clin Orthop 2:82–102, 1986.
11. Sarmiento A: A functional below knee brace for tibial fractures. J Bone Joint Surg 52A:295–310, 1970.
12. Stewart MJ, Hundley JM: Fractures of the humerus: A comparative study in methods of treatment. J Bone Joint Surg 37A:681–692, 1955.
13. Zagorski JB, Zych G, Latta LL, et al: Colles' fracture management using prefabricated braces. Orthop Trans 10:471–472, 1986.
14. Zagorksi JB, Zych GA, Latta LL, McCollough NC III: Modern concepts in functional fracture bracing. The Upper Limb. Instr Course Lect 24:377–401, 1984.
15. Zagorski JB, Schenkman JH, Latta LL, et al: Prefabricated brace treatment for diaphyseal tibial fractures. Orthop Trans 6:88–96, 1987.
16. Zych GA, Zagorski JB, Latta LL: Treatment of isolated ulnar fractures with prefabricated braces. Clin Orthop 291:88–94, 1987.
17. Zych GA, Zagorski JD, Latta LL, McCollough NC III: Modern concepts in functional fracture bracing. The Lower Limb. Instr Course Lect 25:403–442, 1984.
18. Zych GA, Zagorski JB, Latta LL: Current concepts in fracture bracing: Part II. Lower extremity. Orthop Surg 5:18–30, 1986.

THAO T. DUONG, MD

COMPLICATIONS OF FRACTURES

From Denver General Hospital
Denver, Colorado

Reprint requests to:
Thao T. Duong, MD
Director, Rehabilitation Services
Denver General Hospital
777 Bannock Street
Denver, CO 80204-4507

Fractures uncomplicated by serious associated injuries usually unite. However, complications do occur in a small proportion of fractures. These complications may develop due to the fracture itself or as a result of injuries to the surrounding tissues. In the care of patients with fractures, early recognition and treatment of complications is of pivotal importance. Some patients may develop complications while they are on the acute surgical service or during rehabilitation. Since fracture complications can affect both the patients' eventual outcome and their functional recovery, it is important for all professionals involved in rehabilitation to be familiar with diagnosis and management of complications. It should be emphasized that some complications occur as the result of treatment and are therefore iatrogenic. Careful selection of appropriate treatment methods and proper care will prevent unwanted consequences.

In this chapter, different types of complications will be discussed with regard to the time of their occurrence after the initial fracture.

INITIAL AND EARLY COMPLICATIONS

Infection

Infection is the leading cause of a delayed union or nonunion. Except in rare cases, infection occurs exclusively in open, or compound, fractures. In an open fracture, the wound is contaminated by organisms carried in from the outside environment. The infection frequently involves not only the layers of soft tissue, but it also extends to the bone, resulting in osteomyelitis. Gustilo and Anderson found that the infection rate in type 3 open fractures (fractures involving extensive soft tissue damage such as skin flaps, avulsions, muscle and nerve injuries, and major arterial injuries) was 10% versus an overall rate of 2.4% for all fractures.[17] Others have reported osteomyelitis occurring at a rate of 12%[43] to 15%[7] in open fractures. Infrequently, a closed, or simple, fracture may become infected when it is treated via open operative intervention. The femoral shaft, intertrochanteric area, femoral neck, and tibia are the most common fracture sites to develop infection.[2,45]

Malnutrition[42] and immunodeficiency[5] also have been identified as risk factors for musculoskeletal infections. Once bone is infected with pyogenic organisms, chronic infection may be inevitable. A portion of the bone may die through impairment of its blood supply. This dead bone invariably forms a sequestrum within the cavity in the bone, which may require surgical removal. Following an open intraarticular fracture and, less commonly, open surgical repair of an intraarticular fracture, infection of the joint (septic arthritis) may occur. If not treated early and aggressively, septic arthritis can lead to joint cartilage destruction and eventual degenerative arthritis. Meticulous cleansing of the wound with large amount of sterile water or saline, excisions of all devitalized tissue, proper wound closure after the treatment of a fracture, and antibacterial drug treatment are all important in the prevention of infection. The lowest infection rate has been found in patients who are given an antibiotic combination that covers both gram-positive and gram-negative organisms.[34] *Staphylococcus aureus* has been reported as the offending organism in 60–70% of bone infections, 25% of which are mixed infections.[19,45] Other possible bacteria include *Streptococcus, Escherichia coli, Pseudomonas, Klebsiella,* and *Aerobacter.*

With most infections, symptoms occur within 4 weeks of the open wound. In few cases, however, symptoms may be delayed until months later. Pain is commonly the primary finding in association with erythema, swelling, and tenderness. Drainage from the wound may or may not be present. Severity of clinical signs and symptoms often depends on the virulence of the infecting organisms.[19]

Upon routine radiographic examination, findings such as soft tissue swelling, bone destruction, and new periosteal bone formation do not become visible for approximately 2 weeks from the onset of the infection. They may be delayed even further when the patient is being treated with appropriate antibiotics.[19] Currently, bone scintigraphy (gallium-67 citrate and indium-111-labeled leukocytes) is generally recommended as the imaging technique for diagnosis of osteomyelitis if there has been no previous osseous involvement. With continuing research efforts in the evaluation of various diagnostic imaging techniques, radiolabeled polyclonal immunoglobulins and magnetic resonance imaging may prove to be clinically more useful. All of the above techniques are capable of detecting only the inflammatory changes or the bone reactions that are associated with infection but not the infection proper.[47]

Injury to Major Blood Vessels

Minor blood vessels are unavoidably torn at the time of fractures, but injuries to major vessels are relatively uncommon. Vascular injury may result from laceration or angulation of an artery or vein by the fractured and displaced bony fragment, contusion or laceration as a direct consequence of external traumatic forces, or sudden distortion with shearing of the vessels at their point of origin.

In penetrating injuries such as high-velocity gunshot wounds, vessels are commonly damaged from direct contact with the missile or its blast effect.[9] This type of trauma accounts for the majority of civilian arterial injuries, with only 10% of which being attributed to fractures resulting from blunt trauma.[38] The incidence of vascular injuries associated with long-bone fractures and dislocations that require surgery is 0.3–3%.[10] Major arteries are particularly vulnerable to certain specific fractures: axillary artery in fracture-dislocations or dislocations of the shoulder; brachial artery in supracondylar fractures of the humerus; hypogastric, iliofemoral, and sacral vessels in major pelvic fractures; femoral artery in fractures of the shaft of the femur; popliteal artery in fractures of the distal end of femur, proximal end of tibia, and dislocations of the knee; and dorsalis pedis artery in fractures of the forefoot.[30,39] When an artery is completely severed, it usually retracts and stops bleeding spontaneously; however, bleeding continues if it is incompletely torn. Possible consequences of major vessel injuries are numerous and include arterial spasm or occlusion, hemorrhage, pulsating hematoma (false aneurysm), gangrene, ischemic paralysis of nerves, compartment syndrome (also known as Volkmann's ischemia) or limb loss.

Peripheral circulation of an extremity must be observed closely after a long-bone fracture. Severe pain is commonly the first symptom suggesting ischemia. Pain is increased on passive extension of the toes or fingers. Numbness or decreased sensibility distally in the digits also may be noticed by the patient. Perfusion can be further assessed by checking the capillary refill time to compare it with that of the uninjured extremity. A limb with a complete arterial occlusion may be found on examination to be pale in appearance and cool to the touch distally, with loss of arterial pulse. The skin may later become mottled and dark in color, which heralds gangrene. If the presence of peripheral pulses is questionable, a Doppler probe is useful in detecting those that are too weak to be palpable. Doppler signals and even palpable pulses, however, do not positively exclude vascular damage.[10] In the case of an arterial injury resulting from a major pelvic fracture, the patient may present with shock. It has been reported that the mortality rate of hemodynamically unstable patients with pelvic fractures is 42%, whereas the mortality rate of those not presenting in shock is only 3.4%.[31] High-quality, biplane, sequential angiography remains the gold standard in diagnosing vascular injuries. In partial vessel transection, there will be extravasation of contrast material into the adjacent soft tissue. On the other hand, a complete block of flow of the contrast media signifies either a thrombus or a complete transection.[26,27]

Complications from a major vessel injury should always be managed as an emergency, because the effects of ischemia rapidly become irreversible. In the case of shock, restoration of hemodynamic stability should be the highest priority. The treatment of an arterial occlusion varies depending on whether the patient presents with ischemia when first received (primary injury) or after reduction and immobilization of the fracture (secondary injury). If the vascular injury is primary, the clinician should remove any potentially constricting external splint or bandage and reduce the fracture with gentle manipulation of grossly displaced fragments. If these measures fail to restore circulation, an angiogram coupled with an operation may be necessary to determine the nature of the arterial injury so that appropriate surgical vascular repair can be performed. The fracture may also be reduced and fixed internally at this point to prevent further vascular damage from recurrent displacement. If ischemia occurs after reduction and immobilization, the cast and underlying dressing must be immediately split along their entire length. If circulation does not return within half an hour, the artery must be evaluated by an angiogram and repaired, if indicated.

Compartment Syndromes and Reperfusion Injury

Compartment syndrome has been defined as "a condition in which increased pressure within a limited space compromises the circulation and function of the tissues within that space."[28] The increased intracompartmental pressure could be the result of tissue swelling or the increase in interstitial fluid. In crushing trauma with major hemorrhage, compartmental pressure will increase rapidly; however, the onset of compartment syndrome is often delayed relative to the onset of ischemia. This presentation points toward capillary injury as the result of increased vascular permeability and ischemia-reperfusion phenomenon. Although compartment syndrome can develop in any osteofascial compartment, it most commonly occurs in the flexor compartment of the forearm and in the four compartments of the lower leg. Unlike gangrene, the distal skin and subcutaneous tissues are minimally affected in compartment syndrome. They are more resistive to ischemia when compared to skeletal muscle or peripheral nerves. Peripheral nerves and muscles are found to withstand up to only 4 and 6 hours of ischemia, respectively. The main difference between nerves and muscles, however, lies in the fact that necrotic muscles do not regenerate. They eventually are replaced by dense fibrous scar tissue that may shorten and result in classic compartment contracture or Volkmann's contracture.

Signs of impending compartment syndrome include deep, throbbing, and unrelenting pain. Pain may appear out of proportion to the injury.[4] Stretching of the involved muscles produces pain, but in patients with direct trauma to the extremity, this sign may be difficult to assess. Because changes in neuromuscular function also may occur, careful examination will help with early detection. For example, hypesthesia in the cleft between the first and second metatarsal may be an indication of deep peroneal nerve dysfunction from an anterior compartment problem.

Compartment syndrome in an alert and cooperative patient is generally apparent on repeat examination. However, because its diagnosis may be much more difficult in comatose or neurologically impaired patients, techniques to measure compartmental pressures in these situations become invaluable tools. Various methods for tissue pressure measurements have been described[28,29,48] and range from use of a simple central venous pressure manometer attached to an 18-gauge needle to a solid-state transducer small enough to be placed in a catheter tip. Normal muscle compartmental pressure in the leg is less than or equal to 20 mm Hg. Any pressure above 20 mm Hg is considered abnormal. At this time, there is no established agreement on an absolute pressure level above which fasciotomy is always indicated and below which it is not necessary. In general, fasciotomy is recommended when compartmental pressure exceeds 35–45 mm Hg, especially in the face of appropriate clinical symptoms. Blood studies in patients with muscle necrosis may reveal elevated creatinine phosphokinase and hyperkalemia. Myoglobinuria also may occur. Motor nerve conduction studies have been used in patients who cannot cooperate or who sustained direct trauma to the extremity.[28] If a muscle is paralyzed as a result of a nerve injury from a compartment syndrome, nerve stimulation proximal to to the site of increased compartment pressure should not result in a normal evoked response. Measurement of segmental limb blood pressures and calculations of the Doppler-derived ankle:brachial index are of importance in the sequential evaluation of any patient with an injured and ischemic extremity. In a few cases, arteriography has also been used to delineate subtle signs and symptoms of compartment syndrome.

Prompt fasciotomy along the complete length of the compartment (decompression prior to tissue necrosis) is the definitive treatment for compartment syndrome. Cohen et al. advocate lengthening the skin incision to an average of 16 cm in lower extremity compartment syndrome, which has been found to significantly decrease intracompartmental pressure.[8] Precise knowledge of anatomy and care are required to avoid any further peripheral nerve or vascular injury. If muscle necrosis is present, all dead tissue must be debrided to prevent ensuing infection. Postoperatively the incisions are packed open with bulky dressings that are changed frequently, and the limb is then splinted. About 3–5 days after the fasciotomy, delayed primary closure of the wound should be performed. The use of osmotic diuretics such as Mannitol early in the treatment program has also been advocated by some surgeons as a way to prevent the need for fasciotomy.[36] It is of pivotal importance that passive and active range of motion exercise programs are begun immediately and performed throughout the healing period to maintain normal joint motions, to avoid contractures, and to improve venous and lymphatic drainage. Reduction of edema is an integral part of treatment plan because swelling could interfere with blood supply and result in the formation of fibrous scar tissue. Elevation of the involved extremity, proper splinting and bracing, scar management, and early mobilization are indicated. Weightbearing of the affected lower extremity in the presence of a fracture and the use of mechanical compressive devices are generally not recommended.

Fat Embolism and Fat Embolism Syndrome

The term *fat embolism* denotes the presence of fat globules in the lung parenchyma and peripheral circulation after a fracture of a long bone or other major trauma. Fat droplets larger than 20 μm in diameter have been found in more than 90% of patients with long-bone fractures.[25] The term *fat embolism syndrome* (FES) denotes a more serious manifestation of the same phenomenon but is associated with clinical respiratory insufficiency and decreased alveolar diffusion of oxygen. Overall, FES has been reported to occur in only 3–4% of patients with long-bone fractures. The risk of FES increases in bilateral or multiple bone fractures. The risk is 1–3.5% in a single tibia or femur fracture but 5–10% in bilateral or multiple bone fractures.[24,35] Gurd and Wilson have reported that half of cases of FES occur in patients with multiple fractures, 30% occur in femur fracture alone, 10% in tibia fracture alone, and 5% in pelvic fracture alone.[16]

FES has been divided into three groups depending on its severity: subclinical, overt clinical, and fulminating. The subclinical form is detected incidentally by blood gas analysis and is associated with a PaO_2 value of less than 60 mm Hg. The overt clinical form, which usually occurs 24–72 hours following fracture, presents with classic respiratory distress with dyspnea, hemoptysis, tachypnea, and cyanosis. Signs and symptoms of emboli to other organs can also be manifested. For example, cerebral emboli may cause headache and irritability, followed by delirium, stupor, and possibly coma. Cardiac emboli can cause tachycardia and a drop in blood pressure. Multiple emboli to the skin may become apparent as multiple petechial hemorrhages, particularly in the areas of the upper chest, the axillae, and the conjunctivae. The patient also may develop a fever. The severe and fulminant form of FES usually develops within hours of a fracture. It involves multiple organ systems and is frequently fatal despite aggressive respiratory support and other resuscitative measures. This form is thought to be caused by a massive embolism followed by a succession of further massive emboli.

Gurd's criteria for positive diagnosis of FES are commonly used. The criteria are divided into major and minor features. Major features include hypoxemia ($PaO_2 < 60$ mm Hg; $FiO_2 \leq 0.4$), central nervous system depression disproportionate to hypoxemia, pulmonary edema, and axillary or subconjunctival petechia. Minor features are fever (temperature $> 38.5°$ C), tachycardia (heart rate > 110 beats per minute), emboli present in retina on funduscopic examination, fat present in urine, a sudden unexplained drop in the hematocrit or platelet values, increasing erythrocyte sedimentation rate, and fat globules present in sputum.[15] For a diagnosis of FES, the patient must have at least one major and four minor features. In another study, Linque et al. argued that Gurd's criteria can result in underdiagnosing and therefore proposed that the diagnosis of FES can be made if one of the following criteria is met: (a) sustained $PaO_2 < 60$ mm Hg, (b) sustained $PaCO_2 > 55$ mm Hg or pH < 7.3, (c) sustained respiratory rate > 35 breaths per minute even after adequate sedation, and (d) increased work of breathing as manifested by dyspnea, use of accessory respiratory muscles, and tachycardia combined with anxiety.[25]

Mechanical and biochemical theories have been proposed for the genesis of the fat droplets. The mechanical theory proposes that trauma to the long bone releases fat droplets by disrupting fat cells in the marrow of the fractured bones or in adipose tissues. The fat droplets then enter torn veins near the long bone fracture and are subsequently transported to the pulmonary vasculature. There they are deposited and trapped as emboli in the lung capillaries. Some small fat droplets may pass through the lungs and reach systemic circulation, causing embolization in other organs. This theory requires a transient rise in bone marrow pressure above venous pressure to occur to allow fat droplets to enter the torn vessels.[24]

The biochemical theory, which includes two separate hypotheses, is supported by the occurrence of fat embolism in nontraumatic conditions. In the "toxic" hypothesis, the circulating free fatty acids are released at the time of trauma or during the breakdown of fat in the lung. They in turn directly affect the pneumocytes in the lung and cause adult respiratory distress syndrome. In a severe trauma, free fatty acids could also be mobilized from stores of body fat as a result of the release of catecholamines.[3] The "obstructive" theory proposes that a chemical event at the site of the fracture releases mediators that affect the solubility of lipids, thus causing coalescence and subsequent embolization.[24]

Administration of oxygen, supportive pulmonary care, general hemodynamic, and fracture management are the main treatments for FES. Steroids and many other agents have been tried but produced no clear effectiveness. Inadequately stabilized fractures or delayed operative fixation of fractures have been shown to result in an increased incidence of FES.[44] Early operative intervention is recommended.

Deep Venous Thrombosis and Pulmonary Embolism

Immobilization and venous stasis caused by local pressure on a vein in the lower extremities can result in venous thrombosis. Risk factors for venous thrombosis include prior history of venous thromboembolism, age (particularly above 60 years), marked immobility, leg or pelvic trauma or surgery, obesity, chronic congestive heart failure, prior use of estrogen, and the presence of cancer.[28a] Although the risks of thromboembolism have not been well determined for trauma in general population, the estimated incidence of deep venous thrombosis (DVT) in young patients with multiple trauma is 20%.[11] In the orthopedic literature, the incidence of DVT has been reported to vary 45–70% in the absence of prophylaxis in patients undergoing a hip or knee procedure. Clinical significant pulmonary embolism (PE) has been estimated to occur in up to 20% of patients undergoing hip surgery, with 1–3% fatality.[11] When venous thrombosis occurs in the calf, the patient may complain of pain in the lower leg. Distal swelling and tenderness on passive dorsiflexion of the ankle (Homan's sign) are present. If thrombosis occurs more proximally in the leg, the entire lower extremity may be swollen. In most cases, when thrombosis develops unilaterally, there will be a distinct side-to-side difference in calf and thigh circumferences. Noninvasive Doppler ultrasonography[41] and venography of the abnormal extremity are commonly used to diagnose DVT. In good hands, Doppler ultrasound is highly sensitive for detecting occluding thrombi in the popliteal and more proximal veins but less sensitive to calf thrombi. A number of diagnostic criteria have been developed for venographic diagnosis of acute DVT;[22,37] the presence of an intraluminal filling defect, which is constant in all films and in a number of projections, is the most reliable finding. Other techniques that have been used to diagnose venous thrombosis include iodine-125 fibrinogen leg scanning and impedance plethysmography. Radionucleotide venography and thermography also have been used but their diagnostic capabilities require further study. When the thrombus is loosely adherent to the wall of the vessel, it may break off, propagate more proximally, and lodge in the lung, where it may cause PE. Most pulmonary emboli originate from venous thrombi of the iliac or femoral veins.[23] The constellation of symptoms and signs in patients with acute PE includes dyspnea (86%), cough (70%), pleural pain (58%), hemoptysis (38%), syncope (14%), decreased PaO_2 (82%), respiratory rate > 20 breaths per minute (75%), rales (71%), heart rate > 100 beats per minute (67%), fever (47%), sweating (34%), S3 and S4 gallop rhythm (34%), and phlebitis (33%).[40]

Chest x-ray is performed in all patients with cardiopulmonary disorders, including PE. Unfortunately, in most patients with PE, plain films will be "normal" or only show isolated findings, which may be attributed to other diseases. The presence of a pulmonary infiltrate, in combination with an elevated diaphragm on the same side, however, should alert physician to pulmonary embolism/infarction rather than a pneumonia.[40] Findings on electrocardiogram (S1-Q3-T3 or acute cor pulmonale pattern, arrhythmias, QRS abnormalities and ST-T waves changes) are sensitive but not specific in patients with PE. Arterial blood gas may show hypoxemia with an icreased alveolar-arterial oxygen tension difference. Lung scanning with or without the ventilation component is the most frequently used test for the screening of PE. If it is normal on multiple views, pulmonary embolism can be excluded with a high level of confidence. Lung scans with high probability of PE show either multiple defects or lesions having configurations compatible with vascular defects. Simultaneous ventilation study will add specificity to the scanning procedure. A "mismatched" lesion that shows a normal ventilation scan over an area with perfusion defect is highly specific for PE. "Matched" lesions are generally seen in patients with other disorders, such as chronic obstructive lung disease. An intravascular defect or a vessel cutoff seen on selective pulmonary angiogram is diagnostic of PE, and no further studies are necessary. Pulmonary angiogram is most valuable in patients with pulmonary or cardiac disease; clinical symptoms and signs may be nonspecific and V/Q scan nondiagnostic.[40] Even though pulmonary angiogram is the "gold standard" for making the diagnosis of PE, it should be used with caution due to its invasive nature and the potential for serious complications.

Once the diagnosis of deep venous thrombosis and/or pulmonary embolism is made, and if there is no obvious contraindication, the patient should be started on intravenous heparin therapy. Approximately 8–12 days of heparin therapy is generally recommended to allow the thrombus to stabilize and attach firmly to the vein wall. Oral anticoagulants such as warfarin should be started as soon as possible with 3–5 days of overlapping heparin. There is no consensus regarding the optimal duration of chronic oral anticoagulation therapy. About 3–6 months of therapy is generally advised. Supportive pulmonary management is also required in patients with respiratory insufficiency. In cases in which anticoagulation may be contraindicated (concomitant traumatic intracerebral hemorrhage) or discontinued (bleeding complications) or when embolism recurs during adequate heparin therapy, placement of an inferior vena cava filter may be preferable. Pulmonary embolectomy may be indicated in rare cases of massive pulmonary embolism in which maximal medical therapy fails.[40]

During the acute and rehabilitation phases of fracture treatment, noninvasive prophylactic approaches should be used when possible to decrease the risk of thromboembolism and to avoid the potential morbidity/mortality associated with the disease and its treatment. Mechanical methods include early ambulation, use of elastic stockings, and external lower extremity compression. Low-dose anticoagulants such as warfarin and subcutaneous heparin also are frequently advocated and used.

Neurologic Complications

Peripheral nerve injury, although uncommon, may occur in association with a fracture (stretching during actual dislocation or damage by sharp bone fragment) or fracture treatment during closed or open reduction. Delayed onset nerve injury can also occur as a result of nerve being caught in the callus. The specific nerve injury is usually related to the location of the fracture. For example, the circumflex branch of the axillary nerve may be injured in shoulder dislocations; radial nerve in midshaft humeral fractures; ulnar nerve in avulsion fracture-dislocations of the medial epicondyle; sciatic nerve in posterior dislocations and fracture-dislocations of the hip; and tibial and peroneal nerves in dislocations of the knee. Furthermore, the peroneal nerve is also at risk due to external pressure from the cast.

Nerve injuries can be classified into three types according to Seddon's classification: neurapraxia, axonotmesis, and neurotmesis.[1] In neurapraxia, there is conduction loss but no structural change in the axon. The viability of the axon is therefore maintained, and recovery occurs spontaneously within a few weeks. If there is associated demyelination, the conduction velocity will not return to normal until remyelination is completed. In axonotmesis the axon is sufficiently affected to cause loss of axonal continuity. In the first few days, normal nerve conduction continues in the segment distal to the point of nerve injury. However, Wallerian degeneration subsequently occurs in the distal axon segment and results in loss of the axon's ability to conduct. The observed response to electrical stimulations above and below the point of nerve injury, after Wallerian degeneration has occurred, will help distinguish between neurapraxia and axonotmesis. An evoked response can still be elicited with stimulation below the nerve injury in neurapraxia but not in axonotmesis. In the axonotmesis, recovery can occur spontaneously, but the time to recovery depends on the rate of regeneration—typically about 1–3 mm per day. In neurotmesis, the nerve and its supporting structure are either severed by the fractured bone edge or interrupted by severe scarring. Nerve regeneration, if it occurs, is usually incomplete and not well organized.[21] The damaged nerve segment can be repaired by excision of the segment plus end-to-end suture of the nerve stumps or by bridging with nerve grafts. The results, however, are often unsatisfactory.

Nerve conduction studies and electromyography can help to distinguish between the different types of nerve injuries and can assist in following the progress of possible nerve regeneration.[21,46]

In closed fractures, the nerve injury is usually assumed to recover spontaneously. If the signs of recovery are not observed within the expected time (clinically or by electromyography after 3 months), exploration of the nerve may be indicated. Upon exploration, the nerve can be freed or microsurgically repaired if it has been severed or badly scarred.

In open fractures, the nerve is assumed to be severed and the wound should be explored carefully. It has been recommended, although this remains controversial, that the severed nerve not be reattached permanently but instead be connected together with one or two sutures. Secondary nerve repair is subsequently performed at 3–4 weeks after the injury upon sufficient wound healing.[1] The extremity must be protected, properly positioned with the use of splints, and put through a full range of motion on a regular basis by the therapist during the observation and recovery period. These steps will help to avoid further complications such as soft tissue swelling and joint contractures. Tendon transfer can also be performed in cases in which prognosis of neuronal recovery is poor.

Injuries to Viscera

The viscera may be damaged either by the agent causing the fracture, by the fractured bone fragments, or by the severe associated blunt trauma. Examples include laceration of lung or pleura in rib fractures or penetrating injury to the large intestine. Computed tomography and magnetic resonance imaging are used to evaluate the injury or serially follow the improvement over time. The incidence of bladder or urethral injury in pelvic fracture or dislocation has been reported to range from 0.7–25%.[30,33] The injuries are most commonly seen in association with straddle fractures (fractures of pubic rami) and are uncommon in women. Diagnosis of bladder perforation is made by cystogram showing extravasation of contrast material when the bladder is distended. Bladder rupture is documented with either peritoneal or, more frequently, extraperitoneal extravasation.[19]

General surgical principles should be used in the treatment of visceral injuries. Due to the life-threatening nature of these injuries, their treatment may need to precede any treatment of the actual fracture.[1]

Skin Complications

A patient who sustains multiple fractures is at great risk of developing decubitus ulcers due to his/her immobility. Most frequently affected areas are those overlying bony prominences such as the greater trochanters, the sacrum, and the heels. The patient must be turned on regular basis and be mobilized as soon as possible. An incorrectly applied cast also can produce a pressure sore. Attention should be paid to the actual cast application and the patient's complaints after application. Early stabilization of major fractures in polytraumatized patients facilitates early mobilization and decreases the skin complications associated with bedridden patients.

LATE COMPLICATIONS

Delayed Union

There is no absolute amount of time required for fracture healing. If the fractured fragments are still mobile after 3 or 4 months, the union is classified as delayed. At the same time, on radiographic examination, there will be persistence of the fracture line with absent or limited callus formation.[19] Delayed union is generally a result of one or more of the following factors: (1) bone infection, (2) inadequate blood supply to one or both fragments, (3) excessive movement between the two fragments, (4) loss of apposition between the two fragments, (5) interposition of soft tissue between the fragments, (6) dissolution of fracture hematoma by synovial fluid, as in the case of fractures involving the joints, and (7) destruction of bone by tumor as in the case of pathologic fractures.

In most cases of delayed union, treatment is conservative, and union will eventually occur. If union still has not occurred after 6 months or more, surgical intervention may be required, possibly with bone grafting or rigid internal fixation. During rehabilitation, it is important that precautions such as range of motion and weightbearing restrictions be strictly followed by the patient and all rehabilitation personnel. In many cases, the patient initially may not be able to comply with the restrictions due to poor mental status, either premorbid or as a result of concomitant brain injury. The rehabilitation staff, in such instances, will need to educate and remind the patient frequently of the precautions. Various techniques, from repetition to verbal cues and visual demonstration, can be employed. Mobility and activities and training in skills of daily living should be individualized and modified depending on the patient and the type of fractures.

Nonunion

If the fractured fragments are still not united after many months and the radiologic appearance is distinctive of nonunion, the fracture is not likely to heal conservatively. There are two general types of nonunion: hypertrophic and atrophic. In the more common hypertrophic nonunion, the bone ends at the site of fracture appear dense and rounded and have a distinctive fracture line. The medullary canal is occluded by eburnated bone and no callus is seen crossing the fracture line. In atrophic type of nonunion, a fine line of sclerosis usually crosses the medullary canal of the apposing fragments. The healing process has arrested with no further attempt to bridge the fractured fragments with callus. The gap is instead filled with fibrous tissue. Synovial fluid may fill a cavity, which is developed within the fibrous tissue mass in an attempt to form a false joint (pseudarthrosis). The causes of nonunion are the same as those of delayed union, only more severe. The treatment of nonunion depends on the site of fracture and the degree of disability. In some cases, the fracture may be left untreated with minimal residual impairment, such is in certain scaphoid fractures. In the majority of the cases, however, surgical treatment is indicated. In nonunited long-bone fractures, bone grafting with internal fixation has been reasonably successful in promoting union. Electromagnetic stimulation also has been shown to produce unions both with or without bone grafting.[6,12]

Malunion

Malunion occurs when the fractured bony fragments are healed in an unacceptable position—with angulation, rotation, loss of end-to-end apposition, or overlapping with resultant shortening. In most cases, significant malunion deformities can be prevented by proper alignment and immobilization during the treatment period. Due to the severe and comminuted nature of some fractures, a degree of malunion has to be accepted in some cases. If disability is slight, the malunion is best left alone. When indicated, the problem needs to be repaired surgically. In the lower limb, shortening of 2 cm or more can be corrected by a shoe-lift, but in some cases a leg-shortening procedure can be performed in the longer leg to achieve a more level pelvis. An abnormal gait due to leg-length discrepancy can result in chronic low back pain and potential scoliosis. Newer techniques developed in Russia (Ilizarov[2a,40a]) are being used to correct nonunions and malunions using special external fixators and limited osteotomies with slow correction occurring over long times.

Avascular Necrosis

Death of bone resulting from insufficient blood supply is termed *avascular necrosis*. The blood supply to the bone is compromised by a fracture near the joint where the terminal fragment needs to depend on the intraosseous vessels, which were torn at the time of injury, for its nutrition. With dislocations of the joints, the vital blood vessels are torn or occluded and impair the blood supply to the bone fragments. The bone cells subsequently die, and the avascular bone gradually loses the rigid trabecular structure and becomes granular. The bone softens significantly and can easily collapse under the body weight or the stress of muscle pull across the joint. This process occurs slowly and can present up to 3 or more years after injury.

The areas most vulnerable to avascular necrosis include (1) the head of the femur after fracture of the femoral neck or after dislocation of the hip, (2) the proximal half of the scaphoid after a fracture through the waist of the bone, and (3) the body of the talus after a fracture through the neck of the talus.

Avascular necrosis may be diagnosed on x-rays several months after injury. The avascular segment will appear denser than the more osteoporotic surrounding bone. Radioisotope scanning with technetium-99m also may be helpful. Due to the lack of blood supply to the affected fragment, the isotope will not be taken up normally and thus appears as a void. In many cases where avascular necrosis has occurred, early surgical intervention is recommended. It may be necessary to either excise the whole avascular segment and reconstruct the joint with arthroplasty or stabilize and fuse the joint with arthrodesis.[1] In the latter option, the joint mobility will be lost and abnormal biomechanical movement will result. The rehabilitation therapy program will be tailored to the individual patient based on the degree of disability and range of motion restriction.

Chronic Osteomyelitis

Chronic infection results from incomplete treatment of an acute infection. It can occur in open fractures or in closed fractures treated via an open procedure. Purulent drainage from the infected site may persist, and the adjacent bone fragments may separate as sequestra. Chronic osteomyelitis is notoriously resistant to treatment such that a major operation may be required to gain control over the infection.

Posttraumatic Osteoarthritis

In fractures involving the articular surfaces, some degree of osteoarthritis is inevitable. It is very difficult to reduce the fracture so that the joint surface is perfectly smooth. Any slight displacement may result in significant disability, especially in a weightbearing joint. Typical radiographic findings are asymmetric joint space narrowing, subchondral cyst formation, subchondral sclerosis of bone, and joint margin spur formation.[19]

Posttraumatic Ossification

In a small number of patients with fracture, heterotopic ossification (HO), or bone formation at an abnormal site, occurs. Heterotopic ossification also may occur following a central nervous system injury such as traumatic brain injury or spinal cord injury. The incidence of all significant HO has been reported to be about 10–20%.[14] Children and young adults are at increased risk of developing HO. Traumatic HO is noted most frequently in elbow and hip injuries. The site for traumatic HO, however, differs from that of neurogenic HO.[13] If there is severe injury to the joint at the time of trauma or to the muscle, a hematoma results. The hematoma is subsequently invaded by osteoblasts and becomes ossified. When this occurs in the thigh, especially after a quadriceps contusion, the abnormal bone mass is called *myositis ossificans*. This mass initially is radiolucent but will soon appear calcified on radiographic examination.

Limited range of motion is the most common finding on physical examination, and, at times, it is the first sign to indicate the development of HO. The patient may also present with pain, localized swelling, erythema, and warmth. Thrombophlebitis is frequently included in the differential diagnosis, especially if the signs and symptoms occur in the lower extremity. Patients with clinically significant HO also demonstrate elevated levels of serum alkaline phosphatase. This enzyme level appears to rise within 2 weeks after injury but does not become elevated after 3 weeks. The serum level remains elevated for an average of 5 months.[32] The serum alkaline phosphatase level does not appear to correlate with the HO activity or the number of HO lesions.[18] Triple-phase bone scan with Tc-99m has been used commonly for detection and activity observation of HO. The first two phases are most sensitive for early detection (within the first 2–4 weeks after injury).

Traumatic HO begins, and is evident on radiologic examination, much earlier than neurogenic HO. The abnormal bone deposition is also not as exaggerated, and maturation is usually completed by 6 months after injury, allowing for early resection. Treatment modalities include diphosphonates, indomethacin, radiation, range of motion exercises, and surgical excision. The use of manipulation is rather controversial; some authors argue that it may accelerate the formation of HO. Surgical excision is frequently delayed until the HO is deemed mature based on available diagnostic measures.

Refracture

Rarely a second fracture can occur through the same fracture line during healing. The bone may have weakened and become predisposed to fracture by a screw hole, a pin tract, infection, or disuse osteoporosis. The lower extremities are the most common sites of refracture since they are subject to greater stresses than the upper extremities, especially in weightbearing activities such as ambulation.

SUMMARY

This chapter has described the various types of complications that can occur with fractures. Since these complications will affect patients' eventual functional outcome, careful attention to their prevention is critical. In the event that complications do occur, the physician must promptly detect and intervene to minimize the residual disability.

REFERENCES

1. Adams JC, Hamblen DL: Complications of fractures. In Outline of Fractures. 10th ed. New York, Churchill Livingstone, 1992, pp 48–67.
2. Alho A, Koskinen VS, Malberg H: Osteomyelitis in non-operative and post-operative fracture treatment. Clin Orthop 82:123–133, 1972.
2a. Alonso JE, Regazzoni P: The use of the Ilizarov Concept with the AO/ASIF tubular fixateur in the treatment of segmental defects. Orthop Clin North Am 21:655–665, 1990.
3. Baker PL, Pazell JA, Peltier LF: Free fatty acids, catecholamines, and arterial hypoxia in patients with fat embolism. J Trauma 11:1026–1030, 1971.
4. Bourne RB, Rorabeck CH: Compartment syndromes of the lower leg. Clin Orthop 240:97–104, 1989.
5. Brennan PJ, Pia DeGirolamo M: Musculoskeletal infections in immunocompromised hosts. Orthop Clin North Am 22:389–399, 1991.
6. Brighton CT, Pollack SR: Treatment of recalcitrant non-union with a capacitively couples electrical field. J Bone Joint Surg 67A:577–585, 1985.
7. Clawson DK, Dunn AW: Management of common bacterial infections of bones and joints. J Bone Joint Surg 49A:164–182, 1967.
8. Cohen MS, Garfin SR, Hargens AR, Mubarak SJ: Acute compartment syndrome: Effect of dermotomy on fascial decompression in the leg. J Bone Joint Surg 73B:287–290, 1991.
9. Collins HA, Jacobs JK: Acute arterial injuries due to blunt trauma. J Bone Joint Surg 43:193–197, 1961.
10. Cone JB: Vascular injury associated with fracture-dislocations of the lower extremity. Clin Orthop 243:30–35, 1989.
11. Consensus Conference: Prevention of venous thrombosis and pulmonary embolism. JAMA 256:744–757, 1986.
12. Crenshaw AH: Delayed union and non-union of fractures. In Crenshaw AH (ed): Campbell's Operative Orthopaedics. 7th ed. St. Louis, Mosby, 1987, pp 2112–2113.
13. Garland DE: Clinical observations on fractures and heterotopic ossification in the spinal cord and traumatic brain injured populations. Clin Orthop 233:86–101, 1988.
14. Garland DE: A clinical perspective on common forms of acquired heterotopic ossification. Clin Orthop 263:13–29, 1991.
15. Gurd AR: Fat embolism: An aid to diagnosis. J Bone Joint Surg 52B:732–737, 1970.
16. Gurd AR, Wilson RI: The fat embolism syndrome. J Bone Joint Surg 56B:408–416, 1974.
17. Gustilo RB, Anderson JT: Prevention of infection in the treatment of one thousand and twenty five open fractures of long bones: Retrospective and prospective analyses. J Bone Joint Surg 58A:453–458, 1976.
18. Heilburn N, Kuhn WG Jr: Erosive bone lesions and soft tissue ossifications associated with spinal cord injuries (paraplegia). Radiology 48:579–593, 1947.
19. Hendrix RW, Rogers LF: Diagnostic imaging of fracture complications. Radiol Clin North Am 27:1023–1033, 1989.
20. [Reference deleted.]
21. Kimura J: Anatomy and physiology of the peripheral nerve. In Electrodiagnosis in Diseases of Nerve and Muscle: Principles and Practice. Philadelphia, FA Davis, 1986, pp 59–81.
22. Lea Thomas M: Phlebography. Arch Surg 104:145–161, 1972.
23. LeQuesne LP: Relation between deep vein thrombosis and pulmonary embolism in surgical patients (current concepts). N Engl J Med 291:1292–1296, 1974.
24. Levy D: The fat embolism syndrome: A review. Clin Orthop 261:281–286, 1990.
25. Lindeque BG, Schoeman HS, Dommisse GF, et al: Fat embolism and the fat embolism syndrome: A double-blind therapeutic study. J Bone Joint Surg 69B:128–131, 1987.
26. Lord RSA, Irani CN: Assessment of arterial injury in limb trauma. J Trauma 14:1042–1053, 1974.
27. Love L: Arterial trauma. Semin Roentgenol 5:267–283, 1970.

28. Matsen FA, Winquist RA, Krugmire RB: Diagnosis and management of compartmental syndromes. J Bone Joint Surg 62A:286–291, 1980.

28a. Moser KM, Fedullo PF: Venous thromboembolism. Three simple decisions (Part I). Chest 83:117–121, 1983.

29. Mubarak SJ, Hargens AR: Acute compartment syndromes. Surg Clin North Am 63:539–565, 1983.

30. Mucha P Jr, Welch TJ: Hemorrhage in major pelvic fractures. Surg Clin North Am 68:757–773, 1988.

31. Mucha P Jr, Farnell MB: Analysis of pelvic fracture management. J Trauma 24:379–386, 1984.

32. Orzel JA, Rudd TG: Heterotopic bone formation: Clinical, laboratory, and imaging correlation. J Nucl Med 26:125–132, 1985.

33. Palmer JK, Benson GS, Corriere JN Jr: Diagnosis and initial management of urological injuries associated with 200 consecutive pelvic fractures. J Urol 130:712–714, 1983.

34. Patzakis MJ, Wilkins J: Factors influencing infection rate in open fracture wounds. Clin Orthop 243:36–40, 1989.

35. Peltier LF, Collins JA, Evarts CM, Sevitt S: Fat embolism. Arch Surg 109:12–16, 1974.

36. Perry MO: Compartment syndromes and reperfusion injury. Surg Clin North Am 68:853–864, 1988.

37. Rabinov K, Paulin S: Roentgen diagnosis of venous thrombosis in the leg. Arch Surg 104:134–144, 1972.

38. Rose SC, Moore EE: Trauma angiography: The use of clinical findings to improve patient selection and case preparation. J Trauma 28:240–245, 1988.

39. Salter RB: Fractures and joint injuries—general features. In Textbook of Disorders and Injuries of the Musculoskeletal System. 2nd ed. Baltimore, Williams & Wilkins, 1983, pp 394–414.

40. Sasahara AA, Barsamian EM, Cella G, et al: Recognition and management of acute pulmonary embolism. In Grand Rounds in Medicine: Recognition and Management of Thromboembolic Disorders. Professional Postgraduate Service, 1982, pp 17–28.

40a. Schwartsman V, Choi SH, Schwartsman R: Tibial nonunions. Treatment tactics with the Ilizarov method. Orthop Clin North Am 21:639–653, 1990.

41. Sigel B, Felix WR Jr, Popky GL, Ipsen J: Diagnosis of lower limb venous thrombosis by Doppler ultrasound technique. Arch Surg 104:174–179, 1972.

42. Smith TK: Nutrition: Its relationship to orthopedic infections. Orthop Clin North Am 22:373–377, 1991.

43. Stevens DB: Postoperative orthopaedic infections: A study of etiologic mechanisms. J Bone Joint Surg 46A:96–102, 1964.

44. Svenningsen S, Nesse O, Finsen V, et al: Prevention of fat embolism syndrome in patients with femoral fractures—Immediate or delayed operative fixation? Ann Chir Gynaecol 76:163–166, 1987.

45. Waldvogel FA, Medoff G, Swartz MN: Osteomyelitis: A review of clinical features, therapeutic considerations, and unusual aspects. N Engl J Med 282:198–206, 1970.

46. Weber RJ: Motor and sensory conduction and entrapment syndromes. In Johnson EW (ed): Practical Electromyography. 2nd ed. Baltimore, Williams & Wilkins, 1988, p 97.

47. Wegener WA, Alavi A: Diagnostic imaging of musculoskeletal infection: Roentgenography; gallium, indium-labeled white blood cell, gammaglobulin, bone scintigraphy; and MRI. Orthop Clin North Am 22:401–418, 1991.

48. Whitesides TE Jr, Haney TC, Morimoto K, Harada H: Tissue pressure measurements as a determinant of the need of fasciotomy. Clin Orthop 113:43–51, 1975.

JAY V. SUBBARAO, MD, MS
SIDNEY J. BLAIR, MD, FACS

REFLEX SYMPATHETIC DYSTROPHY SYNDROME

From the Department of
  Orthopaedic Surgery
Physical Medicine and
  Rehabilitation Section
Loyola University Medical
  Center, Hines Comprehensive
  Rehabilitative Services
Maywood, Illinois

Reprint requests to:
Jay V. Subbarao, MD, MS
ACOS for Rehabilitation
P.O. Box 5000 (11R)
Hines VA Hospital
Hines, IL 60141

The International Association for the Study of Pain (IASP)[32] defines reflex sympathetic dystrophy as "continuous pain in a portion of an extremity after trauma which may include fractures, but does not involve a major nerve associated with sympathetic activity." IASP defines causalgia as "burning pain, allodynia, and hyperpathia after partial injury of a nerve or one of its major branches."[32] Still another definition (by author SJB) is that of a sensorimotor alteration and trophic changes secondary to injury which produces diffuse limb pain.

Reports of painful disorders associated with injuries of peripheral nerves of the extremities began to appear in the 16th century. However, the most significant article was that of Civil War surgeon Silas Weir Mitchell, who published his findings regarding causalgia in 1864 and 1867.[38]

In 1946, Evans coined the term *reflex sympathetic dystrophy*, and in 1953, Bonica recommended that all the following conditions be considered under reflex sympathetic dystrophy syndrome (RSDS): (1) minor causalgia, (2) posttraumatic pain syndrome, (3) posttraumatic spreading neuralgia, (4) posttraumatic vasomotor disorders, (5) posttraumatic painful arthrosis, (6) Sudek's atrophy, (7) sympathalgia, (8) shoulder-hand syndrome, (9) chronic traumatic edema, (10) posttraumatic edema, (11) reflex dystrophy. Table 1 summarizes the commonly used synonyms. Following the taxonomy of the IASP, Bonica[11] reported that most members of

TABLE 1. Synonyms for Reflex Sympathetic Dystrophy

Causalgia—Mitchell, 1864	Reflex dystrophy of the extremities—DeTakats, 1937
Acute atrophy of bone—1900	
Sudeck's atrophy—Lenggenhager	Minor causalgia—Homans, 1940
Peripheral acute trophoneurosis—Zurverth, 1929	Post infarctional sclerodactyly—Johnson, 1943
Traumatic angiospasm—Morton and Scott, 1931	Reflex neurovascular dystrophy—Steinbrocker, 1947
Posttraumatic osteoporosis—Fontaine and Herrmann, 1933	Reflex sympathetic dystrophy syndrome—Evans, 1947
Traumatic vasospasm—Lehman, 1934	

From Escobar PL: Reflex Sympathetic Dystrophy. Belle Mead, NJ, Excerpta Medica, 1986; with permission.

the IASP committee believed that the term *causalgia* should be reserved for the classical syndrome in which there is a nerve injury and that reflex sympathetic dystrophy should be used in cases in which the injury does not involve a major nerve. Other authors have disagreed with this and included causalgia under reflex sympathetic dystrophy.

THE ETIOLOGIES

Various causes of RSDS include (1) accidental injury and surgery and (2) diseases that include infection and visceral, neurologic, and vascular dysfunction.

The pathophysiologic mechanism is that of tissue damage that initiates a response, which is a dynamic activity involving the vasomotor and thermal regulatory system. Various ideas of the etiology have evolved over a number of years. More recently, many animal models have been developed; however, their applicability in humans has been challenged. It is now believed that a variety of pathophysiologic mechanisms may generate the process. Ochoa presents an in-depth discussion regarding studies in humans.[49]

As Raj[52] has pointed out, any discussion of pathophysiology must be able to explain the burning pain, which is relieved by sympathetic blocks early, and the failure of these sympathetic blocks and surgery in the later phases. The various theories can be divided into the *central* and *peripheral theories.* The central theories include the gate control theory of Melzack and Wall.[48] The idea is that there is an imbalance between the slowly conducted painful impulses. Essentially, this balance is between the large A beta fibers and small A delta fibers and C fibers. The theory is that the A beta impulses modulate the other fibers and, if these modulation activities were not present, the C fiber and A delta fiber activity would be uninhibited. Roberts[55] has suggested that there is sensitization of neurons in substantia gelatinosa of the dorsal horn. The sensitization of these fibers could explain some of the symptoms of hyperalgesia and allodynia.

Livingston[45] proposed that abnormal firing patterns in the internuncial pool could set up a vicious circle of reflexes that distort information processing in the spinal cord and account for some of the symptoms. Peripheral mechanisms, such as the artificial synapse of Doupe,[19] may explain some of the ongoing phenomena. It is believed that there is an artificial synapse between the sensory and the sympathetic, causing the ongoing vasomotor problem. Campbell[13,14] and others have considered the problem in the periphery to be that of an alpha adrenergic disease and have suggested that there is a sensitization of the receptors in the periphery. Deyor,[18] from Israel, developed a neuron model in animals that explains the ongoing symptoms from spontaneous rhythmic discharges from the neuroma or injured axon. This work showed that newly sensitized alpha receptors would be sensitized to adrenergic stimuli.

In the past decade, theories have been proposed under the title of reflex neurogenic inflammation.[43,64] These mechanisms are based on the idea that nerve injury could cause increased production of neuropeptides, which could be transported both centrally and peripherally. These substances could cause vasodilation and edema and sensitization of the nerve endings. Sensitization could occur both peripherally and centrally. Subsequent activation of sympathetics could lower the threshold of mechano receptors (a subpopulation of polymodal with afferent fibers), which would account for the allodynia and hyperalgesia.

In 1991, the potential role of an autoimmunologic mechanism was suggested.[36] This theory proposes that a reactivation of a latent infection occurs in the dorsal root and sympathetic ganglia. Another proposed mechanism is that a sympatho-trophic factor is released during trauma, and this is thought to be a nerve growth factor that has profound effect on stimulating inflammation. In an extensive review of the literature, Schwartzman[63] attempted to correlate the symptoms of RSDS with the present knowledge of the etiologic contributory factors.

INCIDENCE AND DIAGNOSIS

An accurate incidence of RSDS in patients sustaining trauma is not known.[62] About 45% of 125 patients studied by Subbarao[71] were reported to have a history of trauma, 28 of whom sustained fractures involving the wrist. More than half of recognized cases of RSDS do occur after bone fractures. An 11% incidence of RSDS following Colles' fracture has been reported.[56] Table 2 shows the predisposing causes of RSDS of the upper extremity. The frequency of RSDS after peripheral nerve injury is 1–15%. In a study of Vietnam veterans, Rothberg[57] found an incidence of 10–15% in patients 17–34 years old and 47% in patients older than 35. In a prospective study of 100 consecutive patients with brain injury, Gellman et al.[24] found a 12% incidence. They noted that RSDS was present exclusively in the spastic upper extremity, but there was significantly higher incidence of upper extremity injury (75%) associated with dystrophy. Wainapel[78] reported two cases of RSDS involving the upper extremity of patients with traumatic cervical spinal cord injuries.

The clinical syndrome of RSDS affects females more commonly than males. The male-female ratio is 1:2.9 and, although the syndrome has been described in all age groups, the median age at onset is 54 years.[70] The age at onset depends on associated factors such as trauma, surgery, stroke, and myocardial infarction. In a study of 70 children younger than 18 with RSDS, Wilder et al.[80] found that the male-female ratio was 11:59 and that the lower extremity was involved most often. They commented that the syndrome is under-recognized in this age group because of the long time interval from injury to diagnosis. Deitz[16] reiterated the higher incidence in the lower extremities and found noninvasive nonpharmacologic management to be generally successful in children. The precipitating injury or event is not easily identifiable in children, and x-rays show minimal or no osteoporosis. However, the prognosis in children is better than in adults.[16,80]

There are isolated reports of cases of the syndrome involving only part of an extremity, such as the knee.[35,73] Kozin[39] found some cases in which bone scan abnormalities were noted in the opposite side in patients who had symptoms in only one extremity. Schiffenbauer[60] described a patient with four episodes of RSDS involving three limbs over a 4-year period. The case was unusual because the episodes occurred over so long a time.

TABLE 2. Predisposing Causes of Sympathetic Dystrophy of Hand

Causes		Number of Patients	
Cardiac		4	(3%)
Myocardial infarction	1		
Cardiac surgery	3		
Trauma		56	(45%)
Minor trauma	14		
Fracture involving hand	3		
Fracture involving wrist	28		
Injury to forearm	3		
Injury to elbow	1		
Injury to shoulder	5		
Neck injury	2		
Neurologic		36	(29%)
CVA on same side	4		
CVA on opposite side	1		
Head injury	1		
Neoplasm	2		
Brachial plexus lesions	5		
Median neuropathy	18		
Ulnar neuropathy	1		
Other	4		
Other causes		29	(23%)
Periarthritis, shoulder	8		
Surgery on hand	8		
Unknown	13		
TOTAL		125	(100%)

From Subbarao JV: Reflex Sympathetic Dystrophy Syndrome of the Upper Extremity: Analysis of Total Outcome of Management of 125 Cases. Philadelphia, WB Saunders, 1981; with permission.

The information necessary for a precise diagnosis of reflex sympathetic dystrophy syndrome comes through an understanding of the mechanism of injury; an understanding of the history of pain, including psychological, social, and vocational aspects; and a gentle but comprehensive physical examination. RSDS is a multisymptom complex with many causative factors that are poorly understood, and it may involve one or more extremities. In this chapter, discussion of the diagnosis and management will be limited to posttraumatic RSDS. Early diagnosis is critical to avoid permanent structural, functional, and psychological changes. The pathognomonic criteria for clinical diagnosis are pain, vasomotor instability, skin changes, motor dysfunction, and loss of function.

CLINICAL FEATURES

The clinical symptoms and signs vary with the interval from onset to evaluation and are essentially the same in the upper and lower extremities.[47,77]

1. **Pain.** Pain includes the presence of severe, constant burning pain that does not follow any dermatomal distribution, is out of proportion to the initiating injury or initiating factor, and has features of hyperpathia. Allodynia is the common mode of presentation.

2. **Vasomotor Instability.** Patients may complain of hyperhidrosis (increased sweating). The extremity may feel cool to touch and appear pale, suggesting vasoconstriction, or it may be warm and erythematous, indicating vasodilation.

3. **Skin Changes.** In the early stages of RSDS, the skin may appear glossy and dusky and exhibit mottling. However, in the atrophic stage, there is evidence of dryness, scaling, nail changes, and skin atrophy.

4. **Loss of Function.** Because of the swelling and constant pain with allodynia, patients do not use the extremity for functional hand activities, which leads to joint stiffness and further loss of function. The withdrawal from light touch and joint proprioceptin results in sensory deprivation and promotes the persistence of pain.

5. **Motor Dysfunction.** Patients may present with tremor, muscle spasm, dystonia, and inability to initiate movement. The motor symptoms may precede pain and are sometimes seen on the opposite side of the body. These manifestations commonly occur in late stage 2 and stage 3 RSDS but may occur suddenly in any stage. Sympathetic blockade or sympathectomy may control the movements, but recurrences are quite common.[17,63]

Stages of Reflex Sympathetic Dystrophy Syndrome

Patients may present in various stages of this painful condition. The clinical presentation is influenced by the original precipitating factor, such as injury, surgery, or illness, and time from onset to evaluation. About 18–50% of cases of RSDS involving the hand have associated pain and limitation of movement in the shoulder. Three stages of RSDS have been described,[11,70] and they sometimes overlap in presentation and duration.

Stage 1 (acute congestive RSDS). The patient complains of severe burning pain limited to the site of injury. Hyperesthesia accompanied by pitting edema with stiffness and decreased range of movement is common. Vasomotor dysfunction by way of warm, red, dry skin initially changing to a cyanotic, cold, and sweating extremity is noted. Hyperhidrosis is commonly seen. Evidence of some demineralization is seen in x-rays after the fourth week following onset. Average duration of stage 1 is 6 weeks–3 months; however, in mild cases the symptoms respond well to treatment and resolve rapidly.

Stage 2 (dystrophic RSDS). More severe diffuse pain, edema becomes brawny, joint stiffness increases, severe pain occurs when the patient attempts to move the joint. Decreased range and pain in proximal joints such as the shoulder are common. The onset of shoulder pain is insidious and may not be noticed by the patient. Patients may present with redness of the skin, particularly around the joints, with atrophy of subcutaneous tissue, fascitis, hair loss, nails becoming grooved, brittle, and cracked. Hyperhidrosis changes to dryness. The osteoporosis is quite pronounced with involvement of the ends of long bones. This stage may last 3–6 months.

Stage 3 (atrophic RSDS). The severity of pain may decrease. The swelling subsides, but induration remains around the joints. Trophic changes in skin are prominent, with glossy skin, atrophy of subcutaneous tissues and muscles, and fascitis progressing to contractures. Deformities of the joints (mostly flexion deformities) occur. Marked diffuse bone deossification is seen. This stage is considered irreversible.

INVESTIGATIONS

Roentgenographic studies, three-phase bone scans, and thermography are considered adjuncts to the clinical examination but have no specific abnormalities that will confirm the diagnosis of RSDS.

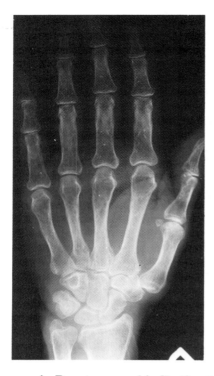

FIGURE 1. X-ray of wrist and hand showing patchy demineralization close to the epiphysis.

1. **Roentgenographic Studies.** In the initial stages, roentgenographic studies may reveal soft tissue swelling and reticulated appearance of the bones. Patchy demineralization close to the epiphyses is noted 3–6 weeks from onset (Fig. 1). In stage 2 there is evidence of subperiosteal bone resorption with a ground glass appearance and tunneling of the cortices and endosteal surface of the bone (Fig. 2). The disadvantage of the roentgenographic studies is that the changes are not seen in the first 3 weeks from onset, and the late changes are not specific for RSDS. In one study,[9] 44 patients with posttraumatic algodystrophy and Colles' fracture and 33 patients with Colles' fracture serving as controls were immobilized in the same manner and for the same duration. Both groups showed loss of bone during immobilization, but the regional skeletal losses, which may be irreversible, were greater in patients with algodystrophy.

2. **Radionuclide Bone Scans.** A three-phase bone scan is performed following injection of 20 mCi of Tc 99m pyrophosphate or Tc 99m medronate sodium. Images are obtained soon after injection, in 10 minutes, and in 2 hours. Characteristic findings of RSDS include diffuse increased asymmetric uptake in the affected limb in the first two phases of the scan and blood flow and blood pooling images and periarticular asymmetric hyperfixation of tracer in the third phase (Figs. 3 and 4). Kozin et al.[40] compared sensitivity and specificity of roentgenographic studies and scintigraphy in the assessment of RSDS. They reported a 71% specificity for roentgenography and 8.6% for scintigraphy, and they found 69% and 60% sensitivity, respectively. Simon[66] and Holder[30] further studied the efficacy of scintigraphy in the diagnosis of RSDS. Criteria for grading

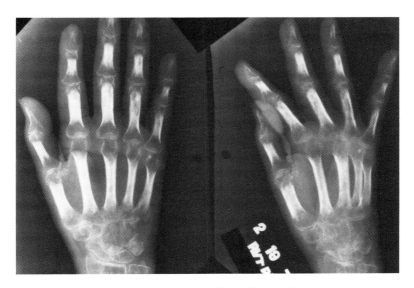

FIGURE 2. Extensive bone resorption with ground glass appearance.

FIGURE 3. Three-phase bone scan revealing diffuse asymmetric uptake in the right wrist and hand.

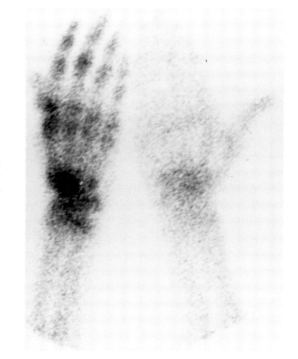

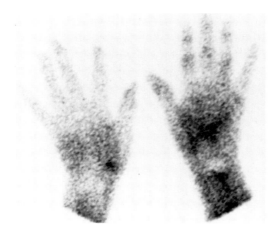

FIGURE 4. Blood pooling and periarticular asymmetric hyperfixation of tracer in the third phase.

positive three-phase radionuclide bone scans of the hand were proposed by Holder.[66] Atkins[5] observed that increased uptake in bone scans at the metacarpophalangeal joints closely correlated with uptake at the metacarpal bones, contrary to the previous reports that the uptake is confined to the periarticular areas. He also found correlation with increased uptake, local tenderness, and dolorimetry, suggesting that the bone scan is not only a diagnostic tool but also provides a quantitative indication of the severity of the condition, which may be useful in planning and assessing treatments. However, although bone scan studies help the clinician confirm the diagnosis, they are not specifically diagnostic of RSDS.

3. **Computed Tomography and Magnetic Resonance Imaging (MRI).** Sambrok and Champion[59] reported "swiss-cheese" bone osteopenia seen in CT studies as characteristic of RSDS. In a study of 25 patients with clinical findings and positive scintigraphy, MRI was normal in 10 patients and showed nonspecific soft tissue changes or bone marrow sclerosis in six. Thus, the authors concluded that MRI fails to detect RSDS.[37]

4. **Thermographic Assessment.** RSDS is especially amenable to thermographic detection because of the autonomic disturbances.[34,58,76] Williams[81] and Rothschild[58] used thermography to follow the clinical course of the rheumatologic and other musculoskeletal disorders. They noted that when there is no clinical response, there is failure of such agents to alter thermographic findings.

5. **Electrodiagnostic Studies.** In most cases, electrodiagnostic studies are used to establish the association of "nerve damage" in patients with RSDS rather than diagnose RSDS.

6. **Diagnostic Blocks.** These fall into the following two categories.

Sympathetic blockage. Some RSDS patients respond to pharmacologic or surgical blocking of the sympathetic innervation of the affected part. In an intravenous phentolamine test to diagnose and prognosticate the response,[3] the authors found that individuals who respond, even transiently, to intravenous phentolamine were very likely to respond favorably to subsequent sympatholytic treatments.

Differential nerve blocks. Differential nerve blocks are used to separate patients with central pain from those who respond to sympathetic blocks. Initially, normal saline is infused, followed by 1% of procaine hydrochloride. If pain relief does not occur, brachial/lumbar plexus blocks are done with 1% procaine hydrochloride. No response to any of these peripheral blocks suggests that the patient has "central pain."

7. **Psychological Assessment.** RSDS may occur more frequently in individuals who have "personality characteristics" that predispose them to the condition. In a retrospective study, Subbarao[71] reported that HS (hysteria), D (depression), and HY (hypochondriasis) scales are abnormal in the Minnesota Multiphasic Personality Inventory (MMPI) in RSDS patients. Some clinicians consider that there are personality traits that predispose for RSDS and that outcomes are not favorable in patients with the above MMPI abnormalities. Each patient must be assessed individually for possible psychological implications, because this greatly influences the patient's management and outcome. A critical analysis of literature to identify "predisposing psychologic factors" in the development of RSDS revealed that depression, anxiety, or life stressors may influence the development of RSDS through their effects on adrenergic activity.[12,46] These analyses stress the need for prospective studies to establish an etiologic significance of these findings.

Shelton et al.[65] summarized signs and symptoms and the stages of RSDS (Table 3). Amadio et al.[2] postulated that early and late stages tend to have fewer significant factors than the middle stages (Fig. 5).

TABLE 3. Staging Classification of Reflex Sympathetic Dystrophy

	Stage 1 (Sympathetic Denervation)	Stage 2 (Sympathetic Overactivity)	Stage 3 (Atrophic)
Onset after injury	3 days–3 wk	3–7 mo	by 8 mo
Duration	1 mo	3–6 mo	Indefinite
Vasculature	Vasodilation	Vasoconstriction	Vasoconstriction
Heat intolerance	+	−	−
Cold intolerance	−	+	+
Temperature	Warm	Cool	Cool; decreased differential of affected and unaffected limb
Color	Erythema; dependent rubor; red knuckles	Pallor; cyanosis; mottled flexure crease erythema (spreading; fusiform)	Pallor; cyanosis; smooth and glossy
Edema	+	+	−
Hair	Increased growth	Decreased growth	Hypertrichosis
Nails	Increased growth and transverse curvature	Brittle	Brittle
Sweating	Anhidrosis; later hyperhidrosis	Hyperhidrosis	Anhidrosis
Pain	+	+ Decreased; spreading neuralgia	Decreased or intractable
Glovelike sensory defect	Hypoesthesia or hyperesthesia	±	±
Subcutaneous tissue atrophy	−	+	Tapered digits +
Osteoporosis	−	Patchy +	Diffuse +
Range of motion	Decreased; muscle spasm	Decreased	Decreased; flexion contractures

+, Present; −, absent; ±, reports of presence and absence both occur in the literature.
Adapted from Shelton RM, Lewis CW: Reflex sympathetic dystrophy: A review. J Am Acad Dermatol 22:513–520, 1990; with permission.

Early: Days to Weeks   Late: Years

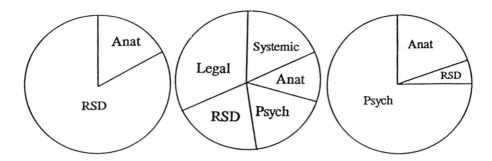

Middle: Months

FIGURE 5. Early and late stages of RSDS tend to have fewer significant factors that may maintain the pain syndrome than the middle stages. *Left,* in the early stages, days to weeks, prognosis is generally good. Evaluation often finds treatable anatomic problems. *Center,* in the middle stages, months, the prognosis is guarded. Multiple problems usually are evident, and the main challenge exists in this phase. Evaluation may find a treatable problem. *Right,* the late stages occur after years of impairment. Prognosis is poor. Evaluation rarely finds a treatable problem. If a treatable problem is found, treatment rarely results in a "cure." The late stage may have little or no active reflex sympathetic dystrophy, but represents an end-stage diffuse fibrosis, ankylosis, atrophy, and, often, psychiatric impairment. (From Amadio PC: Reflex Sympathetic Dystrophy Syndrome: Consensus Report of an Ad Hoc Committee of the American Association for Hand Surgery on the Definition of Reflex Sympathetic Dystrophy Syndrome. Baltimore, Williams & Wilkins, 1991; with permission.)

MANAGEMENT

Early recognition of the symptom complex will enable prompt initiation of treatment, which is most essential for a successful outcome. A number of treatments have been used over the years with varying success. Reported outcomes were related to the managing physician's specialty. For example, good outcomes have been reported with the use of blocks by anesthesiologists, and physiatrists have stressed the need for physical modalities. A complex syndrome such as RSDS requires a multimodality approach and, preferably, a team approach. A management plan can be designed to eliminate main contributory factors such as persistent pain diathesis and abnormal sympathetic reflexes.[54] Escabor[21] summarized treatment of patients by stage of the syndrome.

The treatment can be tailored to individual patients' clinical presentations. The goals are to decrease edema, desensitization, and pain; improve range of movement and functional hand activities; and provide counseling and patient education.

Edema Control

The edema can be reduced by compression glove and friction massage. If the patient has hyperesthesia and cannot tolerate the massage and edema persists, a pneumatic pump with pressure up to 40–60 mm Hg can be used. Following the pump treatment, compression should be continued with a glove or ace wrap. Medications such as prednisone and antiinflammatories will further facilitate edema management. Diuretics are rarely used for control of local edema. The extremity needs to be elevated while at rest to decrease edema.

Modalities

The use of cold or heat depends on the clinical stage in which the patient is seen. Heat generally increases swelling. Patients with hyperesthesia may not tolerate cold well. Patients need to be monitored for skin changes. Contrast baths are effective and commonly used by patients on a long-term basis. In later stages of RSDS, a paraffin bath is quite effective to mobilize soft tissue and the joints. The advantage of a paraffin bath is that it can be done at home, is therefore cost-effective, and patients have better compliance.[71] Heat and cold facilitate reestablishment of vascular tone and decrease muscle spasm. Ultrasound is used in stage 3 RSDS to facilitate stretching of contractures but is rarely of benefit when used alone. Fluidotherapy is commonly used to provide superficial heat while the patient is performing functional activities, and it is more commonly used for the hand. If hydrotherapy is used, special emphasis on edema control is essential because the heat and dependency is likely to increase swelling in early stages.

Splinting

The extremity involved should not be immobilized unless an associated fracture requires immobilization. However, it is common to prescribe a "resting hand splint" to maintain functional hand position, especially at night. When immobilized, the hand should be maintained in 20° wrist extension. The main goals of splinting are to decrease pain, minimize contractures, and maintain a "balanced hand." Patients should be given a "splint wearing schedule" and a list of exercises to maintain the range of movement in the joints. In late stage 2 and early stage 3, dynamic splinting may be used to provide sustained stretch. The splint should be comfortable and should not deprive sensory feedback.

Desensitization Program

Most patients in early stages of RSDS present with a hypersensitivity response to touch and will develop a "protective reflex," thus decreasing the tactile and proprioceptive feedback. The patient should be reassured and educated regarding the desensitization program. Initially, gentle stroking is started with cotton and is advanced to materials with increasing friction and coarseness to touch. The program is more successful when the patient is trained to perform the desensitization under professional guidance and continues at home in frequent but brief sessions. Ice massage may also facilitate desensitization. The control of hyperesthesia and other dysesthesias is a critical step before instituting functional hand activities and a strengthening program.

Exercises

The role of exercise in patients with established RSDS remains controversial.[61] Exercises should not trigger additional pain or apprehension for the patient. Passive exercise should be avoided. Initially, the exercises should be gentle, active, frequent, and of short duration. As the patient improves, the exercises should be modified to incorporate functional hand activities. The modalities are generally prescribed before the exercises. In patients with RSDS involving the hand and foot, range of movement of proximal joints such as the elbow, shoulder, knee, and hip should be maintained. The patients will benefit from general conditioning exercises such as walking, stretching, and swimming. Such activities will prevent deconditioning and shift the focus away from the involved area. Good results have been reported when patients were involved in a "stress loading" program that consisted of active traction and compression exercises that provide stressful stimuli to the extremity without joint motion.[79] The patient should be involved in an individualized intense vocational, athletic, or recreational retraining program with professional guidance to allow them to return to the highest level of productive life.

Transcutaneous Electrical Stimulation

TENS is commonly used for pain control. In our experience, patients with hyperesthesia poorly tolerate TENS over the involved area. Stimulation of the sensory nerve supplying the area or acupuncture points are more often successful. A TENS unit will be a good adjunct for other treatment tools and more so in chronic stage. The relief provided by a TENS unit is postulated to be from "blocking the gate" by artificially generated pulses from large-diameter fibers.[48] The advantages of a TENS unit are that the patient will control its use, and it does not result in any adverse effects.

Medications

Medications used in the management of RSDS include the following:
A. Antiinflammatories
   Corticosteroids
   Nonsteroidal antiinflammatories
B. Analgesics
   Narcotics
   Nonnarcotics
C. Abnormal sympathetic reflex blockade
   Sympatholytic phenoxybenzamine (Dibenzyline)
   Phentolamine (Regitine)
   Reserpine (Serpasil)
   Guanethidine (Ismelin)
D. Muscle relaxants
   Cyclobenzaprine (Flexaril)
   Methocarbamol (Robaxin)
E. Miscellaneous
   Diazepam (Valium)
   Chlordiazepoxide (Librium)
   Amitriptyline (Elavil)
   Fluphenazine hydrochloride (Prolixin)
   Propranolol (Inderal)

Antiinflammatories. Some studies report that prednisone is efficacious in early stages of RSDS. The dosages and duration of treatment are quite variable. The commonly recommended regimen is 60–80 mg/day, gradually tapered over the next 3–4 weeks. In a double-blind study in which some patients took 10 mg of prednisone three times a day and others took a placebo, both for a maximum of 12 weeks, good results were reported in 75% of patients treated with prednisone.[15]

The general contraindications for use of corticosteroids should be considered before starting treatment. Kozin[40] observed that several patients required retreatment following initial therapy due to recurrence of RSDS and that prolonged treatment with high-dose corticosteroids may be beneficial in the treatment of prolonged RSDS. Therapy with corticosteroids should be considered for patients who refuse or cannot tolerate treatments that directly block sympathetic activity. Other nonsteroidal antiinflammatories have been prescribed with varying success, but there are no good studies evaluating the effectiveness of these medications.

Analgesics. Both narcotic and nonnarcotic medications should be used sparingly after the acute stage and, preferably, on a scheduled basis than as needed. Long-term use of narcotic medications may lead to dependency in some patients.

Sympatholytics. The interruption of the abnormal reflex mediated by the sympathetic system is the main rationale for this approach. The blockade can be attempted by intravenous infusion of reserpine or guanethidine or by agents that effectively produce a transient chemical sympathectomy. Driessen[20] modified Hannington-Kiff's method,[29] injecting 20 mg of guanethidine sulphate diluted in 10 ml of 1% lidocaine and 30 ml of 0.9% physiologic saline. Of the 20 patients Driessen studied, 11 had good, 2 had moderate, and 7 had poor results.[20] In a randomized study of 66 RSDS patients, one group received physical therapy and three sprays of 100 IU of calcitonin-salmon by intranasal spray daily, and the other group received three sprays of placebo. Patients treated with calcitonin had decreased pain and an improved ability to return to work.[26] In another prospective randomized study,[8] 400 IU of nasal calcitonin daily was found to have no demonstrable effect on the clinical or skeletal progression of the disorder. Ghostine[25] studied the effect of phenoxybenzamine on patients with RSDS in acute stage and noted complete resolution of symptoms; however, some patients developed orthostatic hypotension.

Arner[3] studied 48 patients with RSDS in whom the upper limb was affected in 38 and the lower limb in 10. Twenty-six patients had "nerve lesion," 22 as a result of trauma. Doses of 5–15 mg of phentolamine were continuously injected over 5–10 minutes. Patients who responded were very likely to respond to other types of sympatholytic treatments.

In another study, 513 regional intravenous guanethidine blocks in 125 patients with RSDS revealed positive results; 22 patients had moderate side effects but continued treatment, and another 22 patients had serious complications requiring interruption of treatment.[22] Although the reported complications with the use of reserpine and guanethidine are few, prolonged orthostatic hypotension, dizziness, somnolence, nausea, and vomiting occur. Guanethidine functions as a false transmitter and competitively blocks the sympathetic nerve endings, thus replacing norepinephrine from its storage sites. Reserpine intraarterially produces similar effects by reducing the storage vesicle reuptake of catecholamines and thus depletes the norepinephrine stores in sympathetic nerve endings.[6] Thomsen[74] demonstrated a threefold increase in total blood flow following guanethidine block, which lasted up to 72 hours.

Favorable results have been reported with propranolol in high oral doses in nonresponsive patients.[67]

Somatic Nerve Blocks and Sympathetic Ganglion Blocks

Peripheral nerve blocks can be done at various levels depending on the extent of involvement. These blocks are aimed at eliminating the sympathetic impulse transmission. Bupivacaine, a longer-acting anesthetic, is usually used with minimal side effects. A Bier block technique is used for regional anesthesia. In a study of blocks with lidocaine hydrochloride and hydrocortisone sodium succinate in 28 patients, 57% achieved good results.[51] In another study, 11 of 16 patients had almost total relief at 6 months. When 15 of the patients were reassessed at an average follow-up of 28 months, none of the patients with an early satisfactory response experienced recurrence.[75]

The use of sympathetic ganglion block was first described by Homans[31] in 1940. A stellate ganglion block is done using 1% lidocaine or 0.25% bupivacaine hydrochloride at the level of the seventh cervical and first thoracic vertebra. A successful block results in Horner syndrome, cool dry hand, and relief of pain. In the lumbar region the level of sympathetic block is determined by initial epidural sensory block. The sympathetic ganglion block is the most logical management approach in patients who have not responded to traditional physical therapy and medications. Patients who do not respond with significant pain relief following a technically successful block should be assessed for conditions other than RSDS. Using laser Doppler flowmetry and thermometry, Irazuzta et al.[33] studied changes in the skin capillary bloodflow (SBF) and temperature before, during, and 1 hour after unilateral lumbar paravertebral sympathetic block. They noted tenfold increase in SBF within 4 minutes and increase of $1°C$ in skin temperature within 11 minutes. One hour later the SBF increased 18-fold, but it significantly decreased in the contralateral toes. Sympathetic ganglion blocks have been found to be more effective than corticosteroids.[69] In a study of 125 patients, 35 patients were successfully treated with sympathetic blocks.[71] Structured therapy programs in conjunction with blocks in series of three injections were given on successive days, with an average of up to three blocks. The number of sympathetic blocks and interval between each block still remains arbitrary.[71]

The guanethidine block has been shown to last longer and to be superior to stellate ganglion block in terms of some early pharmacologic effects. However, at 1-month and 3-month follow-up, a guanethidine block carried out every 4 days up to a total of four blocks is comparable with a stellate block done every day up to 8 blocks.[10] Continuous infusions of local anesthetic by indwelling catheter also have been attempted.[7,10] Linson et al.[44] injected bupivacaine hydrochloride every 8 hours to the stellate ganglion for an average of 7 days. They noted 90% improvement at discharge from hospital and only a 25% relapse rate and marked improvement persisted on long term follow-up for an average 3 years.

Trigger Point Injections

Patients with RSDS may develop multiple tender areas in the involved extremity and sometimes more diffusely even in the paraspinal region. Trigger points are best managed with local injection of 0.5% Marcaine followed by massage and muscle relaxation and stretching. Control of these trigger points will prevent additional tension myalgias that further complicate management and, if not treated in a timely fashion, will lead to poor functional outcomes.

Surgery

Except for sympathectomy, the role of surgery in the management of RSDS is limited. Olcott et al.[50] described the role of surgeon and stressed the need for a team approach in the management. Common surgical procedures include the following:

Surgical cervical or lumbar sympathectomy. Surgical ganglionectomy is recommended for patients who experience effective but transient relief from sympathetic blocks.[4,41,68] A number of techniques of sympathectomy have been described.[50] Rasmussen[53] noted that periarterial sympathectomy is less effective than ganglionectomy.

Reconstructive and rehabilitative surgery. There is a limited role for reconstructive rehabilitative surgery. The most common surgical procedures are performed in the late stages and are aimed at increasing range of movement and decreasing deformities. A majority of them are capsulotomies with or without resection of the volar plate and tenolysis of flexor tendons. *No surgery to gain motion should be considered until abnormal sympathetic reflex is eliminated.* Postoperatively the patient should continue appropriate exercises, splinting, and functional activities described earlier in this chapter.

Cordotomy and rhizotomy. Cordotomy and rhizotomy are rarely considered for patients who have RSDS resulting from trauma but who do not have major neurologic deficit such as brachial plexus or spinal cord injury.

Dorsal column stimulator implantation and implanted pumps. Electrical stimulation for control of chronic pain is based on the same principles as the TENS unit and is aimed at closing the "gate."[48]

Biofeedback and Behavioral Therapy

Alioto[1] and Gainer[23] have proposed supportive, stress reduction psychotherapies and behavioral treatment for this chronic painful disorder. The interdisciplinary team approach such as the one used in chronic pain management places heavy emphasis on patient education. Lifestyle adaptations and counseling may enhance the patient's functional level and increase the return to social and vocational roles in greater numbers.

Subbarao[71] found no strong correlation between litigation and functional outcome. Although litigation is not a medical diagnosis, it is an important variable that has impact on the management.[2]

Amadio et al.[2] postulated that early and late stages tend to have fewer significant factors than the middle stages (*see* Fig. 5).

FOLLOW-UP, OUTCOMES, AND PREVENTION

Greipp[27] studied long-term effects of RSDS in 27 young clients and noted that early diagnosis (less than 6 months' duration) led to no significant difference in the effectiveness of treatments. This is contrary to a majority of the reports and the authors' experience. Wilder,[80] in a study of 70 patients younger than 18 followed for an average of 3 years, observed that "although treatment produced substantial improvement in pain and function in the group as a whole, many patients still had considerable pain and dysfunction at the time of the latest follow-up." Only 46% were free of symptoms and fewer than half who were competing in sports prior to onset of symptoms returned to sports after treatment. A total of 94% reported that the illness had adversely affected their school work. The response to various modalities used was variable; nearly 60% of the patients had some persistent symptoms.[71] Table 4 shows vocational outcomes in these patients. While the patients complained of residual pain, many of them were not taking narcotics and were able to perform their daily activities. Of the 26 patients who were receiving disability payments, only four were taking narcotics and 13 did not take any medications.

TABLE 4. Vocational Outcome*

Work Status	n	Persistent Complaints*				Continuing Medications				Normal Daily Activities*				
		Hand		Shoulder		None	Occasional	Regular	Narcotics	100%	75%	50%	25%	0
		Stiffness	Pain	Stiffness	Pain									
Resumed same job	23	19	11	7	9	17	4	2	0	6	10	3	1	1
Housewife able to do housework	28	19	12	8	11	25	2	2	0	14	11	2	0	2
Retired prior to onset	13	7	7	3	4	6	2	4	1	4	5	2	2	1
Changed occupation	15	11	9	8	8	10	0	4	1	2	4	3	2	6
Retired after onset	23	17	15	8	10	13	3	6	1	6	6	5	2	4
Receiving disability payments	26	21	19	18	14	13	2	7	4	2	4	6	4	9
Housewife unable to do housework	27	24	21	17	16	12	3	9	4	0	4	10	4	8
Student not back to school	10	7	6	5	5	6	2	1	1	4	1	2	0	3

* Based on assessments by patients. Patients often made more than 1 selection.

From Subbarao JV: Reflex sympathetic dystrophy syndrome of the upper extremity: Analysis of total outcome of management of 125 cases. Arch Phys Med Rehabil 62:549–554, 1981; with permission.

Most agree that early recognition of RSDS can prevent the severe sequela. There should be early aggressive therapy that includes decreasing sympathetic activity. Hannington-Kiff,[28] discussing relief and prevention of reflex sympathetic dystrophy, developed a hypothesis of failed opioid modulation and recommended injection of opioid (morphine) into the stellate ganglion. He believed that this would prevent RSDS from developing following a surgical procedure.

When surgical procedures are used to correct stiffness, it is recommended that the condition be quiescent and that there be no pain or swelling.[42] One can use postoperative stellate blocks. Corticosteroids such as hydrocortisone can be given interoperatively and can be used postoperatively, if necessary, as long as there is no contraindication.

SUMMARY

Reflex sympathetic dystrophy is a syndrome in which pain is accompanied by autonomic dysfunction resulting in loss of function. The etiology is still unclear and factors other than the autonomic nervous system should be considered as etiologic basis because of variations in clinical presentations, response to treatment, and results. The accompanying psychologic diathesis, workers' compensation, and medicolegal factors should be fully evaluated while designing a treatment plan. The available investigations are nonspecific but contribute toward an early diagnosis and intervention, which is essential for a good outcome. Treatment should be pain-free, minimize immobilization, and include patient education and active participation. Multiple modalities are commonly used concurrently with blocks and emotional support to the patient and a team approach with positive outlook. There are very few long-term follow-up studies to assess the functional outcome in posttraumatic RSDS patients in whom treatment was instituted fewer than 3 months following onset. The management principles described above should be instituted at the earliest suspicion of the diagnosis but not wait for a definitive diagnosis before initiating treatment.

ACKNOWLEDGMENT

The authors thank Ms. Vaunda Bray of the Hines Comprehensive Rehabilitation Center, Hines, Illinois, for her assistance in the preparation of this chapter.

REFERENCES

1. Alioto JT: Behavioral treatment of reflex sympathetic dystrophy. Psychosomatics 22:539–540, 1981.
2. Amadio PC, Mackinnon SE, Merritt WH, et al: Reflex Sympathetic Dystrophy: Consensus Report of an Ad Hoc Committee of the American Association for Hand Surgery on the Definition of Reflex Sympathetic Dystrophy Syndrome. Plast Reconstr Surg 87:371–375, 1991.
3. Arner S: Intravenous phentolamine test: Diagnostic and prognostic use in reflex sympathetic dystrophy. Pain 46:17–22, 1991.
4. Atkins HJB: Sympathectomy by axillary approach. Lancet 1:538–539, 1954.
5. Atkins RM, Tindale W, Bickerstaff D, Kanis JA: Quantitative bone scintigraphy in reflex sympathetic dystrophy. Br J Rheumatol 32:41–45, 1993.
6. Benzon HT, Chomka CM, Brunner EA: Treatment of reflex sympathetic dystrophy with regional intravenous reserpine. Anesth Analg 59:500–502, 1980.
7. Betcher AM, Bean G, Casten DF: Continuous procaine block of paravertebral sympathetic ganglions. JAMA 151:288–305, 1953.
8. Bickerstaff DR, Kanis JA: The use of nasal calcitonin in the treatment of post-traumatic algodystrophy. Br J Rheumatol 30:291–294, 1991.
9. Bickerstaff DR, Charlesworth D, Kanis JA: Changes in cortical and trabecular bone in algodystrophy. Br J Rheumatol 32:46–51, 1993.

10. Bonelli S, Conoscente F, Movilia PG, et al: Regional intravenous guanethidine vs. stellate ganglion clock in reflex sympathetic dystrophy: A randomized trial. Pain 16:297–307, 1983.
11. Bonica JJ: The Management of Pain, Vol. 1. Philadelphia, Lea & Febiger, 1990.
12. Bruehl S, Carlson CR: Predisposing psychological factors for the development of reflex sympathetic dystrophy: A review of the empirical evidence. Clin J Pain 8:287–299, 1992.
13. Campbell JN, Raja SN, Meyer RA, MacKinnon SE: Myelinated afferents signal the hyperalgesia associated with nerve injury. Pain 32:89–94, 1988.
14. Campbell JN, Meyer RA, LaMotte RH: Sensitization of myelinated nociceptive afferents that innervate monkey hand. J Neurophysiol 42:1669–1679, 1979.
15. Christensen K, Jensen EM, Noer I: The reflex dystrophy syndrome response to treatment with systemic corticosteroids. Acta Chir Scand 148:653–655, 1982.
16. Deitz FR, Mathews KD, Montgomery WJ: Reflex sympathetic dystrophy in children. Clin Orthop 258:225–231, 1990.
17. Deuschl G, Blumberg H, Lucking CH: Tremor in reflex sympathetic dystrophy. Arch Neurol 48:1247–1252, 1991.
18. Devor M, Wall PD: Plasticity in the spinal cord sensory map following peripheral nerve injury in rats. J Neurosci 1:679–684, 1981.
19. Doupe J, Cullen CH, Chance GQ: Post-traumatic pain and the causalgic syndrome. J Neurol Neurosurg Psychiatry 7:33–48, 1944.
20. Driessen JJ, Van DerWerken C, Nicolai JPA, Crul JF: Clinical effects of regional intravenous guanethidine (Ismelin) in reflex sympathetic dystrophy. Acta Anaesthesiol Scand 27:505–509, 1983.
21. Escobar PL: Reflex sympathetic dystrophy. Orthop Rev 15:646–651, 1986.
22. Eulry F, Lechevalier D, Pats B, et al: Regional intravenous guanethidine blocks in algodystrophy. Clin Rheumatol 10:377–383, 1991.
23. Gainer MJ: Hypnotherapy for reflex sympathetic dystrophy. Am J Clin Hypn 34:227–232, 1992.
24. Gellman H, Keenam MA, Stone L, et al: Reflex sympathetic dystrophy in brain injured patients. Pain 51:307–311, 1992.
25. Ghostine SY, Comair YG, Turner DM, et al: Phenoxybenzamine in the treatment of causalgia: Report of 40 cases. J Neurosurg 60:1263–1268, 1984.
26. Gobelet C, Waldburger M, Meier JL: The effect of adding calcitonin to physical treatment on reflex sympathetic dystrophy. Pain 48:171–175, 1992.
27. Greipp MA: Reflex sympathetic dystrophy syndrome: A retrospective pain study. J Adv Nurs 15:1452–1456, 1990.
28. Hannington-Kiff JG: Does failed natural opioid modulation in regional ganglia cause reflex sympathetic dystrophy. Lancet 2:1125–1127, 1991.
29. Hannington-Kiff JG: Intravenous regional sympathetic block with guanethidine. Lancet 1:1019–1020, 1974.
30. Holder L, Mackinnon SE: Reflex sympathetic dystrophy in the hands: Clinical and scintigraphic criteria. Radiology 152:517–522, 1984.
31. Homans J: Minor causalgia: A hyperesthetic neurovascular syndrome. N Engl J Med 222:870–874, 1940.
32. International Association for the Study of Pain, The Subcommittee on Taxonomy, Classification of Chronic Pain: Descriptions of chronic pain syndromes and definitions of pain terms. Pain Suppl 3:S1–S226, 1986.
33. Irazuzta JE, Berde CB, Sethna NF: Laser Doppler measurements of skin blood flow before, during, and after lumbar sympathetic blockade in children and young adults with reflex sympathetic dystrophy. J Clin Monit 8:16–19, 1992.
34. Karstetter KW, Sherman RA: Use of Thermography for initial detection of early reflex sympathetic dystrophy. J Am Podiatr Med Assoc 81:198–205, 1991.
35. Katz MM, Hungerford DS: Reflex sympathetic dystrophy affecting the knee. J Bone Joint Surg 69B:797–803, 1987.
36. Knobler RL: Pathogenesis of reflex sympathetic dystrophy. Presented at Immune and Viral Mechanism symposium. Philadelphia, May 3–4, 1991.
37. Koch E, Hofer HO, Silear G, et al: Failure of MR imaging to detect reflex sympathetic dystrophy of extremities. J Rheumatol 156:113–115, 1991.
38. Koman LA, Poehling GG: Reflex sympathetic dystrophy. In Gelberman RH (ed): Operative Nerve Repair and Reconstruction. Philadelphia, JB Lippincott, 1991.
39. Kozin F, Genant H, Bekerman C, et al: The reflex sympathetic dystrophy syndrome. II. Roentgenologic and scintigraphic evidence of bilaterality and periarticular involvement. Am J Med 60:332–338, 1976.

40. Kozin F, Ryan LM, Carrera GF, et al: The reflex sympathetic dystrophy syndrome. III. Scintigraphic studies further evidence for the therapeutic efficacy of systemic corticosteroids and proposed diagnostic criteria. Am J Med 70:23–30, 1981.
41. Kux M: Thoracic endoscopic sympathectomy in palmar and axillary hyperhidrosis. Arch Surg 113:264–266, 1978.
42. Lankford LL: Reflex sympathetic dystrophy. In Green DP (ed): Operative Hand Surgery. New York, Churchill Livingstone, 1988, pp 633–663.
43. Levine JD, Dardick SJ, Basbaum AI, et al: Reflex neurogenic inflammation. I. Contribution of the peripheral nervous system to spatially remote inflammatory responses that follow injury. J Neurosci 5:1380–1386, 1985.
44. Linson MA, Leffert R, Todd DP: The treatment of upper extremity reflex sympathetic dystrophy with prolonged continuous stellate ganglion blockade. J Hand Surg 8A:153–159, 1983.
45. Livingston WK: Pain Mechanisms. New York, Macmillan, 1943, pp 209–233.
46. Lynch ME: Psychological aspects of reflex sympathetic dystrophy: A review of the adult and pediatric literature. Pain 49:337–347, 1992.
47. McNerney JE: Reflex sympathetic dystrophy: Traumatic and post-operative presentation and management in the lower extremity. Clin Podiatr Med Surg 8:287–307, 1991.
48. Melzack R, Wall PD: Pain Mechanisms, A New Theory. Science 150:971–979, 1965.
49. Ochoa JL, Verdugo R: Reflex sympathetic dystrophy definitions and history of the ideas with a critical review of human studies. In Low PH (ed): Clinical Disorders of Autonomic Function. Boston, Little, Brown & Co, 1943.
50. Olcott E, Eltherington LG, Wilcosky BR, et al: Reflex sympathetic dystrophy—the surgeon's role in management. J Vasc Surg 14:488–495, 1991.
51. Poplawski ZJ, Wiley AM, Murray JF: Post traumatic dystrophy in the extremities. J Bone Joint Surg 65A:642–655, 1983.
52. Raj P, Calodney A, Janisse T: Reflex sympathetic dystrophy. In Browner BD, Jupiter JB, Levine AM, Trafton PG (eds): Skeletal Trauma. Philadelphia, WB Saunders, 1992, pp 471–499.
53. Rasmussen TB, Freedman H: Treatment of causalgia: An analysis of 100 cases. J Neurosurg 3:165–173, 1946.
54. Regional Review Course in Hand Surgery, 1986. The American Society for Surgery of the Hand, Denver, 1986.
55. Roberts WJ: A hypothesis on the physiological basis for causalgia and related pains. Pain 24:297–311, 1986.
56. Rosenthal AK, Wortmann RL: Diagnosis, pathogenesis and management of reflex sympathetic dystrophy syndrome. Compr Ther 17(6):46–50, 1991.
57. Rothberg JM, Tahmoush AJ, Oldakowski R: The epidemiology of causalgia among soldiers wounded in Vietnam. Mil Med 148:347–350, 1983.
58. Rothschild BM: Thermographic assessment of bone and joint disease. Orthop Rev 15:765–780, 1986.
59. Sambrook P, Champion G: Reflex sympathetic dystrophy: Characteristic changes in bone on CT scan. J Rheumatol 17:1425–1426, 1990.
60. Schiffenbauer J, Fagien M: Reflex sympathetic dystrophy involving multiple extremities. J Rheumatol 201:165–169, 1993.
61. Schutzer SF, Gossling HR: The treatment of reflex sympathetic dystrophy syndrome. J Bone Joint Surg 66A:625–629, 1984.
62. Schwartzman RJ, McLellan TL: Reflex sympathetic dystrophy. Arch Neurol 44:555–561, 1987.
63. Schwartzman RJ: Reflex sympathetic dystrophy and causalgia. Neurol Clin North Am 10:953–973, 1992.
64. Schwartzman RJ: Sympathetic dystrophy. In Hachinski VL (ed): Controversies and Challenges in Neurology. Philadelphia, FA Davis, 1988.
65. Shelton RM, Lewis CW: Reflex sympathetic dystrophy: A review. J Am Acad Dermatol 22:513–520, 1990.
66. Simon H, Carlson DW: The use of bone scanning in the diagnosis of reflex sympathetic dystrophy. Clin Nucl Med 5:116–121, 1980.
67. Simson G: Propranolol for causalgia and Sudeck atrophy. JAMA 3:227–327, 1976.
68. Spurling RG: Causalgia of the upper extremity: Treatment by dorsal sympathetic ganglionectomy. Arch Neurol 23:784–788, 1930.
69. Steinbrocker O, Newstadt G, Lapin L: Shoulder hand syndrome: Sympathetic block compared with corticotropin and cortisone therapy. JAMA 153:788–791, 1946.
70. Steinbrocker O: Shoulder hand syndrome: Present perspective. Arch Phys Med Rehabil 49:388–394, 1968.

71. Subbarao JV, Stillwell GK: Reflex sympathetic dystrophy syndrome of the upper extremity: Analysis of total outcome of management of 125 cases. Arch Phys Med Rehabil 62:549–554, 1981.
72. Szenifeld M, Palleres VS: Considerations in the treatment of causalgia. Anesthesiology 58:294–296, 1983.
73. Teitjen R: Reflex sympathetic dystrophy of the knee. Clin Orthop 209:234–243, 1986.
74. Thomsen MB, Bengtsson M, Lassvik C, et al: Changes in human forearm blood flow after intravenous regional sympathetic blockade with guanethidine. Acta Chir Scand 148:656–661, 1982.
75. Tountas AA, Noguchi A: Treatment of post traumatic reflex sympathetic dystrophy with intravenous blocks of a mixture of corticosteroids and lidocaine: A retrospective review of 17 consecutive cases. J Orthop Trauma 5:412–419, 1991.
76. Uematsu S, Hendler N, Hungerford D, et al: Thermography and electromyography in the differential diagnosis of chronic pain syndromes and reflex sympathetic dystrophy. Electromyogr Clin Neurophysiol 21:165–182, 1981.
77. Van Wyngarden TM, Bleyaert AL: Reflex sympathetic dystrophy: Objective clinical signs in diagnosis and treatment. J Foot Surg 31:75–78, 1992.
78. Wainapel S: Reflex sympathetic dystrophy following traumatic myelopathy. Pain 18:345–349, 1984.
79. Watson KH, Carlson L: Treatment of reflex sympathetic dystrophy of the hand with an active "stress loading" program. J Hand Surg 12A:779–785, 1987.
80. Wilder RT, Berde CB, Wolohan M, et al: Reflex sympathetic dystrophy in children: Clinical characteristics and follow-up of seventy patients. J Bone Joint Surg 74A:910–919, 1992.
81. Williams WR: Reflex sympathetic dystrophy. Rheumatol Rehabil 16:119–125, 1977.

SCOTT NAFTULIN, DO
STEVEN NIERGARTH, DO

CONTINUOUS PASSIVE MOTION

From Coordinated Health Systems
Bethlehem, Pennsylvania
  (Naftulin)
    and
Department of Orthopedic
  Surgery
Michigan State University
College of Osteopathic Medicine
East Lansing, Michigan (Niergarth)

Reprint requests to:
Scott Naftulin, DO
Coordinated Health Systems
2775 Schoenersville Road
Bethlehem, PA 18017

Since the days of Hippocrates the controversy of rest versus motion has been a part of medicine. With musculoskeletal injury, this controversy has been the center of great debate. The opinions and general consensus of the medical community have changed dramatically with time. It was Aristotle who first emphasized the principle that "movement is life."[61,89] This opinion was in contradiction to that of his predecessor Hippocrates, who taught: "It is especially needful for the body to be at rest."[61,89]

In the 1950s the Association for Osteosynthesis established as their guiding principle open reduction with rigid internal fixation, no cast, and rapid return to full activity. They coined the term *fracture disease*,[68] referring to the deleterious effects of cast immobilization for the treatment of fractures, including edema, atrophy, joint stiffness, and disuse osteoporosis.[89] In 1955, Dehne described the *spinal adaptation concept*, which stated that repair was an adaptive life process interacting with intrinsic and extrinsic stimuli.[22] This concept could be further divided into three aspects: (1) adverse reaction to excessive external stimuli; (2) favorable response to graduated functional stimulation; and (3) consistent early recovery with decreased incidence of temporary side effects or long range impairment.[22]

Despite the contrasting clinical beliefs concerning the use of motion or rest in the treatment of fractures, there was little or no scientific evidence to support either method. However, experimental investigations in animals eventually demonstrated the detrimental effects of immobilization.

In the 1970s, Salter et al. introduced a new concept: continuous passive motion (CPM).[96] Based on the scientific data accumulated at that time, Salter felt that little controversy remained and that motion was the most logical choice. Furthermore, if more is better, he reasoned, continuous should be superior to intermittent motion.[89,91,93] Thereafter, Salter and others performed numerous experimental investigations using animals to compare immobilization, intermittent active motion, and CPM. Collaboration with engineers eventually yielded continuous passive motion devices for clinical use.[19,89]

In this chapter, the effects of immobilization and continuous passive motion as demonstrated in both basic research animal studies and clinical studies will be reviewed. In addition, the current indications, contraindications, potential complications and risks, and the practical considerations required in the prescription of this modality will be discussed.

EFFECTS OF IMMOBILIZATION

In 1944 Howard Rusk, one of America's most prominent physiatrists, wrote: "Bed rest is often necessary; but bed rest brings about deconditioning and this must be counteracted by specific reconditioning."[89] The deconditioning syndrome results in systemic changes with essentially all organ systems being affected. The complications of bed rest or inactivity are most frequently encountered in the musculoskeletal system.[7,44] If proper measures to prevent these complications are not taken, the complications may become more problematic than the primary disease.[44,53] Subsequently, hospital stays may become unnecessarily prolonged, with increasing use of health care resources.[44] More importantly from a physiatric standpoint, the period of dependency in mobility and activities of daily living is lengthened.[44,65]

Studies both in animals and humans have demonstrated the deleterious effects of immobilization on the musculoskeletal system. Research in rhesus monkeys[71,74] has shown that after 8 weeks of knee immobilization there was an approximately 40% decrease in the maximal failure load in the anterior cruciate ligament-bone complex. After resuming activity for 20 weeks, there was still only partial recovery of strength of the functional ligament unit. In addition, animal studies[5,6,56,71] have demonstrated atrophy and reduction of collagen mass in the medial collateral ligament, reduction of mechanical properties of the lateral collateral ligament, and weakening of the ligament-bone junction of both collateral and the anterior cruciate ligaments after knee immobilization. A prospective, randomized study[43] compared the effects of a standard cylinder cast to a mobile cast brace worn for 4 weeks after reconstruction of the anterior cruciate ligament. The results demonstrated significant atrophy of type 1 muscle fibers as well as a significant reduction in succinate dehydrogenase activity in the vastus lateralis with use of the standard cast. Other human studies[12,58,59] have demonstrated loss of both muscle size and strength in immobilized limbs. Immobility will also lead to disuse atrophy of bone in a brief time.[49,52]

Histologic evaluation of articular cartilage from rat knees after varying periods of immobilization has shown flattening of the cartilage in the contact areas and degeneration of the cartilage in the noncontact areas. Invasion of the peripheral articular cartilage by synovial membrane also occurs.[45] Static compression between small areas of constantly apposed articular cartilage appears to be the major determinant leading to chondrocyte death and cartilage degeneration in the rat.[105] Unilateral immobilization of the rabbit knee for different lengths of time demonstrated that not only long-term immobilization, but short repetitive periods of immobilization, also induce osteoarthritic changes. Interestingly, degenerative changes are also seen both radiologically and histologically in the contralateral nonimmobilized knee.[109]

Using the rat knee, the nature of changes occurring as a result of joint immobilization and the degree of reversibility of these changes has been investigated.[28] Knee immobilization leads to proliferation of intracapsular connective tissue and the formation of adhesions, which, to a limited degree, are reversible. After prolonged immobilization, muscle and capsular contractures form, causing restriction of motion,[28,82] with shortening of muscles being primarily at fault. Rigid immobilization is not essential to produce these structural changes, but the duration of immobilization definitely influences the final range of motion obtained.[28] After forced remobilization of the contracted knee, continued joint motion allows the formation of a cellular layer with synovial membrane characteristics about the knee joint cleft.[28]

Prolonged immobilization of human knees causes intraarticular changes similar to those described in animals.[27] The sequence of intraarticular changes has been summarized: The fibrofatty tissues of the joint proliferate, encroach upon the joint cleft, envelope the cruciate ligaments, become confluent with unopposed articular surfaces, and eventually obliterate the joint cavity. If immobilization continues, there is a gradual absorption of the cartilage by the fibrofatty tissue, which eventually can abut against the subchondral bone and even communicate with the bone marrow.[27]

Changes in the mucopolysaccharide concentrations may be critical in the determination of physical properties of periarticular connective tissue.[3] However, it remains unknown if these changes are the sole cause of contractures.[1] Both in rabbits and dogs, significant amounts of water, hyaluronic acid, and chondroitin-4 and -6 sulfate and smaller amounts of deramatin sulfate are lost from fibrous connective tissue after periods of immobilization.[1,4,114] The loss of these substances is uniform throughout the tendon, capsule, ligament, and fascia.[2,114] The loss of total hexosamine correlates with the degree of joint stiffness.[114] Failure to demonstrate accumulation or increased synthesis of collagen indicates that mechanisms more subtle than fibroplasia and scar formation must explain the contracture resulting from immobility.[114] Alternative hypotheses include the ideas that haphazardly formed collagen interferes with joint mechanics, or loss of water and glycosaminoglycan permits cross-linking between existing collagen fibers.[3,114]

In summary, experimental investigations of the effects of joint immobilization in animals and humans, regardless of the method of immobilization or the weight-bearing status, have demonstrated progressive contracture of the capsule and pericapsular structures and concomitant encroachment on the joint by intra-articular fibrofatty connective tissue with eventual obliteration of the joint cavity by this tissue.[27,28,35,42,45,46,92,105,108,113] Osteoarthritic changes are also induced, including degeneration of articular cartilage and reduction of mechanical properties of ligaments and ligament-bone complexes.

BASIC SCIENCE AND THE DEVELOPMENT OF CPM

The articular cartilage matrix consists of collagen fibers, water, and mucopolysaccharides—mainly chondroitin sulfate. Chondrocytes are responsible for the formation of both collagen and chondroitin sulfate. After the growing period, the metabolism of cartilage is negligible and decreases with advancing years.[13,85,92]

Articular cartilage contains no blood vessels, lymphatics, or nerves.[11,92] The sources of articular cartilage nutrition include synovial fluid and subchondral blood vessels.[92] Normal synovial fluid is important in the prevention of wear and tear of articular cartilage,[8,92] and the process of diffusion of synovial fluid into the articular cartilage is enhanced by joint movement.[26,92] For cartilage to degenerate, either the chondrocyte must die from direct injury or else its metabolism must be seriously impaired.[108]

Salter postulated that articular cartilage receives its primary nutrition through the diffusion of synovial fluid and, therefore, that continuous compression of an area of cartilage would result in the destruction of that cartilage. He hypothesized that joint degeneration associated with immobilization of the joint in a forced position could be explained on the basis of continuous compression of articular cartilage. Furthermore, he knew that the articular cartilage of various animals and humans was quite similar in anatomy, histology, embryology, physiology, and pathology. Thus, he was able to use rabbits to test his assumptions.[91,92] Salter and Field supported the hypothesis by an investigation in rabbits in 1960.[92] Their findings were further supported by Evans et al.,[28] Trias,[108] and others. They described the "pressure necrosis of cartilage," which was felt to be an irreversible lesion. Thus, several pathologic processes, including "subchondral lesion,"[28] pressure necrosis of cartilage,[92] and fibrofatty proliferation and adhesions to the unopposed articular surface[28] resulted from knee immobilization.

In 1961, Trias produced severe articular degenerative changes with compression of the articular cartilage in rabbit knees for up to 6 weeks. Evaluating the pattern of change in collagen and mucopolysaccharide, a greater initial loss of hydroxyproline concentration as compared to hexosamine occurred, which contrasted the chemical changes of cartilage degradation seen with infection.[35] The typical lesions seen resembled human osteoarthritis, exhibiting fibrillation of cartilage, death of chondrocytes, eburnation of joint surfaces, sclerosis of bone, and the production of "bone cysts."[108] In contrast to Salter's and Field's work, however, he noted that the regeneration of cartilage was common and brought about either by deeply situated chondrocytes or by metaplasia of immature bone marrow connective tissue cells.[108]

Destruction of the articular cartilage is the starting point in the evolution of degenerative arthritis, and all subsequent joint changes are secondary.[11,15,92,108] The degeneration of joint cartilage results largely from faulty distribution of pressures across the joint.[108] After only 4 days of constant pressure, the articular cartilage is severely affected.[108] Similar to the pressure necrosis of cartilage, "relief of contact" produces degenerative changes in the articular cartilage.[46] Although these degenerative changes are histologically comparable, differences in regions of compression and relief are present at the bony level. Hypertrophy and localized osteoporosis are seen, respectively.[106]

An experimental model of osteoarthritis was later described in rabbit knees by means of immobilization in extension using a plastic splint. With this rabbit model, degenerative joint disease similar to that seen in advanced osteoarthritis in humans could be fairly easily reproduced.[54]

The deleterious effects of immobilization and abnormal force distribution on the knee joint were elucidated. However, several questions remained. Could these changes be prevented? And after they have occurred, could they be effectively treated? Salter and other investigators set out to answer these questions and, more specifically, to determine the effects of continuous passive motion on articular cartilage and other tissue structures.

They treated experimentally induced full-thickness articular cartilage defects in the distal femurs of rabbits by one of three methods: immobilization; normal cage activity, which simulated intermittent active motion; and continuous passive motion. The healing effects of these three treatments were assessed weekly for up to 4 weeks using both gross examination and light microscopy. Neither immobilization nor intermittent active motion provided adequate stimulus for healing of the full-thickness defects in the articular cartilage. Many joint adhesions were seen in rabbits treated with immobilization. The healing process seen with intermittent active motion was imperfect with combinations of fibrous tissue and poorly differentiated cartilage. While immobilization and intermittent active motion filled significantly fewer defects, the CPM filled more than 50% of the defects within 4 weeks with new hyaline cartilage. This process was called neochondrogenesis.[96,97] CPM also had a stimulating effect on the induction of neochondrogenesis in free autogenous periosteal grafts in a synovial fluid environment.[78] The ability to repair major osteochondral defects in the weightbearing regions of a rabbit's knee by neochondrogenesis after the placement of autogenous periosteal grafts stimulated by postoperative CPM was found later.[79] The cellular origin of the hyaline-like tissue that filled the experimentally induced osteochondral defects was the progenitor cells of the periosteal graft.[116] Further experimental investigation[75] using CPM and free autogenous periosteal grafts to fill large full-thickness osteochondral defects in joint surfaces revealed that the tissue produced resembled articular cartilage grossly, histologically, and biochemically. Thus, "biological resurfacing" for the treatment of large full-thickness osteochondral defects could be achieved. While neochondrogenesis of the free intraarticular periosteal autografts could be obtained in the complete absence of joint motion, the significant beneficial effects of CPM were further substantiated.[23]

CPM subsequently was evaluated in the treatment of intraarticular fracture.[95] Again using rabbits, experimentally induced Salter-Harris type 4 fractures of the medial femoral condyle were treated by open reduction and internal fixation with AO compression screws. Using control groups treated postoperatively by immobilization or normal cage activity, the knees were evaluated at weekly intervals for 1 month and then again at 6 months. Knees treated with CPM showed significantly faster reconstitution of the subchondral bone plate and more frequent healing of articular defects with tissue comparable to hyaline cartilage. More importantly, less development of degenerative arthritis at the 6-month follow-up was seen in the CPM group. Other notable observations included CPM having its greatest effect on the healing articular cartilage in the first postoperative week and being well tolerated by the rabbits when applied to the injured knee.

The efficacy of CPM in the prevention of joint stiffness was assessed after intraarticular injury of the ankles bilaterally. After a treatment duration of 3 weeks, using CPM on one ankle and immobilization on the contralateral side, the posttraumatic difference in joint stiffness between the CPM-treated and immobilized limbs was highly significant and better in the CPM-treated limb.[69] The long-term effects of the CPM, however, remained unknown. In addition, the amount of motion was unclear. In fact, intermittently passively exercised ankles after experimentally induced distal tibial fracture became significantly stiffer when compared to immobilized ankles. The cause of this increased stiffness was also unknown but possibly due to the traumatization of the healing tissue around the fracture site.[40]

In a situation analogous to human patients with early diagnosis and treatment of acute septic arthritis,[90] the beneficial effects of CPM on the protection of the articular cartilage from progressive degeneration was statistically significant when compared to intermittent active motion and immobilization. During this experimental investigation, a range of motion of 40–110° of flexion (arc of 70°) at a rate of 1 cycle per 40 seconds was used.

Additional experimental investigation using animals demonstrated other beneficial effects of CPM, including an accelerated clearance of hemarthrosis,[76] possibly by sinusoidal pressure oscillations;[77] better quality healing of injured tendons in terms of strength, tendon callus, vascularization and range of motion;[32,34,57,88] and reduction of muscle atrophy as compared to postarthrotomy immobilization.[24] Using an avascular model in rabbit knees,[100] CPM did not increase nutrient uptake in the anterior cruciate ligament. However, CPM may have facilitated transport of metabolites out of the joint.

CLINICAL STUDIES

Numerous clinical investigations assessing the efficacy of and determining potential detrimental effects of CPM have been undertaken since the first continuous passive motion device for humans was developed by Salter and his colleagues in Toronto in 1978.[89,97] An uncontrolled study in children[42] used CPM to maintain or gain hip and knee range of motion in 18 patients. In 17 of the patients, range of motion improved and decreased joint pain was reported. The CPM was well tolerated by 16 of the patients. The CPM did not interfere with traction, open wounds, nursing care, or external fixation.[42]

Both retrospective and prospective controlled studies[31,48,98] evaluating CPM and the treatment of elbow contractures reveal a significant improvement in total range of motion after arthrolysis.

Patients undergoing bilateral podiatric procedures were placed in CPM and contralaterally immobilized.[51] The CPM allowed patients to return to wearing normal foot gear an average of 10 days earlier because of reduction in postoperative edema and fibrosis.

The effects of CPM on the venous circulation of the lower extremities in healthy people were evaluated in comparison to pneumatic stockings and during several different leg manipulations.[111] The largest flow in the femoral venous system was obtained by passive straight leg elevation followed by the use of the CPM machine. The CPM device was more effective than active ankle dorsiflexion, pneumatic stocking inflation, manual calf compression, and passive dorsiflexion in increasing the femoral venous flow.

CPM and limb elevation has been found to be more effective than limb elevation alone in reducing hand edema to a statistically significant degree.[36]

In retrospective and uncontrolled studies,[30,41,67,104] CPM has been shown to be effective postoperatively for the treatment of hemophilic arthropathy, patellar dislocation with osteochondral fracture, anteromedialization of the tibial tubercle, and in preventing loss of or restoring range of motion in knees with a variety of disorders.

Prospective, randomized trials also have shown CPM to be of benefit in the treatment of different disorders. CPM was found to be effective for restoring range of motion that was comparable to supervised active and passive motion by an experienced therapist.[20] By adding CPM to the treatment on the fifth postoperative day, no graft disruptions occurred in 10 patients treated for bilateral hand burns. The authors concluded that patients could significantly benefit from the addition of CPM to their treatment, especially if there were extensive burns involving multiple kinetic areas, decreased cognitive function requiring passive motion over long times, and little active motion due to pain or anxiety on the patient's part.

Comparing two groups of nine patients each, beginning CPM either on the second or seventh postoperative day after undergoing anterior cruciate ligament reconstruction,[73] results showed that starting passive motion on the second postoperative day did not increase joint effusion, hemarthrosis, or soft tissue swelling. In addition, no significant difference in the flexion or extension, pain medications used, or length of hospital stays was found. Finally, early knee motion did not stretch the ligamentous reconstruction.

In a prospective, randomized, controlled multicenter clinical study involving 51 patients,[33] CPM was compared to traditional early passive motion in the treatment protocol for rehabilitation after flexor tendon repair. After a mean follow-up of approximately 11 months, the mean active motion for digits in those treated with CPM was significantly increased.[33]

Several studies retrospectively investigating the clinical efficacy of CPM after total knee arthroplasty[21,38,115] have reported conflicting results. Detrimental effects of CPM have included greater suction drainage and requests for more pain medication when CPM was initiated within 48 hours of total knee arthroplasty as compared to immediate immobilization.[21] When comparing the CPM group to the immobilized group after arthroplasty, the CPM group could ambulate and transfer independently sooner, perform straight leg raises earlier, and obtain greater active range of motion on the seventh postoperative day. Nonsignificant findings included differences in length of time to removal of incision staples, duration of hospitalization, and frequency of request for pain medications on the first through third postoperative days. In another retrospective study comparing patients with and without CPM after total knee arthroplasty,[38] the CPM group showed significant decreases in frequency of complications and the length of hospitalization. In contrast, another retrospective study[115] that compared CPM and active assisted range of motion to active assisted range of motion alone, no significant difference in range of motion recovery time and day of discharge between these two interventions was found.

In another study, three modalities, including CPM, used in postoperative inpatient care were evaluated with regard to pain management and unilateral total knee arthroplasty outcomes.[113] The patients were randomized to receive CPM or not to receive CPM. Total pain medication consumption during hospitalization was significantly reduced in the CPM group. However, no significant difference in unilateral total knee arthroplasty outcome using CPM was noted when comparing for postoperative blood drain loss, duration of hospitalization, and range of motion. In a controlled, nonrandomized study evaluating CPM and total knee arthroplasty,[60] no effect on long-term range of motion, knee function scores, or pain relief was found.

In a prospective, controlled, randomized trial comparing CPM to immobilization after a primary total knee arthroplasty in patients with osteoarthritis and rheumatoid arthritis,[50] CPM significantly improved early and late knee flexion. But 1 year later, the difference was significant only in patients with osteoarthritis. The reduction of hospital stay was also significantly decreased in the CPM group; however, the use of prolonged immobilization is not standard rehabilitation protocol after total knee arthroplasty. In the same study, wound viability was determined with direct noninvasive measurement of transcutaneous oxygen tension. Flexion of the knee greater than 40° progressively diminished viability of the wound edges. Yet, speed of the CPM did not significantly affect this parameter.

However, CPM did cause a higher wound complication rate based on the author's definition of "wound complication" in a randomized, controlled, single-blind study evaluating the efficacy of CPM in the postoperative management of both osteoarthritis and rheumatoid arthritis patients undergoing total knee arthroplasty.[62] CPM and standard rehabilitation was compared to standard rehabilitation alone. The conclusions were that CPM was more effective in improving range of motion, decreasing swelling, and reducing the need for manipulation than conventional therapy. Total costs were also lower in the CPM group. CPM, however, did not affect pain, active or passive extension, strength, length of hospital stay, or overall function of range of motion at 6 weeks postoperatively. Although CPM users in this study had slightly more quadriceps strength, this strength difference was not statistically significant, and both groups achieved straight leg raising by the sixth postoperative day. In this study, which is the only study with blinded assessment of outcome, the greatest benefit of CPM appeared to be in avoiding manipulation, which had previously been reported.[18,37,110]

Summarizing these clinical studies, the greatest benefits of CPM after total knee arthroplasty appear to be earlier increases in range of motion and avoiding manipulation. Although there appear to be no long-term benefits in terms of range of motion after total knee arthroplasty when using CPM, the earlier attainment of critical range of motion during the immediate postoperative period may be beneficial in terms of performing more functional activities such as activities of daily living, transfers, and mobility. It also improves circulation and may thus reduce the risks of deep venous thrombosis. These potential benefits must be weighed against the potential risks of increased volume of suction drainage, wound dehiscence, and disruption of any surgical repair.

INDICATIONS

Generally, passive motion can be used for many purposes. As mentioned previously, many studies have been performed to study the efficacy of CPM. CPM has been used in the immediate postoperative management after open reduction and internal fixation of fractures, arthrotomy and/or arthrolysis for posttraumatic arthritis, synovectomy, surgical drainage for septic arthritis, release of extraarticular contractures, metaphyseal osteotomies, total joint replacement, and ligamentous reconstruction.[42,86,93] Specifically in children, indications have included slipped capital femoral epiphysis, juvenile rheumatoid arthritis, fibula hemimelia, proximal focal femoral deficiency, Perthes' disease, posttraumatic synovitis, and congenital femoral shortening.[42]

CPM has been used in the treatment of severe knee flexion contractures as reported in case studies.[102] After debridement of intraarticular and extraarticular knee structures in the treatment of infrapatellar contracture syndrome, CPM has been used postoperatively to maintain range of motion and to afford some pain relief.[80] After intraarticular cruciate reconstruction, CPM is usually applied during the immediate postoperative hospitalization period.[72] Although some practitioners prefer the use of CPM after knee surgery,[9,72,73] others[14,81] prefer no CPM because it is purely passive, can be expensive, and requires meticulous attention to the range of motion settings, which may not represent the patient's actual range of motion. CPM is also used after total knee arthroplasty, as discussed above.[21,50]

Children who had unique problems causing prolonged limitation of joint movement either of the knee or elbow used CPM successfully.[41] As previously discussed, CPM has been demonstrated to accelerate clearance of a hemarthrosis and has been used in both hemophilic arthropathy[41,42,67,70,76] and in traumatic nonhemophilic hemarthrosis.[76]

CPM has also been useful in the treatment of reflex sympathetic dystrophy,[17] talipes equinovarus,[87] the lower extremity after stroke,[112] and range of motion deficits about the elbow, especially after arthrolysis from either the lateral or anterior approach.[48,98] Other uses of CPM have included the treatment of hand burns,[20] treatment after tendon repair based on the dog model,[23,31,33,34,50,51,60,86,98,103,113] reduction of hand edema,[36] postoperative removal of a Morton's neuroma in hopes of preventing postoperative symptomatic plantar fibrosis,[51] and treatment of acute septic arthritis.[66,90]

CPM has had a controversial role in deep venous thrombosis prophylaxis.[51,111] The differing results from studies concerning use of CPM in thrombotic prophylaxis may be due to whether an anatomic or non-anatomic CPM device was used, parameters of the device, and when the CPM was initiated after any surgical procedure.[111]

CPM IN THE TREATMENT OF FRACTURE

As the experimental investigations discussed above demonstrate, CPM can provide several significantly beneficial effects on a joint after injury. These effects can be seen not only in the bone but in articular cartilage, muscle, capsular, and pericapsular structures. The many causative factors of disability after fracture, including limited motion, pain, traumatic arthritis, and muscle weakness,[47] may be positively affected by CPM. Thus, it is not surprising that CPM has been used clinically in the immediate postoperative management of intraarticular fractures of the ankle, knee, hip, elbow, and finger as well as diaphyseal and metaphyseal fractures after open reduction and internal fixation.[51] Specific fractures that have been treated with CPM after open reduction and internal fixation include tibial plateau fractures,[83] nonunion of pseudarthrosis of the humeral shaft supported by hinged or cast braces until union occurs,[84] distal humeral intraarticular fractures,[101] comminuted femur fractures treated in a hip spica cast with a knee hinge,[99] osteochondral fractures from patellar dislocation,[104] and Salter-Harris type 4 medial femoral condyle fractures.[95] The ability of CPM to facilitate "biological resurfacing" makes CPM an ideal therapeutic modality for the treatment of osteochondral defects in a joint surface due to osteochondritis dissecans, osteochondral fractures, and even focal areas of osteoarthritis.[79] However, osteochondral defects approximately 1 mm or smaller heal in a superior manner than the larger defects.[16,79]

CONTRAINDICATIONS, COMPLICATIONS, AND RISK

The few contraindications that exist for the use of CPM are relative rather than absolute and should be assessed individually.[64] The presence of unstable fractures, septic tenosynovitis, or cellulitis are obvious contraindications to CPM.[51] Relative contraindications include a noncompliant patient or a situation in which health care personnel are not familiar with the use of the particular device and, by using it, could place the patient at risk.[64]

The risks of passive motion include the creation of excessive tissue trauma or unwanted joint mobility.[29] Thus, potential specific risks of CPM include disruption of a surgical repair or fracture fixation, or hemorrhage in the immediate postoperative period.[64] Malfunction of the CPM device itself may also cause injury to the patient.[64] The formation of decubiti has been reported in association with the use of CPM.[50] Concerns of wound infection and decreased wound viability have been raised.[50,60] Transcutaneous oxygen tension measurements were compared in patients after knee arthroplasty receiving CPM or immobilization. A significant decrease in the oxygen tension measurement occurred, especially on the lateral edge of the wound at greater than 40° of knee flexion in the CPM group. However, 7 days postoperatively, the viability of the wound determined by oxygen tension measurement was no longer statistically different between the immobilized and CPM groups.[50] The speed of the applied CPM did not seem to affect the oxygen tension measurements. Other studies[50,51] have not demonstrated complications at the surgical site, such as infection or disturbed wound healing, as the result of CPM.

Anterior compartment syndrome after surgical fixation of a tibial plateau fracture and postoperative CPM has been reported in one patient.[39] Notably, the patient was taking full-dose anticoagulant medication for treatment of a deep venous thrombosis at the time. Other reports[48,51] had not demonstrated complications associated with CPM use after podiatric surgery or operative release of a posttraumatic elbow contracture.

CLINICAL USE

CPM devices are available for both the upper and lower extremity, including the hand, wrist, shoulder, elbow, hip, knee, and ankle.[25,93] Two basic designs exist: anatomic and free linkage.[25] The anatomic design supports and mobilizes the joint in a manner as similar as technologically possible to natural anatomic motion.[25,111] The free linkage design provides motion to the adjacent anatomy and allows the joint to seek its own anatomic motion. As a direct result of these designs, the anatomic type usually affords more patient comfort, while the free linkage design is easier to use.[25,111] Since the anatomic design supports the joint, it is safer to use on sensitive ligament repairs such as intraarticular cruciate reconstruction of the knee.[25,107]

The CPM device is composed of three major segments, including the limb carriage, the motor drive, and the controls.[18] Other available components include a built-in goniometer, bed attachment or nonskid base, manual stops, error indicators for a low battery or malfunction, patient safety key, elapsed time meter, built-in neuromuscular electrical stimulator, or add-on orthosis for use in children.[25] Wheels and a carrying handle increase transportability.

When prescribing the CPM device, several factors should be taken into account. The CPM device can be portable or stationary, used at home or in the hospital, purchased or rented.[25] Several parameters must be set when prescribing the device, including the force, rate, and range of motion. In addition, the duration of therapy should be specifically described.[33,93] The rate of motion used is generally one complete cycle every 45 seconds.[91,93] In children, a slower motion of one revolution every 12.5 minutes is advocated based on the concept that very slow motion does not cause pain.[41]

Other factors to consider when prescribing CPM include when to initiate the use of the device especially after surgery, the length of therapy to be used daily, and safety problems that may be specifically encountered in a particular patient population. In one study, increased drainage of the surgical wound after total knee arthroplasty was seen in a CPM group when compared to immobilization in the first 2 days postoperatively. Therefore, recommendations were made not to initiate CPM until the wound stabilizes, that is, at least 2 days postoperatively.[60] Limiting knee flexion to 40° for the first 3 days postoperatively after total knee arthroplasty is supported by measurements of transcutaneous oxygen tension.[50] Controlled animal studies[55] have shown that mechanical stress encourages healing and remodeling of dermal tissue. Nevertheless, the first week of postoperative CPM appears to be the most important in terms of stimulating undifferentiated pluripotential cells of the subchondral bone to differentiate into hyaline cartilage.[94,95] The optimal length of application of the CPM remains unknown.[62] Comparative results have been obtained in groups using CPM either a maximum of 5 hours or minimum of 20 hours daily after undergoing total knee arthroplasty when analyzed for range of motion, edema, pain, and length of hospital stay.[10] Certain CPM machines may be hazardous when used by children due to the accessibility of gears and movable parts to the child's fingers.[42] Limited manual dexterity in patients with rheumatoid arthritis may make self-application of the CPM device difficult when it is necessary to fasten clips. Finally, most patients appear quite comfortable when using a CPM device, possibly due to the "gate control theory" of pain:[89] that continuous proprioceptive mechanoreceptor impulses close the "gate" to pain impulses.[63]

CONCLUSION

The evolution of fracture treatment has progressed from the use of prolonged immobilization based on clinical empiricism to the use of motion based on scientific data. The experimental investigation and subsequent design of CPM devices by Salter and eventual introduction of these devices into the United States by Coutts[18,19] has enabled medical practitioners to minimize the deleterious effects of fracture management. By preventing the complications of immobilization, functional goals can be attained more rapidly.

The indications for CPM now encompass many musculoskeletal entities. Using CPM effectively may allow the rehabilitation team to concentrate on more functional tasks earlier in the patient's course and ultimately improve long-term outcomes. The complications and risks associated with CPM are few, especially if it is used under the direction of informed and experienced personnel.

However, numerous questions remain unanswered regarding the clinical application of CPM. What is the optimal dosage and duration of CPM? What range of motion is best? Is CPM efficacious in the treatment of the various indications reported? It is hoped that future prospective, controlled studies will give us the answers.

REFERENCES

1. Akeson WH, Amiel D, LaViolette D: The connective tissue response to immobility: A study of chondroitin-4 and -6 sulfate and dermatin sulfate changes in periarticular connective tissue in control and immobilized knees of dogs. Clin Orthop 51:183–197, 1967.
2. Akeson WH, Amiel D, LaViolette D: The connective tissue response to immobility: An accelerated aging response? Exp Gerontol 3:289–301, 1968.
3. Akeson WH, Amiel D, Woo S L-Y: Immobility effects on synovial joints. The pathomechanics of joint contracture. Biorheology 17:95–110, 1980.
4. Akeson WH, Soo S L-Y, Amiel D, et al: The connective tissue response to immobility: Biochemical changes in periarticular connective tissue of the immobilized rabbit knee. Clin Orthop 93:356–362, 1973.

5. Amiel D, Akeson WH, Harwood FL, Frank CB: Stress deprivation effect on metabolic turnover of the medial collateral ligament collagen. Clin Orthop 172:265–270, 1983.
6. Amiel D, Woo S L-Y, Harwood FL, Akeson WH: The effect of immobilization on collagen turnover in connective tissue: A biochemical-biomechanical correlation. Acta Orthop Scand 53:325–332, 1982.
7. Arnold JS, Bartley MH: Skeletal changes in aging and disease. Clin Orthop 49:17–38, 1966.
8. Barnett CH: Wear and tear in joints. An experimental study. J Bone Joint Surg 38B:567–575, 1956.
9. Bassett FH, Beck JL, Weiker G: A modified cast brace: Its use in nonoperative and postoperative management of serious knee ligament injuries. Am J Sports Med 8:63–69, 1980.
10. Basso DM, Knapp L: Comparison of two continuous passive motion protocols for patients with total knee implants. Phys Ther 67:360–363, 1987.
11. Bauer W, Ropes MW, Waine H: The physiology of articular structures. Physiol Rev 20:272–312, 1940.
12. Booth FW: Physiologic and biochemical effects of immobilization on muscle. Clin Orthop 219:15–20, 1987.
13. Bywaters EGL: The metabolism of joint tissues. J Pathol Bacteriol 44:247–268, 1937.
14. Cascells SW: Is continuous passive motion useful following cruciate ligament reconstruction? [editorial]. Arthroscopy 7:38, 1991.
15. Collins DH: The Pathology of Articular and Spinal Diseases. London, Edward Arnold & Co., 1949.
16. Convery FR, Avery WH, Keown GH: The repair of large osteochondral defects. An experimental study in horses. Clin Orthop 82:253–262, 1972.
17. Cooper DE, DeLee JE, Ramamurthy S: Reflex sympathetic dystrophy of the knee. Treatment using continuous epidural anesthesia. J Bone Joint Surg 71A:365–369, 1989.
18. Coutts RD: Continuous passive motion in the rehabilitation of the total knee patient, its role and effect. Orthop Rev 15:27–35, 1986.
19. Coutts RD, Craig EV, Mooney V, et al: The use of continuous passive motion in the rehabilitation of orthopaedic problems. Contemp Orthop 16:75–111, 1988.
20. Covey MH, Dutcher K, Marvin JA, Heimbach DM: Efficacy of continuous passive motion devices with hand burns. J Burn Care Rehabil 9:397–400, 1988.
21. Davis D: Continuous passive motion for total knee arthroplasty [abstract]. Phys Ther 64:709, 1984.
22. Dehne E, Torp R: Treatment of joint injuries by immediate mobilization. Clin Orthop 77:218–232, 1971.
23. Delaney JP, O'Driscoll SW, Salter RB: Neochondrogenesis in free intraarticular periosteal autografts in an immobilized and paralyzed limb. An experimental investigation in the rabbit. Clin Orthop 248:278–282, 1989.
24. Dhert WJA, O'Driscoll SW, Van Royen BJ, Salter RB: Effects of immobilization and continuous passive motion on postoperative muscle atrophy in mature rabbits. Can J Surg 31:185–188, 1988.
25. Diehm SL: CPM devices. J Burn Care Rehabil 9:498–504, 1988.
26. Ekholm R: Nutrition of articular cartilage. A radioautographic study. Acta Anat 24:329–338, 1955.
27. Enneking WF, Horowitz M: The intra-articular effects of immobilization on the human knee. J Bone Joint Surg 54A:973–985, 1972.
28. Evans EB, Eggers GWN, Butler JK, Blumel J: Experimental immobilization and remobilization of rat knee joints. J Bone Joint Surg 42A:737–758, 1960.
29. Frank C, Akeson WH, Woo SL-Y, et al: Physiology and therapeutic value of passive joint motion. Clin Orthop 185:113–125, 1984.
30. Fulkerson JP, Becker GJ, Meaney JA, et al: Anteromedial tibial tubercle transfer without bone graft. Am J Sports Med 18:490–496, 1990.
31. Gates HS, Sullivan FL, Urbaniak JR: Anterior capsulotomy and continuous passive motion in the treatment of post-traumatic flexion contracture of the elbow. J Bone Joint Surg 74A:1229–1234, 1992.
32. Gelberman RH, Jayasanker M, Gonsalves M, Akeson WH: The effects of mobilization on the vascularization of healing flexor tendons in dogs. Clin Orthop 153:283–289, 1980.
33. Gelberman RH, Nunley JA, Osterman AL, et al: Influences of the protected passive mobilization interval on flexor tendon healing. A prospective randomized clinical study. Clin Orthop 264:189–196, 1991.
34. Gelberman RH, VandeBerg JS, Lundborg GN, Akeson WH: Flexor tendon healing and restoration of the gliding surface. J Bone Joint Surg 65A:70–80, 1983.
35. Ginsberg JM, Eyring EJ, Curtiss PH: Continuous compression of rabbit articular cartilage producing loss of hydroxyproline before loss of hexosamine. J Bone Joint Surg 51A:467–474, 1969.

36. Giudice ML: Effects of continuous passive motion and elevation on hand edema. Am J Occup Ther 44:914–921, 1990.
37. Goll SR, Lotke PA, Ecker ML: Failure of continuous passive motion as prophylaxis against deep vein thrombosis after total knee arthroplasty. In Rand J, Dorr LD (eds): Total Arthroplasty of the Knee: Proceedings of the Knee Society. Rockville, MD, Aspen Systems Corp., 1987.
38. Gose JC: Continuous passive motion in the postoperative treatment of patients with total knee replacement. Phys Ther 67:39–42, 1987.
39. Graham B, Loomer RL: Anterior compartment syndrome in a patient with fracture of the tibial plateau treated by continuous passive motion and anticoagulants. Clin Orthop 195:197–199, 1985.
40. Grauber D, Kabo JM, Dorey FJ, Meals RA: The effects of intermittent passive exercise on joint stiffness following periarticular fracture in rabbits. Clin Orthop 220:259–265, 1987.
41. Greene WB: Use of continuous passive slow motion in the postoperative rehabilitation of difficult pediatric knee and elbow problems. Pediatr Orthop 3:419–423, 1983.
42. Guidera KJ, Hontas R, Osden JA: Use of continuous passive motion in pediatric orthopaedics. J Pediatr Orthop 10:120–123, 1990.
43. Haggmark T, Eriksson E: Cylinder or mobile cast brace after knee ligament surgery. A clinical analysis and morphologic and enzymatic studies of changes in the quadriceps muscles. Am J Sports Med 7:48–56, 1979.
44. Halar EM, Bell KR: Contracture and other deleterious effects of immobility. In DeLisa JA (ed): Rehabilitation Medicine. Principles and Practice. Philadelphia, JB Lippincott, 1988.
45. Hall MC: Cartilage changes after experimental immobilization of the knee joint of the young rat. J Bone Joint Surg 45A:36–44, 1963.
46. Hall MC: Cartilage changes after experimental relief of contact in the knee joint of the mature rat. Clin Orthop 64:64–76, 1969.
47. Hohl M: Tibial condylar fractures. J Bone Joint Surg 49A:1455–1467, 1967.
48. Husband JB, Hastings H: The lateral approach for operative release of posttraumatic contracture of the elbow. J Bone Joint Surg 72A:1353–1358, 1990.
49. Jenkins DP, Cochran TH: Osteoporosis: The dramatic effect of disuse of an extremity. Clin Orthop 64:128–134, 1969.
50. Johnson DP: The effect of continuous passive motion on wound-healing and joint mobility after knee arthroplasty. J Bone Joint Surg 72A:421–426, 1990.
51. Kaczander BI: The pediatric application of continuous passive motion. J Am Podiatr Med Assoc 81:631–637, 1991.
52. Kharmosh O, Saville PD: The effect of motor denervation on muscle and bone in the rabbit's hind limb. Acta Orthop Scand 36:361–370, 1965.
53. Kottke FJ: The effects of limitation of activity upon the human body. JAMA 196:117–122, 1966.
54. Langenskiold A, Michelsson J, Videman T: Osteoarthritis of the knee in the rabbit produced by immobilization. Acta Orthop Scand 50:1–14, 1979.
55. Langrana NA, Alexander H, Strauchler I, et al: Effect of mechanical load in wound healing. Ann Plast Surg 10:200–208, 1983.
56. Laros GS, Tipton CM, Cooper RR: Influence of physical activity on ligament insertions in the knees of dogs. J Bone Joint Surg 53A:275–286, 1971.
57. Loitz BJ, Zernicke RF, Vailas AC, et al: Effects of short-term immobilization versus continuous passive motion on the biomechanical and biochemical properties of the rabbit tendon. Clin Orthop 244:265–271, 1989.
58. MacDougall JD, Elder GGB, Sale DG, et al: Effects of strength training and immobilization on human muscle fibres. Eur J Appl Physiol 43:25, 1980.
59. MacDougall JD, Ward GR, Sale DG, Sutton JR: Biochemical adaptation of human skeletal muscle to heavy resistance training and immobilization. J Appl Physiol 43:700, 1977.
60. Maloney WJ, Schurman DJ, Hangen D, et al: The influence of continuous passive motion on outcome in total knee arthroplasty. Clin Orthop 256:162–168, 1990.
61. McCarthy MR, O'Donoghue PC, Yates CK, Yates-McCarthy JL: The clinical use of continuous passive motion in physical therapy. J Orthop Sports Phys Ther 15:132–140, 1992.
62. McInnes J, Larson MG, Daltroy LH, et al: A controlled evaluation of continuous passive motion in patients undergoing total knee arthroplasty. JAMA 268:1423–1428, 1992.
63. Melzack R, Wall PD: Pain mechanism: A new theory. Science 150:971–979, 1965.
64. Micheli L, Daniel D, Steadman R: Other modalities: Continuous passive motion, stationary bicycle. In Drez D (ed): Therapeutic Modalities for Sports Injuries. Chicago, Year Book, 1989, pp 81–133.

65. Miller MG: Iatrogenic and neurogenic effects of prolonged immobilization of the ill aged. J Am Geriatr Soc 23:360–369, 1975.
66. Mooney V, Stills M: Continuous passive motion with joint fractures and infections. Orthop Clin North Am 18:1–9, 1987.
67. Mullaji AB, Shahane MN: continuous passive motion for prevention and rehabilitation of knee stiffness. J Postgrad Med 35:204–208, 1989.
68. Muller ME, Allgower M, Schneider R, Willenegger H: Manual of Internal Fixation. New York, Springer-Verlag, 1979.
69. Namba RS, Kabo JM, Dorey FJ, Meals RA: Continuous passive motion versus immobilization. The effect of posttraumatic joint stiffness. Clin Orthop 267:218–223, 1991.
70. Nicol RO, Menelaus MB: Synovectomy of the knee in hemophilia. J Pediatr Orthop 5:330–333, 1986.
71. Noyes FR: Functional properties of knee ligaments and alterations induced by immobilization. A correlative biomechanical and histological study in primates. Clin Orthop 123:210–242, 1977.
72. Noyes FR, Butler DL, Paulos LE, Grood ES: Intra-articular reconstruction. Perspectives on graft strength, vascularization and immediate motion after replacement. Clin Orthop 172:71–77, 1983.
73. Noyes FR, Mangine RE, Barber S: Early motion after open and arthroscopic anterior cruciate ligament reconstruction. Am J Sports Med 15:149–160, 1987.
74. Noyes FR, Torvik PJ, Hyde WB, DeLucas JL: Biomechanics of ligament failure. An analysis of immobilization, exercise, and reconditioning effects in primates. J Bone Joint Surg 56A:1406–1418, 1974.
75. O'Driscoll SW, Keeley FW, Salter RB: The chondrogenic potential of free autogenous periosteal grafts for biological resurfacing of major full-thickness defects in joint surfaces under the influence of continuous passive motion. J Bone Joint Surg 68A:1017–1035, 1986.
76. O'Driscoll SW, Kumar A, Slater RB: The effect of continuous passive motion on the clearance of a hemarthrosis from a synovial joint. Clin Orthop 176:305–311, 1983.
77. O'Driscoll SW, Kumar A, Salter RB: The effect of volume of effusion, knee position and continuous passive motion on intra-articular pressure in the rabbit knee. J Rheumatol 10:360–363, 1983.
78. O'Driscoll SW, Salter RB: The induction of neochondrogenesis in free intra-articular periosteal autografts under the influence of continuous passive motion. J Bone Joint Surg 66A:1248–1257, 1984.
79. O'Driscoll SW, Salter RB: The repair of major osteochondral defects in surfaces by neochondrogenesis with autogenous osteoperiosteal grafts stimulated by continuous passive motion. Clin Orthop 208:131–140, 1986.
80. Paulos LE, Rosenbert TD, Drawbert J, et al: Infrapatellar contracture syndrome. An unrecognized cause of knee stiffness with patella entrapment and patella infera. Am J Sports Med 15:331–341, 1987.
81. Paulos LE, Wnorowski DC, Beck CL: Rehabilitation following knee surgery. Sports Med 11:257–275, 1991.
82. Peacock EE: Some biochemical and biophysical aspects of joint stiffness: Role of collagen synthesis as opposed to altered molecular bonding. Ann Surg 164:1–12, 1966.
83. Perry CR, Evans LG, Rice S, et al: A new surgical approach to fractures of the lateral tibial plateau. J Bone Joint Surg 66A:1236–1240, 1984.
84. Rosen H: The treatment of nonunions and pseudarthroses of the humeral shaft. Orthop Clin North Am 21:725–742, 1990.
85. Rosenthal O, Bowie MA, Wagoner C: Studies in the metabolism of articular cartilage. Respiration and glycolysis of cartilage in relation to its age. J Cell Comp Physiol 17:221–233, 1941.
86. Salter RB: The biologic concept of continuous passive motion of synovial joints. The first 18 years of basic research and its clinical application. Clin Orthop 242:12–25, 1989.
87. Salter RB: Continuous Passive Motion. Baltimore, Williams & Wilkins, 1993.
88. Salter RB: The effect of continuous passive motion on the healing of partial thickness lacerations of the patella tendon in the rabbit [abstract]. Ann RCPSC 14:209, 1981.
89. Salter RB: Motion versus rest: Why immobilize joints? J Bone Joint Surg 64B:251–254, 1982.
90. Salter RB, Bell RS, Keeley FW: The protective effect of continuous passive motion on living articular cartilage in acute septic arthritis: An experimental investigation in the rabbit. Clin Orthop 159:223–247, 1981.
91. Salter RB, Clements ND, Ogilvie-Harris D, et al: The healing of articular tissues through continuous passive motion: Essence of the first 10 years of experimental investigations. J Bone Joint Surg 64B:640, 1982.

92. Salter RB, Field P: The effects of continuous compression on living articular cartilage. J Bone Joint Surg 42A:31–49, 1960.

93. Salter RB, Hamilton HW, Wedge JH, et al: Clinical application of basic research on continuous passive motion for disorders and injuries of synovial joints: A preliminary report of a feasibility study. J Orthop Res 1:325–342, 1984.

94. Salter RB, Harris D, Bogoch E: Further studies in continuous passive motion [abstract]. Orthop Trans 2:292, 1978.

95. Salter RB, Ogilvie-Harris DJ: The healing of intra-articular fractures with continuous passive motion. Instr Course Lect 28:102–117, 1979.

96. Salter RB, Simmonds DF, Malcom BW, et al: The effects of continuous passive motion in the healing of articular cartilage defects [abstract]. J Bone Joint Surg 57A:570, 1975.

97. Salter RB, Simmonds DF, Malcolm BW, et al: The biological effect of continuous motion on the healing of full-thickness defects in articular cartilage. J Bone Joint Surg 62A:1232–1251, 1980.

98. Schindler A, Yaffe B, Chetuit A, et al: Factors influencing elbow arthrolysis. Ann Chir Main Memb Super 10:237–242, 1991.

99. Schouten WR, Van derWerken C: Alternative application of a motorized device for protected continuous passive motion of the knee. Neth J Surg 37:191–192, 1985.

100. Skyhar MJ, Danzig LA, Hargens AR, Akeson YM: Nutrition of the anterior cruciate ligament. Effects of continuous passive motion. Am J Sports Med 13:415–418, 1985.

101. Soffer SR, Yahiro MA: Continuous passive motion after internal fixation of distal humerus fractures. Orthop Rev 19:88–93, 1990.

102. Stap LJ, Woodfin PM: Continuous passive motion in the treatment of knee flexion contractures. Phys Ther 66:1720–1722, 1986.

103. Strickland JW, Glogovac SV: Digital function following flexor tendon repair in zone II: A comparison of immobilization and controlled passive motion techniques. J Hand Surg 5:537–543, 1980.

104. TenThije JH, Frima AJ: Patellar dislocation and osteochondral fractures. Neth J Surg 38:150–154, 1986.

105. Thaxter TH, Mann RA, Anderson CE: Degeneration of immobilized knee joints in rats. J Bone Joint Surg 47A:567–585, 1965.

106. Thompson RC, Bassett CAL: Histological observations on experimentally induced degeneration of articular cartilage. J Bone Joint Surg 52A:435–443, 1970.

107. Trez D, Paine R, Neuschwander D, et al: A three-phase study measuring anterior tibial translation in an ACL-deficient knee. Presented at the 14th annual meeting of the American Orthopedic Society for Sports Medicine, June 1988.

108. Trias A: Effect of persistent pressure on the articular cartilage. J Bone Joint Surg 43B:376–386, 1961.

109. Videman T: Experimental osteoarthritis in the rabbit. Acta Orthop Scand 53:339–347, 1982.

110. Vince KG, Kelly MA, Beck J, Insall JN: Continuous passive motion after total knee arthroplasty. J Arthroplasty 2:281–284, 1987.

111. VonSchroeder HP, Coutts RD, Billings E, et al: The changes in intramuscular pressure and femoral vein flow with continuous passive motion, pneumatic compressive stockings and leg manipulation. Clin Orthop 266:218–226, 1991.

112. VonSchroeder HP, Coutts RD, Lyden PD, et al: The use of continuous passive motion for the rehabilitation of the lower extremity after stroke. Presented at the Third International Symposium on the Rehabilitation of Brain Injured Patients, Anaheim, CA, June 21–23, 1990.

113. Walker RH, Morris BA, Angulo DL, et al: Postoperative use of continuous passive motion, transcutaneous electrical nerve stimulation, and continuous cooling pad following total knee arthroplasty. J Arthroplasty 6:151–156, 1991.

114. Woo SL-Y, Matthews JV, Akeson WH, et al: Connective tissue response to immobility. Correlative study of biomechanical and biochemical measurements of normal and immobilized rabbit knees. Arthritis Rheum 18:257–264, 1975.

115. Young JS, Kroll MA: Continuous passive motion compared to active assisted range of motion [abstract]. Phys Ther 64:721, 1984.

116. Zarnett R, Delaney JP, O'Driscoll SW, Salter RB: Cellular origin and evolution of neochondrogenesis in major full-thickness defects of a joint surface treated by free autogenous periosteal grafts and subjected to continuous passive motion in rabbits. Clin Orthop 222:267–274, 1987.

KENNETH J. McLEOD, PhD
CLINTON T. RUBIN, PhD

CLINICAL USE OF ELECTRICAL STIMULATION IN FRACTURE HEALING

From the Musculo-Skeletal
   Research Laboratory
Department of Orthopaedics
State University of New York
   at Stony Brook
Stony Brook, New York

Reprint requests to:
Kenneth J. McLeod, PhD
Musculo-Skeletal Research
   Laboratory
Department of Orthopaedics
State University of New York
   at Stony Brook
Stony Brook, NY 11794-8181

DEVELOPMENT OF ELECTRICAL BONE HEALING DEVICES

Electrotherapy has a well-established role in the armamentarium of practitioners of physical medicine and rehabilitation, particularly in the treatment of pain.[20] Importantly, the technical foundation supporting electrical stimulation of bone healing differs little from the techniques currently used in electrotherapy. While many electrotherapy modalities rely on relatively high electric field or current values to ensure interaction with the nervous system, this is not always the case. More recently developed techniques, for example, use subsensory, pulsed microampere electrical stimulation for the treatment of pain, inflammation, and edema.[48] It has been suggested that the effectiveness of these low-level stimuli may be explained by the Arndt-Schulz law, which states that weak stimuli will tend to increase physiologic activity while very strong stimuli inhibit or abolish activity. In a similar manner, the electrical devices used to enhance fracture healing also rely on the induction of extremely low-level electric fields into the bone and surrounding tissues.

Endogenous Electrical Currents in Bone

The recent interest in attempting to promote bone healing by the induction of electrical currents arose through the study of bone adaptation. While it had been presumed for more than a century that the skeleton remodeled its architecture in response to usage, the definitive demonstration of this phenomenon had to await the development of the roentgenogram. X-ray images permitted physicians to document the adaptation over time of bone fractures healed in angulation.[13] It soon became clear that functional loading of the bone was requisite for proper healing and adaptation, but the physiologic signaling mechanism by which this occurred was completely unknown. Theories published in 1920[34] suggested that bone should always resorb on a convex surface and new bone would form on a concave surface so that a bone healed in angulation would straighten. But such theories could not account for the remodeling activity that must also occur on the medullary cavity surfaces of the bone.[23] More successful theories were based on transduction "signals" associated with the gradients of the mechanical strains within the bone, but the identity of any such "signal" remained unclear. In the late 1950s, Fukada and Yasuda[25] demonstrated that dry bone tissue had piezoelectric properties. Subsequently, Bassett and Becker[7] measured potentials in moist bone during impact loading (corresponding to average induced fields in the bone on the order of millivolts per centimeter) and suggested that the piezoelectric property of bone was the means by which the mechanical loading of the tissue was converted into a signal that could be detected by the bone tissue cells. Later, Fukada[24] showed that the piezoelectric properties of dry bone were indeed dependent on the strain gradient of the tissue. These results seemed to lend strong support for the importance of piezoelectric currents in the process of bone remodeling.

It has subsequently been shown that the collagen matrix of bone, the organic structure that supports the calcium-hydroxyapatite mineralization process, provides the piezoelectric characteristics of bone tissue.[28] However, because bone tissue is also saturated with fluid at a physiologic salt concentration (~ 300 mM), the piezoelectric potentials generated in moist bone during loading will be efficiently shielded by ion relaxation processes. Therefore, it is impossible to record the piezoelectric potentials in moist bone. The potentials recorded by Basset and Becker were not, therefore, piezoelectric, but electrokinetic in origin: arising from the entrainment of ions due to fluid motion through the bone.[22] Nonetheless, the overall hypothesis that either the piezoelectric potentials or the electrokinetic (streaming) potentials, both of which will naturally occur within bone during usage, could be the intermediate signal through which cells within the bone tissue sense the functional demands being placed on the bone remains valid. In fact, despite 20 years of investigation it remains unclear whether bone tissue is differentially sensitive to the piezoelectric currents or the streaming currents generated within the bone tissue. In particular, observations on the frequency dependence of the bone remodeling response, the electrokinetic response characteristics, and the piezoelectric response characteristics suggest that we do not yet fully understand the role of the various endogenous electrical currents in the bone remodeling process.[45,49,52] To further complicate matters, bone tissue is invariably surrounded by muscle tissue, which also induces relatively large electrical currents into the subjacent bone tissue.[33] None of the research into the role of endogenous electric currents in bone tissue has even attempted to incorporate this additional confounding factor.

Development of Clinical Devices

Concurrent with the physiologic research directed toward determining the source and role of the different endogenous currents, clinicians began to develop and use electromagnetic devices to promote bone healing. These clinical devices initially were designed to promote bone healing by inducing electrical currents that would mimic the endogenous currents in the absence of the normal mechanical loading or as an adjuvant to whatever function the patient could undertake. However, it was found that inducing substantial (mV/cm) electric fields at the low frequencies that would mimic the characteristics of the potentials recorded during impact loading of bone was not practical without using an invasive device. For this reason, the clinical devices that have received FDA approval have relied on less physiologic frequencies. These include magnetic induction devices using waveforms consisting of relatively high-frequency (1–10 KHz) pulses, gated at a relatively low frequency (1–100 Hz) and now commonly referred to as pulsed electromagnetic fields (PEMFs); and capacitively coupled devices using relatively high-frequency (10 KHz–100 KHz) sinusoidal electrical stimulation, where the frequency is sufficiently high to induce substantial transcutaneous current.[16] Despite the fact that none of these FDA-approved commercially available devices actually mimic the endogenous electrical currents, they do appear to be able to promote the bone healing process, particularly with respect to the enhancement of the healing of fractures in situations in which the normal progression of healing is delayed.

It is also important to note that invasive devices have not been abandoned. In addition to the dynamic electrical processes that normally occur in skeletal tissue, there also exist steady, or direct, electrical currents in bone tissue due to ion fluxes, which are caused by the active ion pumping activity of cells. These direct currents continue to be extensively studied.[10] Indeed, the study of injury current in wounds far predates the study of dynamic electrical currents, excluding those in excitable tissues.[30] Correspondingly, there is a long history of development of implantable devices used to induce direct, or pulsating direct, current into fracture tissues,[8,27,39] and numerous such devices are FDA-approved. However, it has not been possible to distinguish the electrochemical and mechanical effects arising at the electrodes used in such a treatment modality from the effects of the actual electrical currents in the tissue. Therefore, in this review, direct current implantable devices will be discussed only briefly.

Clinical Observations and Trials

In the normal process of fracture healing, the rapidly formed hematoma is converted into fibrocartilage in the secondary stages of callus development. The fibrocartilage is subsequently invaded by blood vessels, and the cartilagenous material is removed as the tissue becomes calcified.[12] When this final step in the fracture healing process is delayed for an extended time, a true nonunion or pseudarthrosis will develop. To prevent the development of nonunions, delayed unions or fractures likely to become nonunions (open tibial fractures have a nonunion rate of 15–20%) are conventionally treated through surgical intervention. However, because surgical intervention can actually hinder the healing process, orthopedic surgeons have pursued numerous noninvasive means to enhance fracture healing, including the use of growth hormone, thyroxine, calcitonin, insulin, hyperbaric oxygen, and physical exercise.[12,17] The efficacy of these prophylaxes has not been ideal, leading some investigators to avert nonunions by the induction of electrical currents. However, despite the potential advantages, the inherent risks in undertaking a new technique for treatment of a condition for which so many alternative approaches have failed has precluded the careful study of electrical treatment for delayed union. So, while sufficient anecdotal evidence of successful treatments was collected to obtain FDA approval, starting in 1970, to use electrical devices to treat nonunion fractures in the United States,[5] no double-blind clinical trials have taken place in this country.

Conversely, in Europe, perhaps due to a greater interest in long-term cost reduction or to inherent delays in scheduling surgery, several double-blind trials have been designed to test the efficacy of PEMF treatment. In the earliest trial[4] PEMF treatment was found to be no more effective than conservative treatment in promoting union in patients with fractures that had not healed in 52 weeks. In a subsequent trial, Sharrard[53] showed that for delayed unions (incomplete healing after 16–32 weeks) there was a substantial and significant benefit to PEMF treatment. A significant benefit has been even more evident in the promotion of healing following surgical intervention. A recent double-blind trial in Italy of PEMF effectiveness in enhancing healing following tibial osteotomies (which are designed to change the weightbearing surface of the knee) has shown that PEMF treatment doubles the number of patients at stage 3 or 4 (50–100% healed) within 60 days of treatment.[41] These results were consistent with an earlier double-blind trial on femoral intertrochanteric osteotomies by some of the same researchers.[11]

These latest successes appear to have prompted a reexamination of the efficacy of electrical stimulation in the United States. Several recent studies, for example, have investigated the use of electrical stimulation in the treatment of osteonecrosis of the femoral head, a condition in which the vascular supply to the head of the femur is lost but hip replacement can be delayed if resorption of the bone within the femoral head can be slowed or halted.[3,6,55] In addition, coincident with the increasing use of noncemented prostheses, the possibility of using electrical stimulation to more rapidly stabilize the hip implants[36] and the applicability of electrical stimulation to promote lumbar fusions using bone graft have been investigated.[47]

Electrical stimulation is currently being used in the U.S. and in Europe to treat many musculoskeletal complications. Dermis, ligaments, and tendons heal by fibroplasia, a process distinctly different from the endochondral ossification process of bone healing, but chronic wounds in these tissues are as difficult and frustrating to manage as a nonunion in bone.[1] Not surprisingly, the possibility that soft tissue healing may be electrically stimulated has been studied by numerous groups.[58] In vivo studies have, in fact, shown substantial increases in the tensile strength of healing skin wounds exposed to electromagnetic fields,[26] but it is not clear if animal preparations reflect the considerable diversity associated with chronic skin wounds. Nonetheless, in a placebo-controlled, blinded clinical trial of the efficacy of PEMF to enhance healing of venous stasis ulcers,[32] twice as many patients treated with active devices versus those treated with placebo devices (67% vs. 32%, n = 44, $p < 0.02$) were healed within 90 days. At 1 year follow-up, 42% of controls and 89% of treated patients had healed.

More remarkably, recently published work suggests that PEMF stimulation may be beneficial for osteoarthritis.[57] This work is particularly intriguing both because of the ubiquity of osteoarthritis and the common belief that cartilage heals poorly, if at all. In a double-blind, randomized pilot clinical trial, the investigators found a significant improvement in function in patients treated with a PEMF stimulus for 30 minutes per day, principally in those with osteoarthritis of the knee. However, overall assessment of improvement relied on subjective measures because there was no significant change in any of the laboratory data. In addition, studies are underway to determine the ability of electromagnetic fields to prevent or reverse senile or postmenopausal osteopenia.[43] Here again, though, while bone densitometry can be used to demonstrate a reduced rate of bone loss or even increased bone mass, a definitive demonstration of efficacy will require proof of a decrease in fractures, the definitive symptom of osteoporosis. Studies capable of demonstrating such a decrease will certainly require long-term follow-up and the conclusions will not be known for several, if not many, years.

MECHANISMS OF ELECTRIC FIELD INTERACTION WITH BONE TISSUE

Perhaps no clinically effective treatment is viewed with as much skepticism as treatment of fractures by electromagnetic fields. In part, this is no doubt due to the long delay between the introduction of electrical devices to the medical market and the demonstration of statistically significant efficacy through carefully planned double-blind clinical trials. However, an additional source of consternation is the almost complete lack of understanding of the physical and biologic mechanisms through which electromagnetic fields are capable of stimulating either the enhancement, or reinitiation, of the healing process.

Basic Electrophysiology and Physical Mechanisms of Interaction

It is well established that induced electric fields can alter cell function by inducing changes in the transmembrane potential. Because the lipid bilayer plasma membrane is a poor conductor, extracellular electrical currents within a tissue will induce surface charge on any cells within the tissue and thereby alter the normal membrane potential. Though the membrane potential is kept essentially stable at 50–75 mV, this potential actually represents the equilibrium condition between passive ion fluxes across the permeable plasma membrane (principally sodium and potassium) and the active pumping of these ions by proteins in the membrane.[31] As a result, the membrane potential fluctuates over time. In excitable cells such as muscle and nerve cells, large variations in the membrane potential give rise to propagating membrane potential transients down the length of the cell, which serve as a rapid signalling mechanism. Classical electrotherapy devices undoubtedly alleviate pain by perturbing the membrane potential of excitable cells sufficiently (1–10 mV) to alter normal electrical signaling processes. But in nonexcitable cells such as bone cells, chondrocytes and fibroblasts, typical membrane potential fluctuations are only 10–100 μV. Nonetheless, even these apparently small fluctuations are much greater than any fluctuations that would be induced by the electrical stimulation devices currently used to accelerate bone healing.

The magnitude of the membrane potential perturbations caused by bone healing devices can be estimated because, at the extremely low frequencies (ELF) used in these devices, the plasma membrane appears as a large impedance (membranes typically have a specific resistance of 10^3 Ω-cm^2 and a capacitance of approximately 1 μF/cm^2). An extracellular ELF electric current will diverge around the cell, inducing a surface charge on the membrane[19] that, for a sinusoidal stimulus, will perturb the static field across the membrane by a value of approximately:

$$\Delta V_m = E\ R\ \sin 2\pi ft$$

where E is the field intensity far from the cell, R is the approximate radius of the cell, and f the frequency of the stimulus.

To put the magnitude of these perturbations in perspective, we have recently shown that a 10 μV/cm, 15 Hz, sinusoidal electric field is capable of stimulating substantial new bone formation in animals.[43] For this field intensity, and assuming a typical cell radius of 10 μm, the maximum induced perturbation of the membrane potential will be 10 nV, which is three to four orders of magnitude smaller than the normal membrane potential fluctuations. In fact, even in the electroreceptors of sharks and rays, which are presumedly optimized for the detection of ELF electric fields, the electroreceptive cells require an induced membrane potential perturbation of 1 μV to ensure a response.[56]

It seems unlikely that clinically effective electromagnetic fields interact with cells by perturbing the membrane potential. As a result, numerous other physical mechanisms have been proposed and, because these low-frequency fields are excluded from the interior of the cell, most of the proposed mechanisms incorporate various phenomena that could occur at, or within, the cell membrane.[19] These include classical phenomena such as stimulation of ion transport,[9] collapse of chemical oscillations,[35] and ion interactions dependent on the orthogonal electric and magnetic fields,[40] as well as quantum mechanical phenomena such as amplification of ion tunneling[54] and Zeeman splitting of energy bands in chemical reactants.[37] Our own observations on the frequency dependence and time course of the reponse of cells to exogenously imposed electric fields has led us to propose that ELF electric fields may interact with living cells through the electrical polarization forces arising at the surface of the cell.[46]

Cell Signaling Mechanisms

Independent of the manner in which electromagnetic fields interact with the cell membrane, there remains the question of which cell populations within the bone or fracture callus are responding to the electrical stimulus and which signaling pathways are used by the cells to enhance or reinitiate the healing process. These are remarkably difficult questions to answer due to the large variety of cells involved in the fracture healing process. Clearly, the possible interaction of electric fields directly with the bone cell population, including osteoblasts and osteocytes, must be considered. Correspondingly, a large body of the scientific literature on in vitro cellular responses has been based on osteoblastic-like cell lines.[14] Indeed, we have recently shown that an osteoblastic cell line in vitro will respond to electromagnetically induced electric fields at frequencies and intensities similar to the fields that will promote osteogenesis in vivo.[44]

The observation that bone cells are capable of responding to electromagnetic fields does not in any way demonstrate that this is the pathway by which the fracture healing process is stimulated by electric fields. Conversely, the presence of osteoblasts in the fracture callus suggests that the healing process is proceeding normally in the absence of exogenous stimulation. It is more likely, therefore, that PEMF stimulation affects a cell type that is resident earlier in the fracture healing process. One important cellular component is the chondrocyte; the fracture callus is first replaced by cartilage prior to calcification. However, efforts to stimulate chondrocytes with electric fields[15,38] have been successful only when the fields have been induced at intensities far higher than those required to affect osteoblasts or fibroblasts,[42] suggesting that the chondrocytes are relatively unresponsive to electric fields.

Nonetheless, it has been shown that PEMF treatment has a significant effect on the endochondral ossification process.[2] Because this process must be stimulated before the appearance of osteoblasts, and because chondrocytes are relatively insensitive to PEMF treatment, this stimulation may well represent the response of yet another cell population. One potential candidate is the cells of the periosteum and endosteum. These surfaces of the bone serve as critical sources of osteoprogenitor cells, which can be stimulated to differentiate into osteoblasts.[18] During normal fracture healing the periosteal blastema forms an external callus, and it has long been known that extensive damage to the periosteum, through distraction or surgical intervention, significantly inhibits the fracture healing process. The osteoprogenitor cell population, therefore, may be the principal target of electromagnetic field treatment, but little work has focused on this possibility.

Finally, the stimulation of fracture healing may depend on stimulation of a nonresident cell population. The healing process is largely initiated by the release of platelet-derived growth factors, and PEMF stimulation may be due to a direct effect on circulating platelets in the region of the callus. Alternatively, removal of cartilage during endochondral ossification requires vascularization so that stimulation may be due to enhanced angiogenesis. These possibilities have not been investigated, and the biological mechanism behind the PEMF stimulation of fracture healing remains undetermined.

FUTURE DIRECTIONS

While treatment of osteoarthritis may prove to be the next important clinical area for electromagnetic stimulation, the complex source of this disease will probably exclude any basic understanding of the mechanism of treatment or broad usage of PEMF. A more likely candidate for new treatment opportunities is osteonecrosis. Because the resident cell population is no longer viable, the only objective of any noninvasive treatment is to inhibit the recruitment of osteoclasts, which can resorb the remaining bone tissue. Because osteoclastic recruitment has been shown to be inhibited in vitro by electromagnetic fields,[50] PEMF treatment may come to serve as an effective, focal treatment that will delay surgical treatment.

Remarkably, the devices used for the electrical stimulation of fracture healing have changed little over the past 20 years. However, as our understanding of exact nature of electric field interactions with cells and tissues improves, significant improvements in the devices also can be expected. The most obvious change will be associated with optimization of the stimulus waveform, permitting reductions in the necessary exposure times. Present devices require treatment times up to 8 hours, but devices currently being tested may reduce the necessary exposures to below 1 hour. In addition, improvement in the uniformity of the induced field intensity may be enhanced by applying rotating magnetic fields in place of the stationary field exposure systems that are currently used. Finally, certain groups have suggested that combining PEMF treatment with direct magnetic field exposure may enhance the efficacy of the treatment, and such treatment protocols are now under investigation.

Perhaps some of the most interesting new developments in electrical stimulation are directed toward the induction of electrical currents through stimulation of endogenous mechanisms. By mechanically stimulating the bone tissue or fracture callus, the normal piezoelectric or electrokinetic processes will correspondingly induce electrical currents in the tissue. By defining the optimal field exposure conditions for enhancing fracture healing, the optimal mechanical loading conditions also become evident. Success then becomes a matter of providing the technology to induce these mechanical loads. Specific applications of this approach include the use of pulsed ultrasound devices[29] to enhance fresh fracture healing, and mechanical vibration of bone to promote ingrowth into a noncemented prosthesis.[51]

SUMMARY

Despite its presence in the clinic for more than 20 years, electrical stimulation in the treatment of fractures has been slow to gain broad acclaim. Principally, this has been due to a lack of early, definitive clinical trials and a lack of understanding of the mechanism by which electric fields could stimulate or reinitiate the fracture healing process. As we improve our understanding of electric field interactions with cells and tissues, and as double-blind trials are undertaken for the new applications of electrical treatment (e.g., promotion of ingrowth, osteonecrosis, osteoarthritis and osteoporosis), a more general acceptance of electrical technology in medicine can be expected. In the meantime, improvements in the technology can be expected to result in more specific treatment protocols of shorter duration and greater efficacy.

REFERENCES

1. Aaron RK, Ciombor D McK: Therapeutic effects of electromagnetic fields in the stimulation of connective tissue repair. J Cell Biochem 52:42–46, 1993.
2. Aaron RK, Ciombor D McK, Jolly G: Stimulation of experimental endochondral ossification by low energy pulsing electromagnetic fields. J Bone Miner Res 4:227–244, 1989.
3. Aaron RK, Lennox D, Bruce GE, Ebert T: The conservative treatment of osteonecrosis of the femoral head: A comparison of core decompression and pulsing electromagnetic fields. Clin Orthop 249:209–218, 1989.
4. Barker AT, Dixon RA, Sharrard WJW, Sutcliffe ML: Pulsed magnetic field therapy for tibial non-union. Lancet May 5:994–996, 1984.
5. Bassett CAL: Fundamental and practical aspects of therapeutic uses of pulsed electromagnetic fields (PEMFs). Crit Rev Biomed Eng 17:451–529, 1989.
6. Bassett CAL, Schink-Ascani M, Lewis SM: Effects of pulsed electromagnetic fields on steinberg ratings of femoral head osteonecrosis. Clin Orthop 246:172–185, 1989.
7. Bassett CAL, Becker RO: Generation of electric potentials by bone in repsonse to mechanical stress. Science 137:1063–1064, 1962.
8. Becker RO, Spadaro JA, Marino AA: Clinical experiences with low intensity direct current stimulation of bone growth. Clin Orthop 124:75–83, 1977.
9. Blank M: Theory of frequency-dependent ion concentration changes in oscillating electric fields. J Electrochem Soc 1134:1112–1117, 1987.
10. Borgens RB, Robinson KR, Vanable JW, McGinnis ME: Electric Fields in Vertebrate Repair. New York, Alan R. Liss, 1989.
11. Borsalina G, Bagnacani M, Bettai E, et al: Electrical stimulation of human femoral intertrochanteric osteotomies: A double blind study. Clin Orthop 237:256–263, 1985.
12. Brand RA, Rubin CT: Fracture healing. In Albright JA, Brand RA (eds): The Scientific Basis of Orthopaedics. 2nd ed. East Norwalk, CT, Appleton & Lange, 1989, pp 325–345.
13. Brighton CT: Bioelectrical effects on bone and cartilage. Clin Orthop 124:2–4, 1977.
14. Brighton CT, McCluskey WP: Cellular response and mechanisms of action of electrically induced osteogenesis. In Peck W (ed): Bone and Mineral Research. Vol 4. New York, Elsevier, 1986, pp 213–254.
15. Brighton CT, Unger A, Stambough J: In vitro growth of bovine articular cartilage chondrocytes in various capacitively coupled electrical fields. J Orthop Res 2:15–22, 1984.
16. Brighton CT, Pollack SR: Treatment of recalcitrant nonunion with a capacitively coupled electrical field. J Bone Joint Surg 67A:577–585, 1985.
17. Connolly J, Hahn H, Jardon OM: The electrical enhancement of periosteal proliferation in normal and delayed fracture healing. Clin Orthop 124:97–105, 1977.
18. Dee R: Bone healing. In Dee R, Mango E, Hurst LC (eds): Principles of Orthopaedic Practice. New York, McGraw-Hill, 1988, pp 68–73.
19. Drago GP, Marchesi M, Ridella S: The frequency dependence of an analytical model of an electrically stimulated biological structure. Bioelectromagnetics 5:47–62, 1984.
20. Duncombe A, Hopp JF: Modalities of physical treatment. Phys Med Rehabil State Art Rev 5:493–519, 1991.
21. [Reference deleted.]
22. Eriksonn C: Streaming potentials and other water-dependent effects in mineralized tissues. Ann NY Acad Sci 238:321–338, 1974.

23. Frost HM: The Laws of Bone Structure. Springfield, IL, Charles C Thomas, 1964.
24. Fukada E: Piezoelectricity as a fundamental property of wood. Wood Sci Technol 2:229–307, 1968.
25. Fukada E, Yasuda I: On the piezoelectric effect of bone. J Phys Soc Japan 10:1158–1169, 1957.
26. Glassman LS, McGrath MH, Bassett CAL: Effect of external pulsing electromagnetic fields on the healing soft tissue. Ann Plast Surg 16:287–295, 1986.
27. Hartshorne E: On the causes and treatment of pseudarthrosis and especially that form of it sometimes called supernumerary joint. Am J Med 1:121–156, 1841.
28. Hastings GW, Mahmud FA: Electrical effects in bone. J Biomed Eng 10:515–521, 1988.
29. Heckman JD, Ryaby JP, McCabe J, et al: Acceleration of tibial fracture healing by noninvasive low intensity pulsed ultrasound. J Bone Joint Surg 75A:26–34, 1993.
30. Herlitzka A: Ein beitrag zur physiologie der regeneration. Wilhelm Roux Arch 10:126–158, 1910.
31. Hille B: Ionic Channels of Excitable Membranes. 2nd ed. Sunderland, MA, Sinauer Associates, 1992.
32. Ieran M, Zaffuto S, Magnacani M, et al: Effect of low frequency pulsing electromagnetic fields in skin ulcers of venous origin in humans: A double-blind study. J Orthop Res 8:276–282, 1990.
33. Inbar GF, Noujaim AE: On surface EMG spectral characterization and its application to diagnostic classification. IEEE Trans Biomed Eng 31:597–604, 1984.
34. Jansen M: On Bone Formation: Its Relation to Tension and Pressure. London, Longmans, 1920.
35. Kaczmarek LK: Frequency sensitive biochemical reactions. Biophys Chem 4:249–252, 1976.
36. Kennedy WF, Roberts CG, Zuege RC, Dicus WT: Use of pulsed electromagnetic fields in treatment of loosened cemented hip prostheses. Clin Orthop 286:198–205, 1993.
37. Lednev VV: Possible mechanism for the influence of weak magnetic fields on biological systems. Bioelectromagnetics 12:71–75, 1991.
38. Lee RC, Rich J, Keyyey K, et al: A comparison of in vitro cellular responses to mechanical and electrical stimulation. Am Surg 48:567–574, 1982.
39. Lente FD: Cases of ununited fractures treated by electricity. NY J Med 5:317–319, 1850.
40. Liboff A, McLeod BR: Kinetics of channelized membrane ions in magnetic fields. Bioelectromagnetics 9:39–51, 1988.
41. Mammi GI, Rocchi R, Cadossi R, et al: The electrical stimulation of tibial osteotomies. Clin Orthop 288:246–253, 1993.
42. McLeod KJ, Lee RC, Ehrlich HP: Frequency dependence of electric field modulation of protein synthesis in fibroblasts. Science 236:1465–1469, 1987.
43. McLeod KJ, Rubin CT: The effect of low-frequency electrical fields on osteogenesis. J Bone Joint Surg 74A:920–929, 1992.
44. McLeod KJ, Donahue HJ, Levin PE, et al: Electric fields modulate bone cell function in a density-dependent manner. J Bone Miner Res 8:977–983, 1993.
45. McLeod KJ, Rubin CT: Observations from mechanically and electrically induced bone remodeling. In Blank M (ed): Electricity and Magnetism in Biology and Medicine. San Francisco, San Francisco Press, 1993, pp 698–700.
46. McLeod KJ, Rubin CT: Role of polarization forces in mediating the interaction of low-frequency electric fields with living tissue. In Blank M (ed): Electricity and Magnetism in Biology and Medicine. San Francisco, San Francisco Press, 1993, pp 559–562.
47. Mooney V: A randomized double blind prospective study of the efficacy of pulsed electromagnetic fields for interbody lumbar fusions. Spine 15:708–712, 1990.
48. Picker RI: Current trends: Low-volt pulsed microamp stimulation. Clin Manag 9:10–33, 1989.
49. Pfieffer BH: A model to estimate the piezoelectric polarization in the osteon system. J Biomech 10:487–492, 1977.
50. Rubin CT, Donahue HJ, Rubin JE, McLeod KJ: Optimization of electric field parameters for the control of bone remodeling: Exploitation of an indigenous mechanism for the prevention of osteopenia. J Bone Miner Res 8:S573–S581, 1993.
51. Rubin CT, McLeod KJ: Promotion of bony ingrowth by frequency specific, low amplitude, mechanical strain. Clin Orthop 298:165–174, 1993.
52. Salzstein RA, Pollack SR: Electromechanical potentials in cortical bone. II. Experimental analysis. J Biomech 20:271–280, 1987.
53. Sharrard WJW: A double-blind trial of pulsed electromagnetic fields for delayed union of tibial fractures. J Bone Joint Surg 72B:347–355, 1990.
54. Sheppard AR, Adey WR: The role of cell surface polarization in biological effects of extremely low frequency fields. In Phillips RD, Gillis WR, Kaune WT, Wahlum DD (eds): Biological Effects of Extremely Low Frequency Electromagnetic Fields. Richland, WA, US Dept of Energy, 1979, pp 132–146.

55. Steinberg ME, Brighton CT, Corces A, et al: Osteonecrosis of the femoral head. Results of core decompression and grafting with and without electrical stimulation. Clin Orthop 249:199–208, 1989.
56. Tenforde TS: Electroreception and magnetoreception in simple and complex organisms. Bioelectromagnetics 10:215–221, 1989.
57. Trock DH, Bollet AJ, Dyer RH, et al: A double-blind trial of the clinical effects of pulsed electromagnetic fields in osteoarthritis. J Rheumatol 20:456–460, 1993.
58. Vodovnik L, Karba R: Treatment of chronic wounds by means of electric and electromagnetic fields. Med Biol Eng Comput 30:257–266, 1992.

JEFFREY W. SPYCHALSKI, MD
BERT J. THOMAS, MD

TREATMENT AND REHABILITATION OF PATHOLOGIC FRACTURES

From the Department of
  Orthopaedic Surgery
University of California
Los Angeles, California

Reprint requests to:
Bert J. Thomas, MD
Chief, Division of Orthopaedics
Veterans Administration Medical
  Center (112D)
16111 Plummer Street
Sepulveda, CA 91343-2036

Metastatic disease of bone and pathologic fractures have been areas of great debate with regard to appropriate treatment. The fact that patients are suffering from a terminal disease and often have limited life expectancy tends to favor a more conservative approach. On the other hand, the severe pain and limitation of function often caused by metastatic disease involving the skeleton tends to support an aggressive approach to patient management. This dilemma applies equally to the orthopedic and rehabilitative management of these patients. The purpose of this chapter is to explore past and present strategies for treating pathologic fractures and to identify areas that remain controversial and merit further study.

WORK-UP OF PATIENTS WITH PATHOLOGIC FRACTURES

When a patient presents with a pathologic fracture, great care must be exercised in thoroughly evaluating the patient's overall disease process. Since a hasty, poorly organized treatment program has the potential for disastrous outcome, certain basic principles should be followed in evaluation (Table 1).

Any evaluation first involves a detailed history and physical examination. A pathologic fracture may be the first manifestation of a malignant process, or the patient may have a history of a malignancy that was previously considered cured. A thorough understanding of the patient's current and past medical condition is thus indispensable. Similarly, physical examination should

TABLE 1. Evaluation of Patients with Metastatic Bone Disease

Detailed History and Physical Examination
Radiographic Examination
Plain radiographs of affected area
Bone scan—total body
Skeletal survey
CT scan for lesions of the spine and pelvis or if required for operative planning
Mammography and chest CT if unknown primary
Laboratory Evaluation
CBC, platelet count, differential, reticulocyte count
Sedimentation rate
Urinalysis
Serum chemistries, alkaline phosphatase, acid phosphatase

be targeted at identifying other evidence of metastatic disease, such as lymphadenopathy, and identifying the primary source of tumor.

Radiographic evaluation is the next step in the work-up of patients with metastatic disease of the bone or pathologic fracture. Radiographs of the affected limb vary in their utility. For a patient with a complete pathologic fracture, radiographs have the obvious role of defining the anatomy of the lesion and the requirements for stabilization. For a patient with bone pain alone, the x-rays may show no evidence of a lesion that could indicate impending pathologic fracture.

The characteristics of a lesion on x-ray may also offer clues to the underlying pathologic process. Many nonmalignant processes that can cause pathologic fracture have distinctive appearances on x-ray, such as the ground glass appearance of fibrous dysplasia. Metastatic lesions can be either predominantly lytic or blastic. Lytic lesions are more commonly associated with carcinoma of the lung, kidney, breast, thyroid, gastrointestinal tract, and neuroblastoma. Blastic lesions are most commonly associated with carcinoma of the prostate, breast, bladder, and the gastrointestinal tract.[37]

In the case of an unknown primary, chest x-ray, breast exam, and mammography should be performed to look for breast and lung carcinoma—the most common tumors that metastasize to bone. The thyroid, kidneys, and prostate also should be examined. A technetium-99 bone scan is also indicated in the evaluation of these patients. Sensitivities of 95–97% in localizing metastatic disease have been reported widely in the literature.[41] One must remember that multiple myeloma and some highly aggressive metastatic lesions can give false negative bone scans. Positive areas on bone scan should be further evaluated with plain radiographs to determine the extent of bony destruction and to plan intervention.[41]

Finally, laboratory studies including complete blood count, sedimentation rate, platelet count, reticulocyte count, urinalysis, alkaline and acid phosphatase and serum chemistries, including liver and renal function tests, should be obtained. These studies are indicators of general body and bone metabolism, and some studies are markers for specific tumors, i.e., acid phosphatase for prostatic cancer.

Of particular concern when evaluating laboratory studies is serum calcium. Hypercalcemia is a frequent complication arising in the presence of skeletal metastases, and it must be recognized early because it can become fatal quickly. Beyond the immediate risks of hypercalcemia, it is a poor prognostic sign. About 60% of patients with hypercalcemia will not survive longer than 1 year.[41] Early treatment aimed at reduction of bone resorption is indicated. Drugs such as mithramycin, calcitonin, indomethacin, and glucocorticoids have been used to decrease osteoclast activity.

BONE HEALING AND MECHANISM
OF SKELETAL METASTASES

The skeleton ranks third among common sites for tumor metastasis. It has been demonstrated both by autopsy studies and bone scan studies that 60% of patients with nonskeletal tumors will show evidence of bony metastasis. Tumors most likely to show skeletal involvement are breast, 67%; lung, 64%; and prostate, 62%.[42] Table 2 shows a more complete list of primary tumors and their likelihood of metastasizing to bone. Approximately 10–15% of patients with skeletal metastases will develop pathologic fracture; therefore, pathologic fracture is a significant concern of physicians who treat cancer patients.[18]

Considering that the skeleton receives only 5–10% of the cardiac output, the relative frequency of skeletal metastasis appears difficult to explain. Additionally, tumor cells show a preference for metastases to central portions of the skeleton— the spine, ribs, pelvis, proximal femur, and proximal humerus. Metastasis to the distal extremities is exceedingly rare.[3] Table 3 shows the common sites for skeletal metastasis and their frequency of involvement. Two theories of metastasis, by Ewing and Paget, have been used to explain these findings.

Ewing's mechanical theory proposed that the distribution of metastases was largely determined by the specific vascular system that is invaded by the primary tumor cells.[3] In support of this theory, Batson demonstrated that the venous system surrounding the prostate was connected to the veins of the spine through a valveless venous plexus. Periods of recumbency or increased abdominal pressure could allow retrograde flow from the prostate to the spine. Similarly, he also demonstrated vascular connections between the mammary veins and the paravertebral plexus. This theory, however, does not explain the frequency of skeletal metastasis outside the spine, which is still disproportionate to the blood flow to the skeleton.[3]

Paget proposed the seed-and-soil hypothesis, which suggests that different organs have different susceptibilities to metastasis. Because metastases occur in the red marrow, it is not surprising that metastases are found disproportionately

TABLE 2. Tumors that Commonly Metastasize to Bone[42]

Tumor Type	Percentage that Metastasize to Bone
Breast	67%
Lung	64%
Prostate	62%
Rectum	61%
Kidney	60%
Colon	57%
Melanoma	57%
Cervix	56%
Rhabdomyosarcoma	56%
Hodgkin's lymphoma	50%
Bladder	43%
Thyroid	43%
Lymphoma	38%

TABLE 3.   Common Sites of Skeletal Metastasis[42]

Anatomic Site	Frequency of Involvement
Thorax	54%
Vertebra	52%
Pelvis	38%
Extremities	34%
Skull	22%

in bones rich in red marrow. The marrow sinusoids are especially permeable, allowing tumor cells to cross easily.[3] Additionally, a chemotactic factor may be involved in the mechanism. Type 1 collagen peptides as well as a resorbing bone factor have been demonstrated to be present and are chemotactic for tumor cells.[3] Finally, there is some evidence that some tumor cells have surface properties that cause them to adhere to marrow elements.[3] It appears that both mechanical factors and seed-and-soil factors are involved in determining the patterns of skeletal metastasis.

The ultimate success of treatment of pathologic fractures depends on the ability of the diseased bone to heal, because any type of fracture fixation will eventually fail in the absence of healing. It was long believed that healing could not occur, but this belief has been more recently disproven. Gainor and Buchert have reported that healing occurs in 35% of pathologic fractures.[19] Factors influencing healing were tumor type, life expectancy, method of fixation, and radiation therapy. Length of survival was most significant, with 75% of fractures healing if the patient lived longer than 6 months. Radiation therapy has been demonstrated to be of great assistance in controling localized metastatic disease, and radiation of less than or equal to 3,000 rads has no detrimental effects on healing, with a union rate of 78% in patients who lived at least 6 months.[4,19,36] Finally, internal fixation combined with radiation of 3,000 rads or less resulted in a healing rate of 90% in patients surviving at least 6 months.[19] In light of the fact that average survival has improved to 18.8 months after a patient's first pathologic fracture, operative treatment of these fractures appears to be of great benefit.[39]

PRINCIPLES OF TREATMENT

Completed Fractures

Several goals are involved in the treatment of pathologic fractures. First is the relief of pain, which can be quite debilitating. Beyond pain, early mobilization and independent ambulation are important. Treatment should result in decreased need for nursing care. All of these factors ultimately influence the patient's emotional well-being and improve the quality of life.[7,20,33,45]

Ultimately, the decision to treat pathologic fractures must be individualized to each patient. Several factors are important in guiding the decision. The patient's general condition must be considered as well as location of the fracture, amount of bony involvement, and life expectancy. A patient's life expectancy, however, is extremely difficult to assess accurately, and this has led many surgeons to advocate intervention in any patient whose general condition will allow an operation.[31,39] The location of a fracture is important because many fractures, such as in the clavicle and dome in the humerus, can be quite effectively treated nonoperatively.

Four basic principles of operative management have been proposed by Sherry:[37]

1. One should perform the best procedure first and avoid a second procedure, which is frequently less satisfactory.
2. One should remove as much diseased bone as possible; therefore, endoprosthetic treatment is often preferred to open reduction and internal fixation.
3. Time in the hospital should be kept to a minimum.
4. Early return to function is essential. Immobilization is poorly tolerated.

Immediate rigid stabilization goes toward satisfying the above four principles. The bone quality is often so poor that internal fixation devices cannot offer the stability needed. The addition of methylmethacrylate, or bone cement, as an adjunct to fixation has been reported extensively. Pain relief and ambulation have been significantly improved in patients treated with methylmethacrylate in addition to internal fixation, and the incidence of implant failure has been significantly reduced.[1,25,32,34,40,44]

Impending Pathologic Fractures

The use of prophylactic internal fixation has been widely advocated for some lytic lesions of bone that have not yet fractured. Fidler reported that lesions in which at least 50% of the cortical bone is destroyed have a 50% risk of progressing to completed fracture.[17] Many surgeons now advocate prophylactic fixation of lytic lesions greater than 3 cm in diameter and involving 50% of the cortex.[39] Others advocate prophylactic operative treatment for lesions that remain painful despite radiation therapy.[39]

Additional factors such as location of the lesion are important when deciding whether to operate on metastatic lesions. Even a small lesion in a high stress area such as the subtrochanteric region of the femur may be best managed with operative stabilization.[10,39] The risk of creating a less stable situation appears to be small considering that bone healing has been demonstrated to be better for impending fractures than for completed fractures.[5]

ORTHOPEDIC MANAGEMENT

Fractures of the Spine

The spine is the most common site of skeletal metastasis. Metastases are often asymptomatic and only become symptomatic when fractures occur, invasion of nerve roots or cord compression occurs, when paravertebral soft tissue extension occurs, or when instability develops due to involvement of the posterior elements.[6,21] Symptomatic metastatic disease requiring intervention is most likely to occur in the thoracic spine, where the room available for the cord is significantly small compared to the cervical and lumbar spine. Because the vertebral body is usually involved first, neurologic symptoms usually start with weakness due to anterior cord compression followed later by sensory changes as the posterior cord is compressed against the lamina.[13,24] Diagnosis of metastatic disease in the spine is similar to diagnosis of all skeletal metastases. Bone scanning is very sensitive in localizing metastatic disease. In the spine, CT scanning is particularly useful for gauging the extent of bony destruction and impingement of the canal.

Treatment of skeletal metastases involves a number of factors. Harrington advocates categorizing patients as described in Table 4. Class 1 patients have no

TABLE 4.   Classification of Spinal Metastases[23]

Class	Characteristics
Class 1	No significant bone involvement No neurologic involvement
Class 2	Bony involvement without collapse or instability Minimal neurologic involvement
Class 3	Major neurologic compromise Minimal bone involvement
Class 4	Vertebral collapse or instability No significant neurologic involvement
Class 5	Vertebral collapse or instability Severe neurologic deficit

significant neurologic involvement. Class 2 patients have bone involvement without collapse or instability. Class 3 patients have major neurologic compromise but minimal bone involvement. Class 4 patients have vertebral collapse and instability causing pain but no significant neurologic involvement. Finally, class 5 patients have collapse and severe neurologic deficit.[24]

Treatment of class 1 and 2 patients involves chemotherapeutic or hormonal manipulation only. No radiation or surgery is indicated. This treatment will not restore bone integrity, but it has been demonstrated to increase longevity.[24]

Class 3 patients are best treated by radiation therapy alone. Radiation therapy alone has been demonstrated to be equally effective as decompressive laminectomy in these patients.[21]

Class 4 and 5 patients should undergo surgical intervention. Additionally, patients who exhibit progressive neurologic compromise in a radioresistant tumor or a previously radiated tumor should undergo surgical treatment.[24]

Anterior decompression and stabilization is the recommended approach because it allows direct access to the tumor and allows correction of the kyphotic deformity.[15,16,23] Posterior decompression and stabilization should be added with significant involvement of the posterior elements causing progressive shear deformity of the spine.[24]

Recommended methods of anterior stabilization have included anterior interbody fusion with corticocancellous graft,[27] the advantage of which is that once healing occurs, permanent stabilization is achieved. Drawbacks are lack of immediate stabilization and failure to heal due to poor bone and a debilitated physical condition.

Use of a methylmethacrylate and metallic construct allows both for immediate stabilization and correction of kyphotic deformity.[23] A drawback is that the construct does not guarantee permanent stabilization; therefore, anterior grafting should be added to the procedure if life expectancy is greater than 2 years.[24] Figure 1 shows surgical stabilization for metastatic disease of the lumbar spine.

Fractures of the Humerus

Clain has reported that 20.2% of metastatic lesions occur in the upper extremity, with 9.6% involving the humerus.[12] Treatment of metastatic disease to the humerus without pathologic fracture involves radiation therapy. Radiation reportedly offers effective palliation in 80% of patients.[38]

Indications for the operative treatment of fractures of the humerus remain somewhat unclear. Closed treatment of pathologic humerus fractures has been

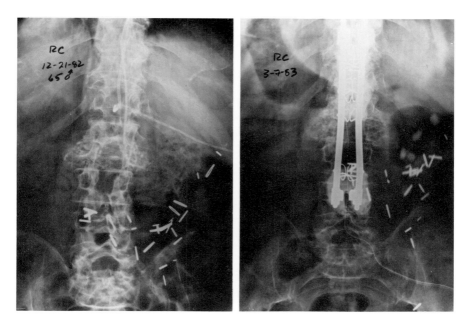

FIGURE 1. Preoperative (left) and postoperative (right) radiographs demonstrating surgical stabilization in a 65-year-old man with metastatic colon carcinoma to the spine.

used with reported good results.[11,26] Other studies have shown less satisfactory results with regard to pain control in nonoperated patients.[43] The decision to operate, therefore, remains an individual decision.

Various types of surgical intervention are possible in humerus fractures. The type of surgical procedure depends on location of the tumor and the extent of bone destruction. In pathologic fractures of the proximal humerus, if adequate bone stock is available, surgical treatment may involve plating alone or plating with supplementation with methylmethacrylate. Figure 2 illustrates treatment with internal fixation and methylmethacrylate.

When extensive bone destruction has occurred, treatment can be undertaken using a proximal humeral endoprosthesis (Fig. 3), which completely replaces the proximal end of the humerus, thus allowing surgical removal of all diseased bone.

Fractures of the humeral shaft are usually easily managed using various internal fixation techniques. Intramedullary rods can be used with or without methylmethacrylate. Additionally, compression plating can be performed. Again, plating can be combined with methylmethacrylate for a more stable construct. When the fracture site is exposed, all tumor tissue should be thoroughly removed before placement of internal fixation devices.

As in proximal humerus fractures, distal humerus fractures may be plated or treated with a distal humerus endoprosthesis if bony destruction is extensive. Again, the key is to remove all malignant tissue and create the most stable and functional reconstruction possible.

A number of studies have looked at surgical management of pathologic humerus fractures, and they have supported operative treatment as superior to

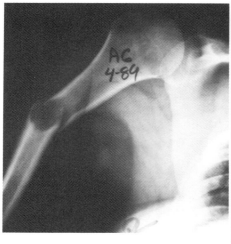
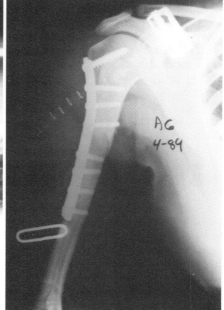

FIGURE 2. Pathologic fracture of the right humerus secondary to metastatic breast carcinoma. The fracture has been treated with internal fixation and supplementation with methylmethacrylate.

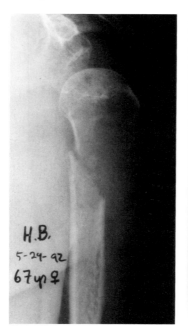
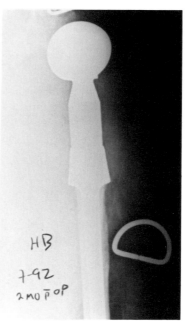

FIGURE 3. Pathologic fracture of the left humerus secondary to metastatic breast carcinoma in a 67-year-old woman. Destruction of the proximal humerus was extensive, requiring endoprosthetic reconstruction with a proximal humerus replacement.

nonoperative management. Most studies also have found that methylmethacrylate augmentation is superior to internal fixation alone.[18,38,43]

Fractures of the Femur

The treatment of pathologic fractures of the femur is similar to that of the humerus except that indications for surgical intervention are much clearer because of the weightbearing function of the lower extremity. Immediate rigid internal fixation offers a clear benefit to patients in terms of mobility and avoidance of the complications of immobilization. Even in previously nonambulatory patients, operative treatment is indicated for pain relief.[35] The only relative contraindication to surgical management is hematopoietic suppression, and this may be sufficiently treatable to allow an operation.[35]

Pathologic fractures about the hip generally require treatment with some type of endoprosthesis. If the acetabulum shows involvement, generally a total hip prosthesis is used to reconstruct both the acetabular and femoral sides.[2,28,29] If the femoral head and neck alone are involved, treatment can be carried out with endoprosthetic replacement of the femoral side only, as shown in Figure 4. Results of these forms of treatment have been quite satisfying with regard to pain relief and restoration of function. In his series of 167 patients, Lane reported that pain was relieved in all patients and ambulation was restored in 72% of patients who were ambulatory prior to their fractures.[28]

Subtrochanteric fractures and femoral shaft fractures can be treated with a variety of internal fixation devices augmented with cement. Intramedullary rods and other intramedullary devices such as Zickel nails can effectively offer immediate rigid stabilization. Figure 5 is representative of intramedullary fixation of a femoral diaphyseal fracture. Occasionally, severe destruction of the subtrochanteric region will require a proximal femoral endoprosthesis.[22]

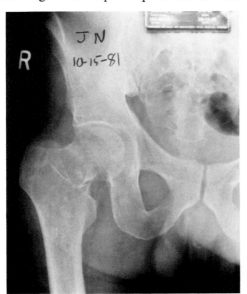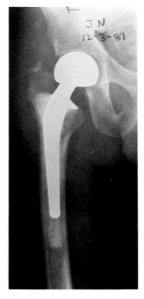

FIGURE 4. Pathologic fracture of the femoral neck secondary to metastatic basal cell carcinoma. Treatment consisted of a cemented bipolar hemiarthroplasty.

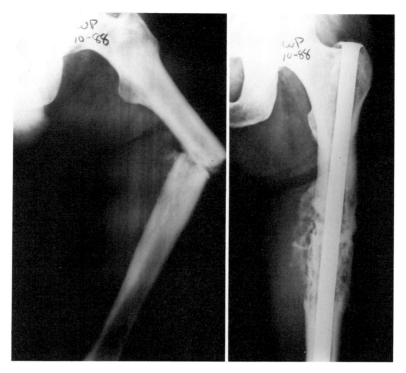

FIGURE 5. Pathologic fracture of the femoral shaft secondary to metastatic melanoma. Surgical reconstruction consists of an intramedullary femoral rod.

Distal femoral fractures of the condylar and supracondylar regions again may be treatable with internal fixation; however, severe destruction may require a distal femoral endoprosthesis.[22] Figures 6 and 7 illustrate these two surgical approaches to metastatic disease of the distal femur.

In general, treatment of femoral fractures is quite successful. Reporting on 283 pathologic fractures and 23 impending fractures of the femur, Habermann found that pain relief and ambulation were significantly improved; 90% had good to excellent pain relief, and 90% of patients who were ambulatory preoperatively regained their ability to walk.[22]

REHABILITATION OF PATHOLOGIC FRACTURES

Whereas operative management of pathologic fractures often takes a narrow view of the specific surgical problem and the function of the affected limb postoperatively, rehabilitation must consider the whole person. The focus of patient rehabilitation encompasses a multitude of factors, including both physical and emotional ones, all of which affect the patient's quality of life. In terms of patient rehabilitation in metastatic bone disease, not only is it important to deal with the physical problem but also the many psychologic, economic, and sociologic factors involved in cancer treatment.

It has long been recognized that patients with bony metastases might significantly benefit from intensive rehabilitation programs. The risk of producing

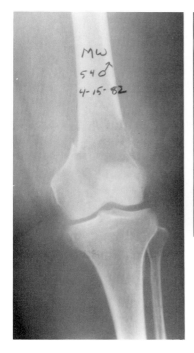

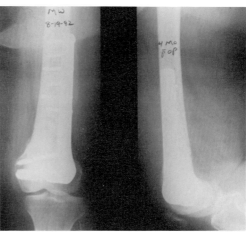

FIGURE 6. Supracondylar fracture of the femur secondary to renal cell carcinoma. The distal femur is stabilized with internal fixation.

pathologic fractures in these patients, however, has been a concern to many clinicians. Bunting et al. looked specifically at the risk of causing pathologic fracture during rehabilitation that emphasized mobilization.[8] Their results suggested that the risk of producing a fracture was actually quite small. Eventually, 16 fractures occurred in 12 patients, but only one fracture occurred in 54 patients during the actual rehabilitation program.

This study also looked at specific characteristics of the patients in an attempt to identify risk factors. A higher risk of fracture was found in females, patients with more advanced disease, younger patients, and patients treated previously for pathologic fractures. The study also suggested that fractures developed in immobilized patients as well as mobilized patients. Ultimately, the risk of rehabilitation causing pathologic fracture appears insignificant in light of the obvious benefits of rehabilitating patients.[8]

Similar to the surgical management of pathologic fractures from metastatic disease, indications for rehabilitation following pathologic fractures have been unclear in the past. Clearly, these patients have significant functional deficits; it has been reported that 40% of patients who underwent surgical stabilization of proximal femur fractures did not regain functional ambulation within a month.[9] Because these patients have limited life expectancy, some people have questioned the utility of rehabilitation programs. Bunting looked at the functional outcome of patients who had suffered pathologic fracture and had been treated in a rehabilitation hospital.[9] Out of 58 patients, 34 patients (59%) were discharged to home, 7 patients were transferred, and 17 patients died. For patients who went home, the average length of stay in the rehabilitation unit was

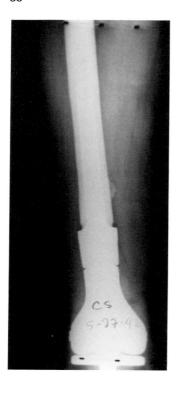

FIGURE 7. A distal femoral endoprosthesis is used to treat metastatic renal cell carcinoma to the distal femur.

37 days, which was 3 days longer than for patients with nonpathologic fractures. None of the patients were able to transfer or ambulate on admission, but 26 could transfer and 23 could walk at discharge. Significant improvement in performing activities of daily living, as measured by Kenny scores, was documented in 27 patients. Bunting concluded that despite limited life expectancy, the patients significantly benefited from treatment with reasonably good functional outcome.

Bunting's study further identified two statistically significant factors that indicated poor prognosis. First, the development of hypercalcemia proved to be a poor prognostic factor; all 11 patients who developed hypercalcemia died. Patients who required parenteral administration of narcotics for pain control also had a poorer outcome. Eleven of 13 patients died, and two required transfer to an acute care setting. Therefore, hypercalcemia and the requirement for parenteral narcotics may be contraindications to multidisciplinary rehabilitation.[9] Aside from this one study, little information on outcome is available, and the authors point out the obvious need for further study.

In general, the rehabilitation process must accomplish two goals.[30] First, the patient must learn to cope with the disease and its characteristics, including pain, limitation of function, and weakness. Second, the patient must learn to cope with life as it has been altered by the dynamics of the disease process. This second goal involves issues such as family dynamics, financial matters, and employment. The rehabilitation process should develop goals in all of these areas and strategies to allow a patient to achieve the goals. As the patient gradually achieves the goals in a controlled setting, a new sense of self-control and independence is developed, and the patient's quality of life is improved tremendously.

Multidisciplinary Approach to Rehabilitation

The goals and strategies discussed above can easily be implemented using a multidisciplinary rehabilitation team.[30] Each team member has specific tasks in the rehabilitation process.

The physiatrist is responsible for directing the overall care of the patient. The physiatrist performs the initial evaluation of the patient's medical, psychologic, and social issues. The position of the physician is then to guide other members of the team and to maintain a focused rehabilitation program. A social worker should assess all of the resources available to the patient, including family and financial resources. The social worker is important in creating a smooth transition from the hospital to home.

Because the nursing staff has a great deal of contact with the patient, it is a great resource for patient and family education. Additionally, the nursing staff can reinforce skills taught by therapists, thereby playing an integral role in fostering the patient's independence.

Physical therapists set mobility goals and help the patient develop the strength necessary to meet the goals. They determine needs for assistive equipment and offer therapeutic modalities that can be useful in the control of pain. Occupational therapists similarly are important in identifying adaptive devices and specialized splinting that will improve pain or function. They develop goals and strategies for self-care and offer the important service of home environment evaluation. The services of a dietitian or religious counselor may be important for some patients. Clearly, cancer patients, who are often anorexic, can benefit from dietary counseling. Religious counseling may offer great comfort to selected patients.

Specific Issues in Rehabilitation of Metastatic Bone Disease

Because these patients suffer from a terminal disease, they will present for rehabilitation with a wide array of needs and perhaps in very different states of physical health. The idea that differences in presentation and need require a system that can be tailored to meet the varying goals for each patient has led to a rehabilitative approach using "functional staging."[14] Patients suffering from metastatic cancer can be categorized in four basic functional stages: preventive, restorative, supportive, and palliative (Table 5).

Patients in the preventive group have metastatic disease to bone that has not yet fractured. These patients benefit from simple interventions such as protective weightbearing and crutches. The goal is to prevent fracture while patients receive appropriate therapy such as radiation.[30]

TABLE 5. Functional Staging in Rehabilitation of Patients with Metastatic Disease[14]

Stage	Characteristics
Preventive	Metastatic disease of bone without fracture
Restorative	Pathologic fracture has occurred. Only minimal residual functional deficit is expected.
Supportive	Pathologic fracture has occurred. Major residual functional deficit is expected.
Palliative	Disseminated end-stage disease

Patients in the restorative group have suffered a pathologic fracture and need restoration to a level of function. These patients are expected to have only minimal functional deficits following a full rehabilitative program as described previously.

Patients are categorized in the supportive group when they have functional limitation that will be ongoing as a result of the disease process. This group includes patients with permanent neurologic injury due to pathologic fracture of the spine. Patients need to learn entirely new self-care strategies, which will be required for the remainder of their lives.[30]

Finally, patients with disseminated end-stage disease are members of the palliative group. Important issues in this group include pain control, bed and wheelchair positioning, and transfer training. The goal is comfort and dignity in the final stage of life.

Rehabilitative Management for Specific Fractures

METASTATIC DISEASE OF THE SPINE

The goals of rehabilitative treatment in metastatic disease of the spine include pain relief, prevention of new fractures, control of muscle weakness, and ambulation.[30] In addition to physical therapy and occupational therapy, various types of braces can be used to help achieve these goals. When prescribing a brace, one must recognize that increased size causes increased energy consumption and affects mobility; therefore, one must balance the requirements for pain control and support with the need for mobility and patient compliance.[30]

In addition to bracing, various modalities including hot packs, ultrasound, and transcutaneous electrial nerve stimulation (TENS) units can offer significant pain relief. These are important in reducing the need for medication.

A major concern in pathologic spine fractures is the risk of neurologic compromise. Studies have demonstrated a 5% incidence of spinal cord compression in widespread cancer.[24] For patients with spinal metastases, the rehabilitation team must always be aware of the risk of cord compression and be alert to signs and symptoms, including progressive pain, changes in walking or transfer ability, and changes in bowel or bladder function.

When neurologic injury has already occurred, the rehabilitation program must address new issues. Joint contracture must be prevented. Emphasis on mobility may change to wheelchair; however, minor bracing may allow mildly weak patients to walk. Patients will require extensive home evaluation to maximize their potential for self care.[30]

UPPER EXTREMITY FRACTURES

Pathologic fractures of the upper extremity usually involve the clavicle, scapula, or humerus. Rehabilitative treatment depends on whether the fracture has been surgically stabilized. Pain control and stabilization are key for nonoperated patients. Restoring full range of motion, strength, and upper extremity function is important in all patients, but it may begin earlier in surgically stabilized fractures. Special adaptive devices may be required in some cases.[30]

LOWER EXTREMITY FRACTURES

Lower extremity pathologic fractures are more likely to have been treated operatively. Clearly, the goals are to restore strength, range of motion, and function. The final goal for many patients will be walking with or without assistance, but for others, simple wheelchair training and transfer training will be the goal. After surgery, a key goal is to get patients mobilized within a few days to avoid the complications of extended immobilization.[30]

Disseminated Disease

For patients with extensive metastatic disease involving the spine and extremities, the goals are much more limited. Pain control and bed and wheelchair comfort become the key goals. Simple mattress modification with sheepskin or air and water mattresses can improve comfort and facilitate sleep. Family members can be instructed in the techniques of positioning, and the patient can be successfully cared for at home with an appropriate family support system.[30]

SUMMARY

The care of patients with metastatic bone disease and pathologic fracture creates many challenges to health care professionals on many levels. Indications both for operative intervention and rehabilitative management remain unclear in many situations. The goal of this chapter has been to review what is known about pathologic fractures, their biology, clinical presentation, treatment, and rehabilitation. In addition, many of the continuing dilemmas and unanswered questions have been identified. Certainly, surgical and rehabilitative treatment can offer great benefit to many patients with pathologic fractures. Further study is required, however, to develop better methods of assessing patients and to develop clearer indications for treatment so that the medical community can provide the optimal benefit for the maximum number of patients.

REFERENCES

1. Anderson JT: Pathologic femoral shaft fractures comparing fixation techniques using cement. Clin Orthop 131:273–278, 1978.
2. Behr JT, Dobozi WR, Badrinath K: The treatment of pathologic and impending pathologic fractures of the proximal femur in the elderly. Clin Orthop 198:173–178, 1985.
3. Berrettoni BA, Carter JR: Current concepts review: Mechanisms of cancer metastasis to bone. J Bone Joint Surg 68A:308–312, 1986.
4. Blake D: Radiation treatment of metastatic bone disease. Clin Orthop 73:89–100, 1970.
5. Bonarigo BC, Rubin P: Non union of pathologic fracture after radiation therapy. Radiology 88:889–898, 1967.
6. Boland PJ, Lane JM, Sundaresan N: Metastatic disease of the spine. Clin Orthop 169:95–102, 1982.
7. Bremner RA, Jelliffe AM: The management of pathological fracture of the major long bones from metastatic cancer. J Bone Joint Surg 40B:652–659, 1958.
8. Bunting R, Laqmont-Havers W, Schweon D, Kliman A: Pathologic fracture risk in rehabilitation of patients with bony metastases. Clin Orthop 192:222–227, 1985.
9. Bunting RW, Boublik M, Blevins FT, et al: Functional outcome of pathologic fracture secondary to metastatic disease in a rehabilitation hospital. Cancer 69:98–102, 1992.
10. Chao EYS, Sim FH, Shives TC, Pritchard DJ: Management of pathologic fracture: Biomechanical considerations. In Sim FH (ed): Diagnosis and Management of Metastatic Bone Disease: A Multidisciplinary Approach. New York, Raven, 1988, pp 171–181.
11. Cheng DS, Seitz CB, Eyre HJ: Non operative management of femoral, humeral and acetabular metastases in patients with breast carcinoma. Cancer 45:1533–1537, 1980.
12. Clain A: Secondary malignant disease of bone. Br J Cancer 19:15–29, 1956.
13. Constans JP, de Vitiis E, Donzelli R, et al: Spinal metastases with neurological manifestations. J Neurosurg 59:111–118, 1983.
14. Dietz JH (ed): Rehabilitation Oncology. New York, John Wiley & Sons, 1981.
15. Fidler MS: Anterior decompression and stabilisation of metastatic spinal fractures. J Bone Joint Surg 68B:83–90, 1986.

16. Fidler MS: Pathologic fractures of the cervical spine. J Bone Joint Surg 67B:352–357, 1985.
17. Fidler MW: Prophylactic internal fixation of secondary neoplastic deposits in long bones. BMJ 1:341–343, 1973.
18. Flemming JE, Beals RK: Pathologic fracture of the humerus. Clin Orthop 169:83–94, 1982.
19. Gainor BJ, Buchert P: Fracture healing in metastatic bone disease. Clin Orthop 178:297–302, 1983.
20. Galasko CSB: Skeletal metastases. Clin Orthop 210:18–30, 1986.
21. Gilbert RW, Kim JH, Posner JB: Epidural spinal cord compression from metastatic tumor: Diagnosis and treatment. Ann Neurol 3:40–51, 1978.
22. Habermann ET, Sachs R, Stern RE, et al: The pathology and treatment of metastatic disease of the femur. Clin Orthop 169:70–82, 1982.
23. Harrington KD: Anterior decompression and stabilization of the spine as a treatment for vertebral collapse and spinal cord compression from metastatic malignancy. Clin Orthop 233:177–185, 1988.
24. Harrington KD: Current concepts review: Metastatic disease of the spine. J Bone Joint Surg 68A:1110–1115, 1986.
25. Harrington KD, Sim FH, Enis JE, et al: Methylmethacrylate as an adjunct in internal fixation of pathological fractures. J Bone Joint Surg 58A:1047–1054, 1976.
26. Hersterberg L, Johnasen TS: Treatment of pathological fractures. Acta Orthop Scand 50:787–790, 1979.
27. Johnson JR, Leatherman KD, Holt RT: Anterior decompression of the spinal cord for neurological deficit. Spine 8:396–405, 1983.
28. Lane JM, Sculco TP, Zolan S: Treatment of pathologic fractures of the hip by endoprosthetic replacement. J Bone Joint Surg 62A:954–959, 1980.
29. Levy RN, Sherry HS, Siffert RS: Surgical management of metastatic disease of bone at the hip. Clin Orthop 169:62–69, 1982.
30. Lie MR: Principles of rehabilitation. In Sim FH (ed): Diagnosis and Management of Metastatic Bone Disease: A Multidisciplinary Approach. New York, Raven, 1988, pp 91–97.
31. Marcove RC, Yang DJ: Survival times after treatment of pathologic fractures. Cancer 20:2154–2158, 1967.
32. Miller GJ, Vander Griend RA, Blake WP, et al: Performance evaluation of a cement-augmented intramedullary fixation system for pathologic lesions of the femoral shaft. Clin Orthop 221:246–254, 1987.
33. Parrish FF: Surgical treatment for secondary neoplastic fractures. J Bone Joint Surg 52A:665–686, 1970.
34. Pugh J, Sherry HS, Futterman B, Frankel VH: Biomechanics of pathologic fractures. Clin Orthop 178:297–302, 1983.
35. Ryan JR, Rowe DE, Salciccioli GG: Prophylactic internal fixation of the femur for neoplastic lesions. J Bone Joint Surg 58A:1071–1074, 1976.
36. Schocker JD, Brady LW: Radiation therapy for bone metastasis. Clin Orthop 169:38–43, 1982.
37. Sherry HS, Levy RN, Siffert RS: Metastatic disease of bone in orthopedic surgery. Clin Orthop 169:44–52, 1982.
38. Sim FH, Pritchard DJ: Metastatic disease in the upper extremity. Clin Orthop 169:83–94, 1982.
39. Sim FH: Operative treatment: General considerations. In Sim FH (ed): Diagnosis and Management of Metastatic Bone Disease: A Multidisciplinary Approach. New York, Raven, 1988 pp 161–170.
40. Sim FH, Daugherty TW, Ivins JC: The adjunctive use of methylmethacrylate in fixation of pathological fractures. J Bone Joint Surg 56A:41–48, 1974.
41. Springfield D, Jennings C: Pathologic fractures. In Rockwood CA, Green DP, Bucholz RW (eds): Rockwood and Green's Fractures in Adults. 3rd ed. Philadelphia, JB Lippincott, 1991.
42. Tofe AJ, Francis MD, Harvey WJ: Correlation of neoplasms with incidence and localization of skeletal metastases: An analysis of 1,355 diphosphonate bone scans. J Nucl Med 16:986–989, 1975.
43. Vail TP, Harrelson JM: Treatment of pathologic fracture of the humerus. Clin Orthop 268:197–202, 1991.
44. Wang G, Reger SI, Maffeo C, et al: The strength of metal reinforced methylmethacrylate fixation of pathologic fractures. Clin Orthop 135:287–290, 1978.
45. Yazawa Y, Frassica FJ, Chao EYS, et al: Metastatic bone disease. Clin Orthop 251:213–219, 1990.

STEVE R. GEIRINGER, MD

REHABILITATION OF STRESS FRACTURES

From Wayne State University
and
The Rehabilitation Institute of
Michigan
Detroit, Michigan

Reprint requests to:
Steve R. Geiringer, MD
The Rehabilitation Institute of
Michigan
261 Mack Boulevard
Detroit, MI 48201

Stedman's Medical Dictionary[63] characterizes stress fractures as "occurring usually from sudden, strong, violent endogenous force ... usually at the point of muscular attachment." Physiatric practitioners of musculoskeletal medicine, particularly sports medicine, recognize stress fracture as a common consequence of overloading the dynamic process whereby bones adapt to increased load. Starting a new exercise or rapidly increasing from the previous exercise level is a common precursor to the development of a stress fracture.

Stress fractures were widely recognized first in members of the military.[22,24,44,47,57,64] Because long-distance walking with heavy packs often caused the problem, they were sometimes labeled "march fractures." Currently, stress fractures are typically associated with athletes, including dancers, runners, and participants in running sports.[4,11]

PATHOPHYSIOLOGY AND LOCATION

Stress fractures can be subdivided into insufficiency and fatigue types.[4,11] Insufficiency fractures occur when normal muscular activity acts on an abnormal bone, usually a mineral-deficient bone. Fractures arising from osteoporosis are discussed elsewhere in this volume. Fatigue fractures, the subject of this chapter, usually result from abnormal muscular stress to a previously normal bone and are found primarily in athletes. The contribution of direct impact forces to bone is now felt to be of less importance, if any, in the pathophysiology of most stress fractures.

It is well known that both muscle and bone will respond to increased activity. Among other changes, muscles undergo hypertrophy and contract in greater synchrony and thereby grow stronger. Bones restructure according to the forces imparted to them, becoming denser and altering their internal architecture. As these changes occur early in training, muscle adapts more quickly than bone,[11] resulting in a mechanical imbalance.[10,14,45,71] If training occurs slowly over time, bone density and structure accommodate the increased muscle strength. When training is advanced too quickly, though, the intrinsic elasticity of bone no longer compensates for the deformations caused by the more powerful muscular contractions, and a stress fracture may develop.

Simply stated, bone is a dynamic structure, with the competing elements of resorption and laying down of new bone ideally in equilibrium. If physical activity is increased too aggressively, the laying down of new bone does not accelerate quickly enough and lags behind the resorption process. Rarely, if activity is not then limited, a complete fracture may occur.[10,14]

The three most common sites of stress fractures are the tibia, especially proximal,[1,53] the fibula, especially distal,[11] and the metatarsal bones.[8] While any of the metatarsal bones can be involved, the second and third are injured most frequently.[24,54,57,71] Fracture at the base of the fifth metatarsal can occur from stress overload or with an acute injury, the latter of which is referred to as a Jones fracture.[37] Recent observations[5,62] point out the importance of this distinction, because the Jones fracture often leads to nonunion if standard stress fracture treatment is used.

Stress fractures of the femur[19,29] and calcaneus[71] are also common, with the latter being prevalent in the military. Femoral neck stress fractures are particularly troublesome and are discussed in more detail later. Other lower body locations and some associated activities include the tarsal navicular bone,[52] the patella,[35,60] the pelvis in runners,[59,67] and the pubic ramus in swimmers.[40] While less common, upper body stress fractures have been reported in the olecranon process in throwers;[33,51] the scaphoid in gymnasts;[16] the ulnar diaphysis in pitchers, weightlifters, and throwers;[2,7,66] the ribs, from rowing,[30] using exercise machinery,[49] or pitching;[25] the clavicle after radical neck dissection;[55] the distal radius in a pool player;[56] and the sternum in a wrestler.[38]

Defects of the vertebral pars interarticularis in adolescents have also been characterized as stress fractures.[3,28,43] They are more common in girls, especially in association with repetitive hyperextension of the lumbosacral region,[42,43] as with gymnastics, cheerleading, and many forms of dance.

CAUSATIVE FACTORS

The underlying pathomechanics of stress fractures have already been described. As with other musculoskeletal injuries, the factors causing the abnormal mechanics in the first place are either intrinsic or extrinsic to the muscle-bone system. A higher incidence of stress fractures has been correlated with narrow and short tibiae, increased hip external rotation, increased knee valgus, and right leg dominance.[17,21] Height has also shown a positive correlation.[65] While these relationships are based on studies of large cohorts, the clinical significance of any one of these findings in an individual athlete is uncertain. Metabolic factors such as eating disorders, dietary calcium, bone density, and menstrual irregularities have shown no consistent positive or negative association.[6,18,50] Finally, single case reports highlight stress fractures caused by altered mechanics at another location, such as at the femoral neck following total knee arthroplasty.[27,41]

Extrinsic causes of stress fractures, especially overuse, are much more common in athletes.[23] Too rapidly increasing the duration, intensity, or difficulty of athletic activity can trigger the mechanical imbalance that precedes a stress fracture. That training error represents the single most common factor in the development of stress injuries. Additionally, equipment or environmental errors can be causative—for example, using ill-fitting shoes or always running on concrete. In these cases, the role of direct impact forces arising from each stride might be primary. In the elderly, commencement of a walking or low-impact aerobic program has led to stress fractures.[9,13,58,61] As mentioned earlier, repeated hyperextension forces of the spine have been implicated in pars interarticularis stress fractures, or spondylolysis, sometimes followed by spondylolisthesis.[42,43]

CLINICAL PRESENTATION AND DIFFERENTIAL DIAGNOSIS

The primary symptom of a stress fracture is pain with activity. One study[26] found that an average of 2.7 months elapsed between the onset of hard training and initial symptoms. On the other hand, with a dramatic increase in physical activity, symptoms can occur within a few days to weeks. Initially, pain is relieved simply by rest, although if the offending activity continues, pain during rest will develop. The athlete may also notice mild local swelling and edema.[39] When pain follows a recent increase in activity, even without other symptoms, a high index of suspicion for stress fracture is warranted. Stated another way, stress fracture cannot be considered only a "diagnosis of exclusion."

Physical examination findings typically include severe point tenderness spanning a very short bone segment directly over the defect and, occasionally, swelling and erythema. Careful study of the underlying biomechanics is also undertaken, in particular to uncover deficiencies in flexibility, or in muscle balance and strength. A rigid, supinated foot, or a hyperlordotic lumbar spine are noted. Running shoes are inspected for abnormal wear patterns and structural integrity. Some stress fractures, even potentially serious ones as in the femoral neck, have few physical examination correlates and, once again, a heightened suspicion is appropriate.

Tibial shaft stress fracture is to be distinguished from deep posterior calf enthesitis ("shin splints") and from anterior compartment syndrome.[23] Differentiation among these three common entities is virtually always possible with the clinical history and physical examination alone. Other bony abnormalities must also be considered, including metastatic or primary bone tumor, Ewing's tumor, osteoid osteoma, and osteomyelitis.[11] In many of the locations noted previously, common musculoskeletal disorders such as tendinitis, strain, or sprain are included in the differential diagnosis.

RADIOLOGIC TESTING

The first study generally ordered when pain arises from physical activity is a plain radiograph. The x-ray abnormalities suggesting a stress fracture may not be apparent for 1–2 weeks after onset of symptoms, however, and in some cases no abnormality is seen even late in the course. One classification of initial radiographic findings is summarized as follows,[71] with examples of each type.[39]

Type 1: Fracture line visible, no callus or periosteal reaction (metatarsals, femoral neck) (Fig. 1)

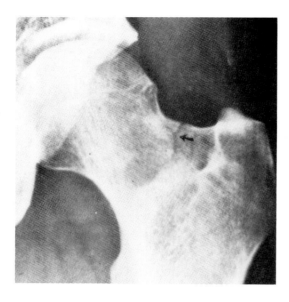

FIGURE 1. Radiographic appearance of a type 1 stress fracture: fracture line visible without callus or periosteal reaction. (From Keats TE (ed): Radiology of Musculoskeletal Stress Injury. Chicago, Year Book, 1990; with permission of Mosby-Year Book.)

Type 2: Focal bone sclerosis, endosteal callus (tibial plateau, calcaneus) (Fig. 2)
Type 3: Periosteal reaction and callus (long bones) (Fig. 3)
Type 4: Combination of the above

Of these, type 3 is most likely to be radiographically confused with a malignant bone tumor.

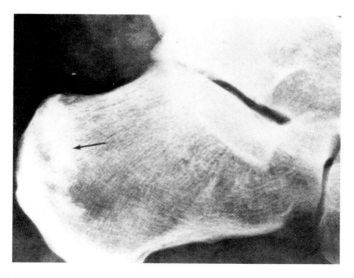

FIGURE 2. Radiographic appearance of a type 2 stress fracture: focal bone sclerosis with endosteal callus. (From Keats TE (ed): Radiology of Musculoskeletal Stress Injury. Chicago, Year Book, 1990; with permission of Mosby-Year Book.)

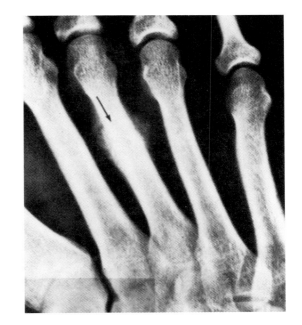

FIGURE 3. Radiographic appearance of a type 3 stress fracture: periosteal reaction and callus. (From Keats TE (ed): Radiology of Musculoskeletal Stress Injury. Chicago, Year Book, 1990; with permission of Mosby-Year Book.)

X-ray of the healing stress fracture shows progression to a fusiform area of maturing callus, eventual disappearance of the fracture line, and bone condensation.[39] Earliest radiologic confirmation of a stress fracture, often within 24 hours of symptoms, is generally possible with radionuclide bone scanning (Fig. 4). The initial dynamic phase of a three-phase scan, with images obtained in the first minutes following isotope injection (using technetium-99m methylene diphosphonate), is particularly sensitive.[39] The gradations of isotope uptake correlate with the degree of underlying pathologic change. A bone scan carries the added advantage of revealing multiple stress fractures, if present, in locations remote

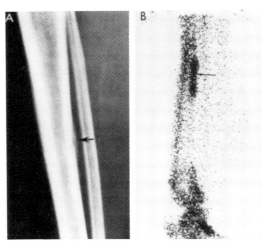

FIGURE 4. Radionuclide bone scan confirmation of a stress fracture in the tibial shaft. (From Keats TE (ed): Radiology of Musculoskeletal Stress Injury. Chicago, Year Book, 1990; with permission of Mosby-Year Book.)

from the presenting symptoms. The bone scan abnormality typically persists from 5 months up to 2 years or longer.[39]

Computed tomography (CT) scanning can also be helpful, especially to reveal endosteal callus, and in sacral or pelvic stress fractures.[39] Single photon emission computed tomography (SPECT) improves the diagnostic power of bone scanning by allowing spatial separation of overlapping bony shadows.[3] SPECT has been shown to be useful in detecting pars interarticularis and pedicle stress injuries.[3,68]

Magnetic resonance imaging (MRI), diagnostic ultrasound, and thermography have also been used in the diagnosis of stress fractures[39] but are less widely accepted than radionuclide scanning (Fig. 5).

TREATMENT

The great majority of stress fractures arising from athletic activity are successfully treated with standard physiatric measures. Initial treatments include icing, oral antiinflammatory medications, and relative rest.

The goal of the first stage of treatment is controlling inflammation and pain. A program of regular application of ice carries the dual benefits of analgesia and reduction of soft tissue swelling. Cold packs are administered for 15–20 minutes at a time, up to four times daily. At least 90 minutes should elapse before re-applying ice, to allow warming of the tissues. As with many other musculoskeletal injuries, when treating an acute stress fracture there is no good physiologic reason to have

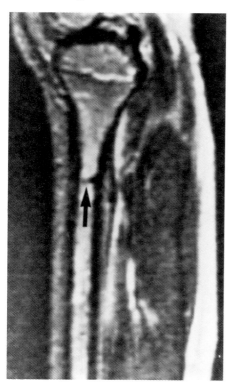

FIGURE 5. Magnetic resonance imaging (MRI) appearance of a stress fracture. (From Keats TE (ed): Radiology of Musculoskeletal Stress Injury. Chicago, Year Book, 1990; with permission of Mosby-Year Book.)

the patient switch to using superficial heat after a fixed time. As symptoms improve, ice can be applied less often.

An oral antiinflammatory agent might also be useful in full doses for several days up to several weeks. After that time, the medication typically can be discontinued or at least reduced to an "as needed" analgesic dosage.

In most cases, the presence of a stress fracture does not require cessation of the contributing physical activity. The clinical history routinely reveals that activity was rapidly increased recently. Bone healing usually occurs satisfactorily if training is reduced to just below the previously pain-free level and maintained at that lower level for at least a few weeks. This illustrates the concept of relative rest,[20] which is applicable for most common lower extremity stress fractures— metatarsal, fibular, and tibial shaft fractures. For most fatigue type injuries, relative rest allows the laying down of new bone to "catch up" with the resorption. Complete rest may be necessary in the few cases where pain persists despite the recommended initial reduction in activity.

Another reported treatment early in the course of lower extremity stress fracture is application of a pneumatic leg brace.[15,70] The brace is applied acutely, with resumption of light training after an average of 1 week. Athletes so treated are generally able to return to high-level competition.

Shock absorbing shoe inserts are of possible benefit in the prevention of lower extremity stress fractures.[46,48] In runners with a supinated, inflexible foot, an arch support may be helpful in preventing metatarsal stress injuries.

The intermediate step in the rehabilitation of stress fractures encompasses the return to usual sporting or other activity. The starting point for this phase is determined using the principle of relative rest. The duration and intensity of exercise are then advanced slowly and without symptoms. In this way, bone restructuring is allowed to take place, keeping in mind that overzealous athletes will often suffer a recurrence. The weekly increase in the duration of each exercise session will range from about 50% in mild cases to a low of 10% in severe or recalcitrant cases. To illustrate the most conservative of these guidelines, a patient recovering from a stress fracture might jog pain-free for 20 minutes, three times the first week, increasing only to 22 minutes, three times the next week, then to 24 or 25 minutes the following week, and so on, to allow bone restructuring. Further counseling about regulating the intensity of exercise is tailored to the individual situation. This process continues throughout recovery, with adjustments made as needed to the training schedule, depending on symptoms, physical examination findings, and, if needed, follow-up radiographic studies.

Prevention of recurrent stress fractures, the third and final step of rehabilitation, is an ongoing process lasting indefinitely but which starts during the second or even first stage of treatment. The physiatrist undertakes a careful study of contributing intrinsic and extrinsic factors in each injury and then counsels accordingly. Any of the factors that might have predisposed to the stress fracture are addressed. Individually determined exercise programs are designed, comprising appropriate flexibility and strength training to optimize muscular balance. Typically, though, the most germane advice to the athlete is to avoid dramatic upturns in duration or intensity of exercise that occur over a short time. Additionally, the adoption of cross-training techniques, whereby varied types of exercise are included in the weekly routine, is helpful, because repeated muscular or impact force to one area of bone is not applied as frequently. Ideally, through educational efforts, the physiatrist will be in a position to furnish information about prevention of stress fractures and other musculoskeletal disorders before any injury arises.

The most common complications of stress fracture treatment are delayed union, nonunion, and displacement. Delayed union or nonunion are associated with a lag in arriving at the correct diagnosis, or with too early a return to vigorous athletic activity. They are more likely to occur following stress fractures of the mid-tibial shaft, fifth metatarsal base, and the tarsal navicular bone, among others.[31] Operative intervention may be warranted, including wiring for delayed union or bone grafting for nonunion.[12,32,34]

The diagnosis of stress fracture of the femoral neck can be difficult early in the course of symptoms, given the nonspecific presentation of hip or groin pain. Objective abnormalities are scarce, and initial radiographic studies may be normal (Fig. 6). A missed diagnosis in this area, however, could lead to disastrous results. Several studies of athletes[19,36,39] point out, first of all, that femoral neck involvement is quite frequent, representing up to 5% of all stress fractures. The predisposing athletic activity typically is running. Once the diagnosis is established, if no displacement is found, initial treatment is nonweightbearing for at least 6–8 weeks. Operative treatment, including internal fixation, has usually followed displacement, and total hip replacement has been needed following the onset of avascular necrosis.[36] Virtually all elite athletes with a stress fracture of the femoral neck have been forced to end their careers as a consequence, regardless of whether initial treatment was operative. Clearly, a high level of clinical awareness is mandatory when an athlete presents with symptoms in the femoral neck.

This chapter has dealt with fatigue type stress fractures, which usually arise after accelerated athletic activity. The physiatrist plays a key role in the diagnosis, early and late treatment, and education about prevention of these injuries. Most

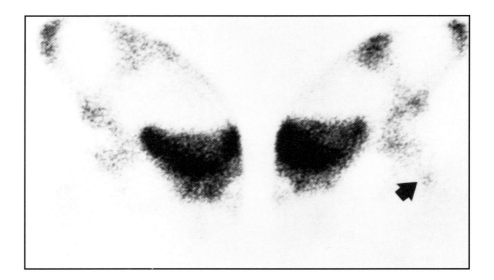

FIGURE 6. Subtle bone scan abnormality in an early femoral neck stress fracture. (From Keats TE (ed): Radiology of Musculoskeletal Stress Injury. Chicago, Year Book, 1990; with permission of Mosby-Year Book.)

such injuries are successfully managed with straightforward physiatric interventions, including relative rest, an individualized exercise program, and monitored return to sports. One needs to remain aware, though, of complications arising from certain stress fractures—most importantly, displacement at the femoral neck.

REFERENCES

1. Beals RK, Cook RD: Stress fractures of the anterior tibial diaphysis. Orthopedics 14:869–875, 1991.
2. Bell RH, Hawkins RJ: Stress fracture of the distal ulna. A case report. Clin Orthop 209:169–171, 1986.
3. Bellah RD, Summerville DA, Treves ST, Micheli LJ: Low-back pain in adolescent athletes: Detection of stress injury to the pars interarticularis with SPECT. Radiology 180:509–512, 1991.
4. Berquist TH, Cooper KL, Pritchard DJ: Stress fractures. In Berquist TH (ed): Imaging of Orthopedic Trauma. 2nd ed. New York, Raven, 1992, pp 881–894.
5. Byrd T: Jones fracture: Relearning an old injury. South Med J 85:748–750, 1992.
6. Carbon R, Sambrook PN, Deakin V, et al: Bone density of elite female athletes with stress fractures. Med J Aust 153:373–376, 1990.
7. Chen WC, Hsu WY, Wu JJ: Stress fracture of the diaphysis of the ulna. Int Orthop 15:197–198, 1991.
8. Childers RL, Meyers DH, Turner PR: Lesser metatarsal stress fractures: A study of 37 cases. Clin Podiatr Med Surg 7:633–644, 1990.
9. Cooper KL, Beabout JW, Swee RG: Insufficiency fractures of the sacrum. Radiology 156:15–20, 1985.
10. Daffner RH: Stress fractures: Current concepts. Skeletal Radiol 2:221–229, 1978.
11. Daffner RH, Pavlov H: Stress fractures: Current concepts. AJR 159:245–252, 1992.
12. DeLee JC, Evans JP, Julian J: Stress fracture of the fifth metatarsal. Am J Sports Med 11:349–353, 1983.
13. DeSmet AA, Neff JR: Pubic and sacral insufficiency fractures: Clinical course and radiologic findings. AJR 145:601–606, 1985.
14. Devas MB: Stress Fractures. London, Churchill Livingstone, 1975.
15. Dickson TB, Kichline PD: Functional management of stress fractures in female athletes using a pneumatic leg brace. Am J Sports Med 15:86–89, 1987.
16. Engel A, Feldner-Busztin H: Bilateral stress fracture of the scaphoid: A case report. Arch Orthop Trauma Surg 110:314–315, 1991.
17. Finestone A, Shlamkovitch N, Eldad A, et al: Risk factors for stress fractures among Israeli infantry recruits. Mil Med 156:528–530, 1991.
18. Frusztajer NT, Dhuper S, Warren MP, et al: Nutrition and the incidence of stress fractures in ballet dancers. Am J Clin Nutr 51:779–783, 1990.
19. Fullerton LR: Femoral neck stress fractures. Sports Med 9:192–197, 1990.
20. Geiringer SR, Bowyer B, Press JM: Sports medicine: The physiatric approach. Arch Phys Med Rehabil 74:S428–S432, 1993.
21. Giladi M, Milgrom C, Simdin A, Danon Y: Stress fractures: Identifiable risk factors. Am J Sports Med 19:647–652, 1991.
22. Gilbert RS, Johnson HA: Stress fractures in military recruits—A review of twelve years' experience. Mil Med 131:716–721, 1966.
23. Gooch JL, Geiringer SR, Akau CK: Sports medicine: Lower extremity injuries. Arch Phys Med Rehabil 74:S438–S442, 1993.
24. Greaney RB, Gerber FH, Laughlan RL: Distribution and natural history of stress fractures in US Marine recruits. Radiology 146:339–346, 1983.
25. Gurtler R, Pavlov H, Torg JS: Stress fracture of the ipsilateral first rib in a pitcher. Am J Sports Med 13:277–279, 1985.
26. Ha KI, Hahn SH, Chung MY, et al: A clinical study of stress fractures in sports activities. Orthopedics 14:1089–1095, 1991.
27. Hardy DC, Delince PE, Yasik E, Lafontaine MA: Stress fracture of the hip: An unusual complication of total knee arthroplasty. Clin Orthop 281:140–144, 1992.
28. Hensinger RN, MacEwen CD: Congenital anomalies of the spine. In Rothman RH, Simeone FA (eds): The Spine. 2nd ed. Philadelphia, WB Saunders, 1982, pp 263–284.
29. Hershman EB, Lombardo J, Bergfeld JA: Femoral shaft stress fractures in athletes. Clin Sports Med 9:111–119, 1990.

30. Holden DL, Jackson DW: Stress fracture of the ribs in female rowers. Am J Sports Med 13:342–348, 1985.

31. Hullko A, Orava S: Diagnosis and treatment of delayed and non-union stress fractures in athletes. Ann Chir Gynaecol 80:177–184, 1991.

32. Hullko A, Orava S, Nikula P: Stress fracture of the fifth metatarsal in athletes. Ann Chir Gynaecol 74:233–238, 1985.

33. Hullko A, Orava S, Nikula P: Stress fractures of the olecranon in javelin throwers. Int J Sports Med 7:210–213, 1986.

34. Hullko A, Orava S, Peltokallio P, et al: Stress fracture of the navicular bone. Nine cases in athletes. Acta Orthop Scand 56:503–505, 1985.

35. Iwaya T, Takatori Y: Lateral longitudinal stress fracture of the patella: Report of three cases. J Pediatr Orthop 5:73–75, 1985.

36. Johansson C, Ekenman I, Tornkvist H, Eriksson E: Stress fractures of the femoral neck in athletes. The consequence of a delay in diagnosis. Am J Sports Med 18:524–528, 1990.

37. Jones R: Fracture of the base of the fifth metatarsal bone by indirect violence. Ann Surg 35:696–700, 1902.

38. Keating TM: Stress fracture of the sternum in a wrestler. Am J Sports Med 15:92–93, 1987.

39. Keats TE: Radiology of Musculoskeletal Stress Injury. Chicago, Year Book, 1990, pp 4–9.

40. Kim SM, Park CH, Gartland JJ: Stress fracture of the pubic ramus in a swimmer. Clin Nucl Med 12:118–119, 1987.

41. Kottmeier SA, Hanks GA, Kalenak A: Fibular stress fracture associated with distal tibiofibular synostosis in an athlete. Clin Orthop 281:195–198, 1992.

42. Krenz J, Troup JDG: The structure of the pars interarticularis of the lower lumbar vertebrae and its relation to the etiology of spondylolysis. J Bone Joint Surg 55B:735–741, 1973.

43. Letts M, Smallman T, Afanasiev R, Gouw G: Fracture of the pars interarticularis in adolescent athletes: A clinical-biomechanical analysis. J Pediatr Orthop 6:40–46, 1986.

44. Linenger JM, Shwayhat AF: Epidemiology of podiatric injuries in US Marine recruits undergoing basic training. J Am Podiatr Med Assoc 82:269–271, 1992.

45. Matheson GO, Clement DB, McKenzie DC, et al: Stress fractures in athletes: A study of 320 cases. Am J Sports Med 15:46–58, 1987.

46. Milgrom C, Finestone A, Shlamkovitch N, et al: Prevention of overuse injuries of the foot by improved shoe shock attenuation. A randomized prospective study. Clin Orthop 281:189–192, 1992.

47. Milgrom C, Giladi M, Chisin R, Dizian R: The long-term followup of soldiers with stress fractures. Am J Sports Med 13:398–400, 1985.

48. Milgrom C, Giladi M, Kashtan H, et al: A prospective study of the effect of a shock-absorbing orthotic device on the incidence of stress fractures in military recruits. Foot Ankle 6:101–104, 1985.

49. Mintz AC, Albano A, Reisdorff EJ, et al: Stress fracture of the first rib from serratus anterior tension: An unusual mechanism of injury. Ann Emerg Med 19:411–414, 1990.

50. Myburgh KH, Hutchins J, Fataar AB, et al: Low bone density is an etiologic factor for stress fractures in athletes. Ann Intern Med 113:754–759, 1990.

51. Nuber GW, Diment MT: Olecranon stress fractures in throwers. A report of two cases and a review of the literature. Clin Orthop 278:58–61, 1992.

52. Orava S, Karpakka J, Hullko A, Takala T: Stress avulsion fracture of the tarsal navicular. An uncommon sports-related overuse injury. Am J Sports Med 19:392–395, 1991.

53. Orava S, Karpakka J, Hulkko A, et al: Diagnosis and treatment of stress fractures located at the mid-tibial shaft in athletes. Int J Sports Med 12:419–422, 1991.

54. Orava S, Puranen J, Ala-Ketola L: Stress fractures caused by physical exercise. Acta Orthop Scand 49:19–27, 1978.

55. Ord RA, Langdon JD: Stress fracture of the clavicle. A rare late complication of radical neck dissection. J Maxillofacial Surg 14:281–284, 1986.

56. Orloff AS, Resnick D: Fatigue fracture of the distal part of the radius in a pool player. Injury 17:419, 1986.

57. Pester S, Smith PC: Stress fractures in the lower extremities of soldiers in basic training. Orthop Rev 21:297–303, 1992.

58. Rawlings CE, Wilkins RH, Martinez S, Wilkinson RH: Osteoporotic sacral fractures: A clinical study. Neurosurgery 22:72–76, 1988.

59. Rockett JF: Three-phase radionuclide bone imaging in stress injury of the anterior iliac crest. J Nucl Med 31:1554–1556, 1990.

60. Rockett JF, Freeman BL: Stress fracture of the patella. Confirmation by triple-phase bone imaging. Clin Nucl Med 15:873–875, 1990.

61. Satku K, Kumar VP, Chacha PB: Stress fracture around the knee in elderly patients: A cause of acute pain in the knee. J Bone Joint Surg 72A:918–922, 1990.
62. Seitz WH, Grantham SA: The Jones' fracture in the nonathlete. Foot Ankle 6:97–100, 1985.
63. Stedman's Medical Dictionary. 22nd ed. Baltimore, Williams & Wilkins, 1972.
64. Stoneham MD, Morgan NV: Stress fractures of the hip in Royal Marine recruits under training: A retrospective analysis. Br J Sports Med 25:145–148, 1991.
65. Taimela S, Kujala UM, Osterman K: Stress injury proneness: A prospective study during a physical training program. Int J Sports Med 11:162–165, 1990.
66. Tanabe S, Nakahira J, Bando E, et al: Fatigue fracture of the ulna occurring in pitchers of fast-pitch softball. Am J Sports Med 19:317–321, 1991.
67. Thorne DA, Datz FL: Pelvic stress fracture in female runners. Clin Nucl Med 11:828–829, 1986.
68. Traughber PD, Havlina JM: Bilateral pedicle stress fractures: SPECT and CT features. J Comput Assist Tomogr 15:338–340, 1991.
69. Volpin G, Hoerer D, Groisman G, et al: Stress fractures of the femoral neck following strenuous activity. J Orthop Trauma 4:393–398, 1990.
70. Whitelaw GP, Wetzler MJ, Levy AS, et al: A pneumatic leg brace for the treatment of tibial stress fractures. Clin Orthop 270:301–305, 1991.
71. Wilson ES, Katz FN: Stress fractures: An analysis of 250 consecutive cases. Radiology 92:481–486, 1969.

MEHRSHEED SINAKI, MD

REHABILITATION OF OSTEOPOROTIC FRACTURES OF THE SPINE

From the Department of Physical
Medicine and Rehabilitation
Mayo Clinic and Mayo Foundation
Rochester, Minnesota

Reprint requests to:
Mehrsheed Sinaki, MD
Mayo Clinic
200 First Street SW
Rochester, MN 55905

Osteoporosis, or the "silent epidemic," is a costly disease. Osteoporosis consists of a heterogeneous group of syndromes in which bone mass per unit volume is reduced, resulting in more porous bone and increasing the likelihood of fracture.[29] In the adult skeleton there is a continuous process of remodeling in which bone resorption is coupled with bone formation. At each remodeling cycle, a stereotyped sequence of events occurs. The cells of bone consist of osteoclasts, osteoblasts, and osteocytes. The entire remodeling cycle, from activation to complete repair, takes about 100 days. Multinucleated osteoclasts, bone-resorbing cells that originate in the monocyte-macrophage cell line, resorb an apparently predetermined volume of bone. After this, the osteoclasts disappear and are replaced by osteoblasts, which lay down osteoid, refilling the cavity. After the osteoid is mineralized, the repair process is completed.

Bone resorption and formation are coupled. In ideal homeostasis, the amount of bone at the initiation of a remodeling cycle is expected to be equal to the amount of bone at the completion of the same cycle. In osteoporosis the ratio of mineral to matrix is normal; in contrast, the amount of mineral is significantly reduced in osteomalacia. Osteopenia is a reduction of bone mass without the occurrence of fractures. Osteoporosis becomes clinically significant only when the bone fractures. There are several types of clinical osteoporosis. The two recognized clinical categories are primary and secondary (Table 1). The most common form is primary osteoporosis, which includes involutional osteoporosis

TABLE 1.   Common Causes of Osteoporosis

Hereditary, congenital: osteogenesis imperfecta, neurologic disturbances (myotonia congenita, Werdnig-Hoffmann disease), gonadal dysgenesis

Acquired (primary and secondary)
  1. Generalized
        Idiopathic (premenopausal women and middle-aged or young men; juvenile osteoporosis)
        Postmenopausal (type 1)
        Senile (type 2)
        Secondary (type 3)
              Nutrition
                    Malnutrition, anorexia nervosa
                    Vitamin deficiency (C or D)
                    Vitamin overuse (D or A)
                    Calcium deficiency
                    High sodium intake
                    High caffeine intake
                    High protein intake
                    High phosphate intake
                    Chronic alcoholism
                    Sedentary life-style
              Gastrointestinal diseases (liver disease, malabsorption syndromes, alactasia, subtotal gastrectomy)
              Nephropathies
              Chronic obstructive pulmonary disease
              Malignancy (multiple myeloma, disseminated carcinoma)
              Immobility
              Drugs: phenytoin, barbiturates, cholestyramine, heparin
              Endocrine disorders
                    Acromegaly
                    Hyperthyroidism
                    Cushing's syndrome (iatrogenic or endogenous)
                    Hyperparathyroidism
                    Diabetes mellitus (?)
                    Hypogonadism
  2. Localized
        Inflammatory arthritis
        Fractures and immobilization in cast
        Limb dystrophies
        Muscular paralysis

From Sinaki M: Metabolic bone disease. In Sinaki M (ed): Basic Clinical Rehabilitation Medicine. 2nd ed. St. Louis, Mosby-Year Book, 1993, pp 209–236; with permission of Mayo Foundation.

(postmenopausal, or type 1; and age-associated, or type 2 forms).[19] Another form of primary osteoporosis is idiopathic osteoporosis, which occurs in premenopausal women and young or middle-aged men, or idiopathic juvenile osteoporosis. Secondary osteoporosis results from an identifiable cause, such as early oophorectomy in women, hypogonadism in men, immobilization, pharmacologic doses of glucocorticoids or thyroid hormones, subtotal gastrectomy, and chronic obstructive pulmonary disease. Osteopenia and osteoporosis associated with multiple myeloma, disseminated carcinoma, or a long history of alcohol abuse are among some of the commonly missed diagnoses. There is no clear-cut distinction between postmenopausal and senile osteoporosis because men lose trabecular bone as they age and cortical bone loss accelerates after menopause. The rate of bone remodeling increases in estrogen-deficient women.[1]

Fractures associated with osteoporosis are not uncommon, particularly in elderly white women. This age-related bone loss is more pronounced in women, who by age 90, have lost about 47% of their maximal young adult bone mass in the axial skeleton and about 30% in the appendicular skeleton.[21] The fractional rate of total skeleton loss is about 0.3% per year in men. In women, this rate of loss is initially the same but increases to 2–3% per year beginning in the perimenopausal period and continuing for 5–8 years after menopause.[22] After skeletal maturity is reached, bone loss begins and persists until age 85–90. Because more significant bone loss occurs from the axial rather than the appendicular skeleton, the disfiguring effect of compression fractures related to the spine needs special care.[22,32]

DIAGNOSIS

For diagnosing osteoporosis, a thorough history and physical examination, including family history of osteoporosis, musculoskeletal pain, general dietary calcium intake, and level of physical activity, are recommended. In addition, the laboratory and radiographic evaluations outlined in Table 2 are required.

Objectives of Different Laboratory Tests

The objectives of laboratory tests for osteoporosis are as follows:

Radiographs of the chest: rule out lymphomas and rib fractures.

Complete blood cell count: rule out anemias of malignancies, especially in multiple myeloma.

Chemistry group tests: assess the level of alkaline phosphatase, which can increase in osteomalacia, bony metastasis, and new fracture (these tests also demonstrate an increase in phosphorus and calcium in hyperparathyroidism).

Urinalysis: check for proteinuria caused by nephrotic syndrome and for low pH resulting from renal tubular acidosis that is causing osteopenia.

24-hour urine test: exclude hypercalciuria.

Radiographs of the lumbar and thoracic spine: evaluate osteoporotic changes and fractures.

Determination of the erythrocyte sedimentation rate: elevated in multiple myeloma and in the presence of an inflammatory process.

Serum protein electrophoresis: determine changes indicative of multiple myeloma.

Thyroxine concentration: an increased total thyroxine concentration may be a cause of osteoporosis because of increased bone turnover.

In addition, optional procedures for further confirmation of the diagnosis of osteoporosis can include quantitative evaluation of bone density and bone biopsy.

TABLE 2.   Diagnostic Evaluations for Osteoporosis

Radiographs of chest
Complete blood cell count
Blood chemistry group
Determination of total thyroxine level
Urinalysis
24-Hour urinary calcium excretion test
Radiographs of thoracic and lumbar spine
Determination of erythrocyte sedimentation rate
Serum protein electrophoresis
Optional: determination of bone mineral density of spine, iliac crest biopsy, bone marrow examination

Adapted from Sinaki M: Osteoporosis. In DeLisa JA, Gans BM (eds): Rehabilitation Medicine: Principles and Practice. 2nd ed. Philadelphia, JB Lippincott, 1993, pp 1018–1035; with permission.

Dual energy absorptiometry and quantitative computed tomography to determine the bone density of the lumbar spine are rapidly becoming available at several medical centers[37] for the evaluation of the risk of fracture. Iliac crest biopsy (after tetracycline double labeling for bone histomorphometry) is recommended for high turnover bone loss and therapeutic decision making. Bone marrow examination is performed to exclude multiple myeloma and metastatic malignancy.[19]

Axial Radiographs

Radiographic findings consist of increased lucency of the vertebral bodies with loss of horizontal trabeculae and increased prominence of the cortical endplates and vertically oriented trabeculae, reduction in cortex thickness, and anterior wedging of vertebral bodies.[2,7] The degree of wedging that indicates a true fracture varies from a 15% to 25% reduction in anterior height relative to the posterior height of the same vertebra. There are other morphologic changes, such as bioconcavity of vertebral bodies and complete compression fractures (reduction in both the anterior and the posterior height by at least 25% compared with the adjacent normal vertebrae).[4,26]

Other Axial Radiographic Findings

Other axial skeletal fractures such as fractures of the sacral alae and pubic rami may also be detected (Fig. 1). Pelvic fractures are particularly common in patients with osteoporosis. Fractures of the pubic rami can occur with minimal strain, and most patients hardly recall severe strain. Healing occurs without invasive techniques. Ambulatory activities are reduced, and a wheeled walker is initially recommended for decreasing pain. Later, crutches and a cane are used. Weightbearing is limited, as dictated by the level of pain in the pelvic area. Fracture of the sacrum with minimal trauma also can occur, and the goal of management is to decrease weightbearing pain with the use of proper assistive devices for ambulation.

SYMPTOMS AND MANAGEMENT

Pharmacologic interventions to reduce bone loss and increase bone mass are discussed extensively in the medical literature. There is no known mechanism to reverse the postural changes of osteoporosis without the use of rehabilitative measures.[25]

When osteoporotic bone is exposed to trauma beyond its biomechanical competence, fractures occur. Osteoporosis is asymptomatic until fractures occur. Limb or pelvic fractures usually necessitate acute medical care. Osteoporosis is commonly diagnosed in patients whose reduction of bone mass is so advanced that vertebral compression fractures have resulted in extensive loss of height or are radiographically identifiable. Such fractures occur most frequently in the weightbearing vertebrae (T7, T8, and below).[27] Cervical and upper thoracic vertebrae are rarely, if ever, involved.

Spinal Compression Fractures

Most spinal compression fractures are asymptomatic at the time of onset and are usually found on routine radiographs of the spine. Acute vertebral fractures may be painful, and the pain may last 2–6 weeks.

Compression fractures of vertebral bodies cause pain at the involved level of the spine. In patients with symptomatic osteoporosis, back pain is usually a major complaint and can be acute or chronic. The pain may develop gradually or occur

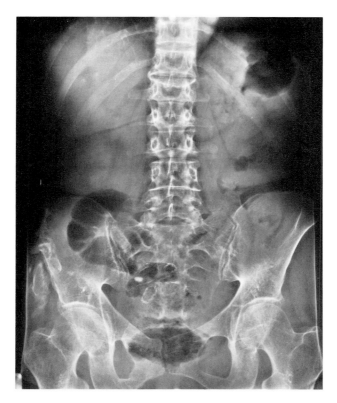

FIGURE 1. Radiograph from a 60-year-old woman with compression of the body of T6 and L1 shows healed fractures of superior and inferior pubic rami on the right and posttraumatic deformity of the right iliac wing.

suddenly when a patient falls, lifts a heavy object, or performs some other activity. Any acute back pain in a patient with osteoporosis that occurs in the absence of a previously known fracture strongly suggests a vertebral compression fracture, especially if osteoporosis has previously been diagnosed. The trauma that induces fracture does not have to be extensive; a minor fall or even an affectionate hug may lead to fracture of a vertebra or rib. Some vertebral fractures may not be apparent on radiographs for up to 4 weeks after the injury,[18] but radiographic or other evidence is necessary for a firm diagnosis of fracture.[4] Fortunately, compression rather than displacement of vertebral bones is the rule. Treatment of compression fractures must focus on relief of pain and prevention of further fractures. The fractures will heal in time, although the resulting bone deformity will remain.

ACUTE PAIN

The management of acute pain in patients with osteoporosis is outlined in Table 3.

Vertebral fracture or crush fracture can develop with minimal or no trauma. Acute back pain is usually due to a recent vertebral fracture and does not radiate,

TABLE 3.   Management of Acute Pain in Patients with Osteoporosis

Bed rest (less than 1 week). Significant aggravation of bone loss is unlikely
   to occur during 3–4 days of bed rest
Analgesics
Avoidance of constipation
Avoidance of exertional exercises
Proper positioning principles to avoid undue strain on spine
Physical therapy: mild heat and stroking massage

From Sinaki M: Metabolic bone disease. In Sinaki M (ed): Basic Clinical Rehabilitation Medicine. 2nd ed. St. Louis, Mosby-Year Book, 1993, pp 209–236; with permission of Mayo Foundation.

is aggravated by weightbearing, and may be accompanied by local tenderness. Pain may be referred to the paravertebral structures and is aggravated by physical activities that involve motion of the spine. It is self-subsiding and resolves in a few days or weeks. Bed rest for up to 3–4 days (on a hard mattress with a soft covering such as synthetic sheepskin or a 2-inch foam pad) can help to reduce the pain. Prolonged bed rest is not recommended because it can aggravate bone loss. The patient should be in the supine position with a thin pillow under the head and a pillow of regular thickness under the knees to avoid undue strain on the spine. Instruction in proper positioning principles to decrease pain is important (Fig. 2).

At the onset of acute pain, cold packs (in some cases), usually moderate superficial heat,[14] and a gentle massage[11] to the paraspinal muscles help decrease pain resulting from muscle spasms. Application of heat for 20 minutes with an infrared lamp is usually recommended. The distance between the lamp and the area to be treated should be 18–24 inches. This type of heat application is inexpensive

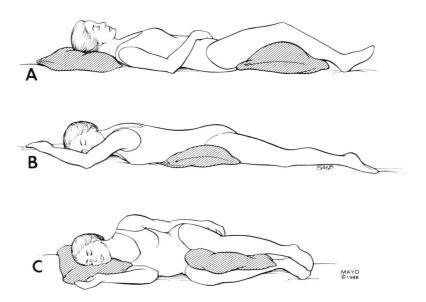

FIGURE 2.   Lying posture. *A,* on back with pillow under the knees. *B,* on abdomen with use of pillow. *C,* lying on side with pillow between knees. (From Sinaki M, Dale DA, Hurley DL: Living with Osteoporosis: Guidelines for Women Before and After Diagnosis. Toronto, BC Decker, 1988; with permission of Mayo Foundation.)

and easy to use. Massage should be done exclusively with gentle stroking because deep massage and heavy pressure may exacerbate the pain.

During this stage, mild analgesics may also be used when needed to relieve pain, but dependence on strong analgesics should be avoided. They are used only in the most refractory cases, and then only for brief periods. Constipation resulting from codeine sulfate or its derivatives can be especially distressing to a patient with back pain. Therefore, steps should be taken to avoid this problem; if constipation occurs, it should be managed appropriately.

If pain persists despite a brief trial of bed rest, prescribing a back support for the patient to wear during ambulatory activities needs to be considered. To expedite the patient's ambulatory activities and reduce the period of bed rest, a properly fitted back support is appreciated more than any other treatment measure by most patients. Full-support, rigid polypropylene braces (or bivalved body jacket, as shown in Figure 3) are preferred by younger patients and usually give the best relief.[28]

The purpose of supporting the spine is to permit ambulation while allowing reduction of motion for the painful area of the back. The application of supports for prolonged periods, depending on the type of back support, can result in atrophy of the back muscles.[12,17] However, in a recent pilot study, an increase in back strength was demonstrated in people who used the Posture Training Support (PTS) and complied with the designated program.[9] Physical therapists can assist with progressive ambulatory activities and physiotherapy to reduce pain. The rehabilitation program should include exercises that strengthen the trunk muscles

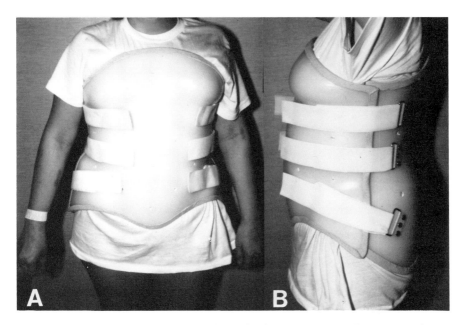

FIGURE 3. *A,* anterior and *B,* lateral views of rigid back support (bivalved body jacket). The brace, made of polypropylene, is custom fitted. (From Sinaki M: Postmenopausal spinal osteoporosis: Physical therapy and rehabilitation principles. Mayo Clin Proc 57:699–703, 1983; with permission of Mayo Foundation.)

and provide muscular support. Good results can be obtained by instructing patients to perform isometric exercises while they are wearing back supports. The rigid back braces are not well tolerated by some overweight people and elderly patients, and they are rarely accepted by patients with orthopnea. These braces are obviously confining, and some of the jackets may weigh as much as 4 pounds. The hyperextension braces that prevent spinal flexion without abdominal contact are used for patients with orthopnea (Figs. 4–6). Rigid back braces, which are usually better tolerated by young patients, provide stronger support.[15,29]

CHRONIC PAIN

One of the most common symptoms of spinal osteoporosis is chronic back pain; its management in patients with osteoporosis is outlined in Table 4. Multiple compression fractures result in loss of height and, in most cases, a thoracic kyphosis and exaggerated cervical lordosis. Postural changes with activities of daily living and abnormal stress on spinal muscles and ligaments result in chronic, dull aching, or burning pain. Attachment pain of highly stretched paravertebral muscles and intervertebral ligaments is the major cause of discomfort. This pain can be particularly prominent in the lower thoracic and lumbar area. The dull pain

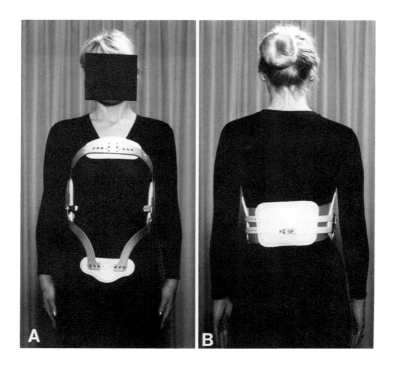

FIGURE 4.   Jewett brace, which is used to prevent lumbar and thoracic flexion when the patient has acute pain due to recent compression fracture of spine. Proper fitting requires proper contact at the base of sternum and over pubic bone. *A,* anterior view. *B,* posterior view. (From Sinaki M: Exercise and physical therapy. In Riggs BL, Melton LJ III (eds): Osteoporosis: Etiology, Diagnosis, and Management. New York, Raven, 1988, pp 457–479; with permission of Mayo Foundation.)

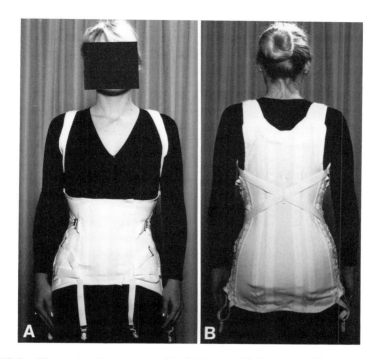

FIGURE 5. Thoracolumbar support with rigid or semirigid stays applied on each side of the spine. Addition of shoulder straps would further decrease kyphotic posture or remind the patient to avoid severe stooping. Proper padding can be added to the shoulder straps to decrease pressure over bony prominences. *A,* anterior view. *B,* posterior view. (From Sinaki M: Exercise and physical therapy. In Riggs BL, Melton LJ III (eds): Osteoporosis: Etiology, Diagnosis, and Management. New York, Raven, 1988, pp 457–479; with permission of Mayo Foundation.)

in the flank and lower rib cage area can be due to iliocostal friction syndrome.[6] Severe kyphosis results in pressure of the lower part of the rib cage over the pelvic rim, which causes significant flank tenderness (Fig. 7).[36] This type of chronic pain needs to be treated with measures that improve posture and increase iliocostal space. As a general rule, patients do not tolerate any pressure over the ribs and upper abdominal area. Therefore, proper back extension exercises and use of a posture training program and Posture Training Support (Fig. 8) are encouraged. An occupational therapist can provide instruction in measures to decrease spinal strain during activities of daily living.

Improving the muscular support of the spine through proper back extension exercises should be tried as soon as tolerated. Extension exercises are recommended (Figs. 9 A–E), as are exercises to reduce lumbar lordosis (Fig. 9 F). Weak abdominal muscles add to the problem of increased lumbar lordosis. Thus, back extension exercises should be complemented by isometric abdominal muscle strengthening exercises (Figs. 9 G and H). Exercises should not increase pain. Figures 9 D and E demonstrate an exercise program whose feasibility we have researched and evaluated extensively for the care of patients with an osteoporotic spine.[27,32] The exercise program should be individualized for each patient according to the

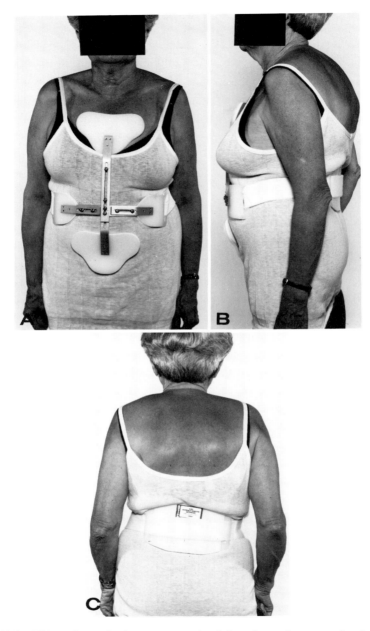

FIGURE 6. This patient, who has osteoporosis of the spine and compression fractures, was unable to tolerate increased intraabdominal pressure with the use of abdominal support because of hiatal hernia. The patient could wear a Jewett brace satisfactorily. *A,* anterior view. *B,* lateral view. *C,* posterior view. (From Sinaki M: Exercise and physical therapy. In Riggs BL, Melton LJ III (eds): Osteoporosis: Etiology, Diagnosis, and Management. New York, Raven, 1988, pp 457–479; with permission of Mayo Foundation.)

TABLE 4. Management of Chronic Pain in Patients with Osteoporosis

Improve faulty posture, if possible
If beyond correction, apply a back support to decrease inappropriate stretch of ligaments
Avoid physical activities that increase vertical compression forces on bodies of vertebrae
Prescribe a sound therapeutic exercise program
Start appropriate medical treatment, as indicated

From Sinaki M: Metabolic bone disease. In Sinaki M (ed): Basic Clinical Rehabilitation Medicine. 2nd ed. St. Louis, Mosby-Year Book, 1993, pp 209–236; with permission of Mayo Foundation.

severity of bone loss and the patient's ability, ranging from back extension exercises while prone to pectoral stretching and back extension while sitting. Axial compression over the osteoporotic spine through flexion exercises is highly discouraged.[32] With different orientation of vertebral bodies to the biomechanical load and stress during recreational and daily physical activities, the risk of fracture can decrease or increase.[3]

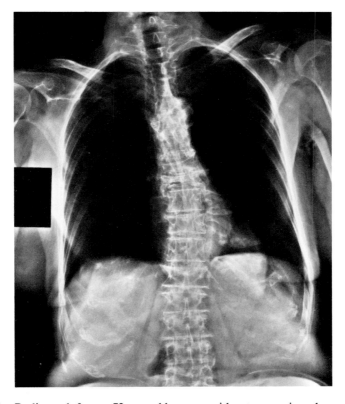

FIGURE 7. Radiograph from a 72-year-old woman with osteoporosis and compressions of T7, T8, T9, and the visualized lumbar vertebrae and anterior wedging of T11. Note iliocostal contact in standing posture. (From Sinaki M, Nicholas JJ: Metabolic bone diseases and aging. In Felsenthal G, Garrison SJ, Steinberg FU (eds): Rehabilitation of the Aging and Elderly Patient. Baltimore, Williams & Wilkins, 1993, pp 107–122; with permission.)

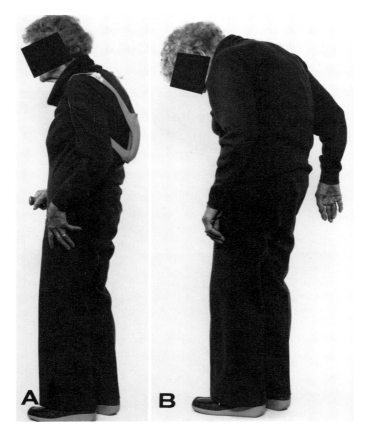

FIGURE 8. An 86-year-old woman with severe kyphotic posturing and osteoporosis, with *(A)* and without *(B)* Posture Training Support.

Scoliosis develops in 58% of patients with idiopathic osteoporosis, and osteoporosis develops in 76% of patients with idiopathic kyphoscoliosis.[5] Therefore, preventive methods such as orthotics that distribute the weight evenly over the vertebral endplates are desirable and can be helpful for decreasing the incidence of vertebral disfiguration.

Spinal Supports

In addition to treatment of acute compression fractures of the spine, spinal supports and exercise can be considered and modified according to the severity of the osteoporosis.

The objectives of bracing in osteoporosis are (1) to reduce the incidence of kyphosis, (2) to decrease the uneven distribution of compressive forces on the anterior half of the fragile vertebral bodies,[2,4] and (3) to provide a backup system for the weak erector spinae muscles, which are the anatomic extrinsic support of the spine during activities of daily living.

The spinal supports are designed on the principle of three-point contact. For avoidance of further flexion of the spine, the three points of contact are the base of the sternum, symphysis pubis, and lumbar spine, as in a Jewett brace (Fig. 4). The conventional thoracolumbar supports assist with extension of the spine through shoulder straps and paraspinal bars and by increasing intraabdominal pressure (Fig. 5).

In a study of osteoporotic patients with back pain, it was demonstrated that facet lesions were more common in patients with higher numbers of collapsed vertebrae.[24] The study suggested that in some patients with osteoporosis and chronic back pain, collapse of the vertebral body or degenerative disk disease is the cause of pain. Therefore, in these situations, the application of appropriate back supports can reduce vertebral motion and decrease pain.

The efficiency of lumbar supports was studied by Morris et al.,[16] who found that lumbar braces increase the intraabdominal pressure of the wearer at rest by compressing the abdomen and turning the abdomen into a semirigid cylinder. This pressure within the abdominal cavity is believed to influence the load on the spine by supporting the trunk anteriorly. When such a support is worn, the weight of the upper half of the body rests both on the vertebral column and on the semirigid cylinder. According to the law of Laplace, the tension in the wall of a container necessary to contain a given pressure on the contents is inversely proportional to the curvature of the wall and directly proportional to the radius of curvature at any point.[35] Thus, the tension in the wall of a container required to exert a particular pressure must be greater if the radius of the curvature is greater. To provide an overweight patient with a sufficient amount of intraabdominal pressure to support the lumbar spine, the tightness of the support must be increased. This by itself contributes to orthopnea and exacerbates problems with diaphragmatic and inguinal hernias. Because the overweight patient would be very uncomfortable, the improper kyphotic posturing that exposes the spine to undue strain can be eliminated through rigid bracing that does not have any abdominal contact but prevents the patient from bending by two-point contact at the sternum and pubis (*see* Fig. 6).

When back supports function through increasing the intraabdominal pressure, certain contraindications such as hiatal hernia or inguinal hernia, orthopnea caused by chronic obstructive pulmonary disease, and obesity limit their use. Severe kyphoscoliosis is also a limiting factor to the use of conventional thoracolumbar supports. For certain cases in which osteoporosis has resulted in the development of severe kyphosis, it may be necessary to use a custom-made plastic jacket to shorten the duration of bed rest (*see* Fig. 3). Although plastic jackets are helpful for acute compression fractures, they are reported to be too confining and not well tolerated in ordinary situations.

For posture training, back supports that decrease kyphotic posturing through counteracting the anterior compressive forces exerted on vertebral bodies can be helpful without increasing intraabdominal pressure. Therefore, use of conventional supports is limited by short stature (shorter than 147 cm, or 58 inches), presence of dyspnea or chronic obstructive pulmonary disease, presence of hiatal hernia or inguinal hernia, moderate to severe obesity, scoliosis resulting from osteoporosis, and compression fractures. The Posture Training Support, which functions through the principle of weight application below the scapulae (Fig. 10) and biofeedback techniques through contact of the weighted pouch and tactile stimulation above the waistline, is better tolerated and does not immobilize the patient. The weight is positioned below the inferior angles of the scapulae and may be increased by quarter-pound increments according to the patient's needs, up to

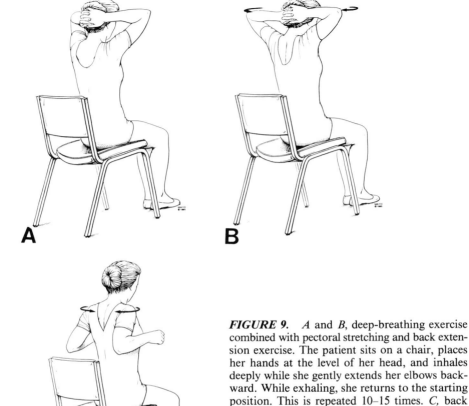

FIGURE 9. *A* and *B*, deep-breathing exercise combined with pectoral stretching and back extension exercise. The patient sits on a chair, places her hands at the level of her head, and inhales deeply while she gently extends her elbows backward. While exhaling, she returns to the starting position. This is repeated 10–15 times. *C,* back extension exercise in sitting position. This position avoids or minimizes pain in patients with severe osteoporosis.   *(Continued on facing page)*

a maximal weight of 2.0 pounds. If the weight application is used for axial stability of gait, the amount can be increased up to 2.5 pounds. Compressive forces applied to the spine during flexion can be multiplied five- to tenfold.[17] Therefore, through shifting the body weight backward, the anterior forces on the spine are decreased by several times.

In general, back supports can be used at three stages in the management of osteoporosis: (1) for reduction of vertebral motion and pain during the acute stage, (2) for postural and ligamentous strain and pain and to compensate for truncal muscle weakness at the chronic stage, and (3) for improving temporal mobility, encouraging proper use of back muscles, and expediting ambulatory activities.

For acute compression fracture with pain, reducing kinetic stress on the spine will decrease paraspinal muscle spasm, prevent overuse, and protect the painful

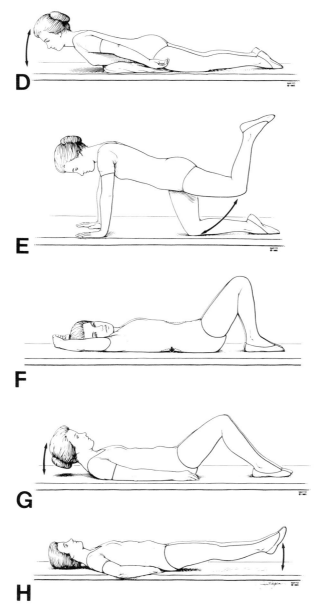

FIGURE 9 *(Continued).* *D*, back extension exercise in prone position. *E*, exercise for improving strength in lumbar extensors and gluteus maximus muscles. *F*, exercise to decrease lumbar lordosis with isometric contraction of lumbar flexors. *G*, technique of isometric exercise to strengthen abdominal muscles with minimal cervical and thoracic flexion. *H*, isometric exercise to strengthen abdominal muscles, which does not involve thoracic flexion. (From Sinaki M: Exercise and physical therapy. In Riggs BL, Melton LJ III (eds): Osteoporosis: Etiology, Diagnosis, and Management. New York, Raven, 1988, pp 457–479; with permission of Mayo Foundation.)

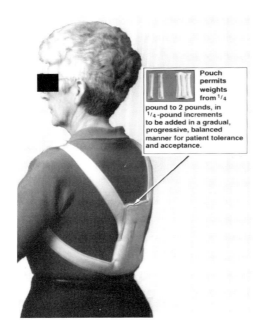

Pouch permits weights from ¹/₄ pound to 2 pounds, in ¹/₄-pound increments to be added in a gradual, progressive, balanced manner for patient tolerance and acceptance.

FIGURE 10. Posture Training Support. Touch-close, acromioclavicular closure with elastic extension for easy, one-hand application and removal. The biomechanical approach appropriately positions weights below the inferior angles of scapulae to counteract the tendency to bend forward. Pouch permits weights from ¼ pound to 2 pounds, in ¼-pound increments, to be added in a gradual, progressive, balanced manner for patient tolerance and acceptance. (From PTS Posturing brochure A838. Jackson, MI, Camp International, 1991; with permission of BISSELL Healthcare Corporation.)

compression fracture area until periosteal edema subsides. Movement of the spine increases pain, and pain induces further overuse of secondary muscles. Bracing becomes helpful and decreases the duration of the patient's confinement to bed because of pain.

Vital capacity can decrease with the use of corrective bracing of the spine.[10] Corrective orthopedic bracing, which is an established form of management for patients with progressive idiopathic scoliosis, results in a significant reduction of vital capacity (14%), functional residual capacity (22%), and total lung capacity (12%). In the erect position, the pattern of chest wall movement is altered; lower rib cage movement is reduced 96%, abdominal wall movement is reduced 39%, and upper rib cage movement is increased 43%. It is suggested that the current indication for bracing be reviewed in view of doubts concerning the influence of bracing on the natural course of idiopathic scoliosis and the substantial reduction of respiratory function caused by bracing.

Therefore, temporary application of rigid bracing of the spine for acute pain due to compression fracture seems appropriate for pain relief in patients with osteoporosis, but justification of rigid bracing for chronic pain needs to be scrutinized.

Therapeutic Exercise

Proper exercise and rehabilitative measures have the potential to build bone mass, decrease the rate of bone loss, or decrease the frequency of falls. Strong back muscles contribute to good posture and skeletal support.[23] A recent study comparing back extension strength in osteoporotic versus normal women age 40–85 demonstrated that although the level of physical activity was comparable in both groups, back extensor strength was significantly lower in osteoporotic than normal women (Fig. 11).[32] Therapeutic exercise programs that improve the natural extrinsic support of the spine can contribute to the maintenance of posture.[8,34]

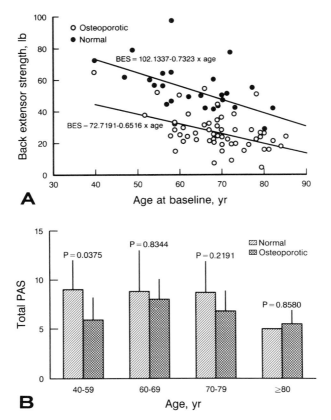

FIGURE 11. *A,* relationship of back extensor strength (BES), in pounds with age for normal and osteoporotic subjects, with least-square regression lines fitted separately to each group. Slopes are not significantly different, but intercepts are (*p* < 0.001). *B,* total physical activity score (PAS) in normal and osteoporotic women. (From Sinaki M, Khosla S, Limburg PJ, et al: Muscle strength in osteoporotic versus normal women. Osteoporosis Int 3:8–12, 1993; with permission of the European Foundation for Osteoporosis.)

Mechanical loading and muscle contraction play a significant role in promoting bone formation and preventing osteopenia caused by immobility.[13,29] Spinal extensor strength correlates with the prevention of vertebral wedging or kyphosis.[23] In the past few years, several therapeutic exercise programs for patients with osteoporosis have been evaluated (*see* Fig. 9). Recreational physical activities that do not overstrain the spine, especially in flexion posturing, are desirable and recommended.[3,33]

SUMMARY

In view of the magnitude of the problem of osteoporosis of the spine, it is imperative to look at the patient's condition as a whole and not only fractures of the spine. Careful assessment of the patient's family history of osteoporosis and risk factors is necessary.[30] The patient's level of physical activity, including recreational and sports activities, needs to be evaluated.[3] Improvement of the biomechanical competence of the skeletal structure and prevention of falls and further fractures are the main objectives of a rehabilitative program.[25,31] In addition to implementation of proper management of the fractures and pain, it is imperative to evaluate the patient for appropriate up-to-date pharmacologic intervention.

REFERENCES

1. Christiansen C, Christensen MS, Larsen N-E, Transbøl IB: Pathophysiological mechanisms of estrogen effect on bone metabolism. Dose-response relationships in early postmenopausal women. J Clin Endocrinol Metab 55:1124–1130, 1982.
2. Doyle FH, Gutteridge DH, Joplin GF, Fraser R: An assessment of radiological criteria used in the study of spinal osteoporosis. Br J Radiol 40:241–250, 1967.
3. Ekin JA, Sinaki M: Vertebral compression fractures sustained during golfing: Report of three cases. Mayo Clin Proc 68:566–570, 1993.
4. Genant HK, Vogler JB, Block JE: Radiology of osteoporosis. In Riggs BL, Melton LJ III (eds): Osteoporosis: Etiology, Diagnosis, and Management. New York, Raven, 1988, pp 181–220.
5. Healey JH, Lane JM: Structural scoliosis in osteoporotic women. Clin Orthop 195:216–223, 1985.
6. Hirschberg GG, Williams KA, Byrd JG: Medical management of iliocostal pain. Geriatrics 47(9):62–67, 1992.
7. Hurxthal LM, Vose GP, Dotter WE: Densitometric and visual observations of spinal radiographs. Geriatrics 5:93–106, May 1969.
8. Hoi E, Sinaki M: Effect of back-strengthening exercise on posture in healthy women 49 to 65 years of age. Mayo Clin Proc 69:1054–1059, 1994.
9. Kaplan RS, Sinaki M: Osteoporotic patients' compliance with use of back supports [abstract]. In Proceedings of the 9th European Congress of Physical Medicine and Rehabilitation. Gent, Belgium, June 1–4, 1993.
10. Kennedy JD, Robertson CF, Hudson I, Phelan PD: Effect of bracing on respiratory mechanics in mild idiopathic scoliosis. Thorax 44:548–553, 1989.
11. Knapp ME: Massage. In Kottke FJ, Lehmann JF (eds): Krusen's Handbook of Physical Medicine and Rehabilitation. 4th ed. Philadelphia, WB Saunders, 1990, pp 433–435.
12. Lane JM, Cornell CN, Healey JH: Orthopaedic consequences of osteoporosis. In Riggs BL, Melton LJ III (eds): Osteoporosis: Etiology, Diagnosis, and Management. New York, Raven, 1988, pp 433–455.
13. Lanyon LE: Control of bone architecture by functional load bearing. J Bone Miner Res 7(suppl 2):S369–S375, 1992.
14. Lehmann JF, De Lateur BJ: Diathermy and superficial heat, laser, and cold therapy. In Kottke FJ, Lehman JF (eds): Krusen's Handbook of Physical Medicine and Rehabilitation. 4th ed. Philadelphia, WB Saunders, 1990, pp 283–367.
15. Lucas DB: Spinal bracing. In Licht S (ed): Orthotics: Etcetera. New Haven, CT, Elizabeth Licht, 1966, pp 274–305.
16. Morris JM, Lucas DB, Bresler B: Role of the trunk in stability of the spine. J Bone Joint Surg 43A:327–351, 1961.
17. Nachemson AL: Orthotic treatment for injuries and diseases of the spinal column. Phys Med Rehabil 1:11–24, 1987.
18. Nordin BEC, Horsman A, Crilly RG, et al: Treatment of spinal osteoporosis in postmenopausal women. BMJ 280:451–454, 1980.
19. Riggs BL: Practical management of the patient with osteoporosis. In Riggs BL, Melton LJ III (eds): Osteoporosis: Etiology, Diagnosis, and Management. New York, Raven, 1988, pp 481–490.
20. Riggs BL, Melton LJ III: Evidence for two distinct syndromes of involutional osteoporosis. Am J Med 75:899–901, 1983.
21. Riggs BL, Wahner HW, Dunn WL, et al: Differential changes in bone density of the appendicular and axial skeleton with aging: Relationship to spinal osteoporosis. J Clin Invest 67:328–335, 1981.
22. Riggs BL, Wahner HW, Melton LJ III, et al: Rates of bone loss in appendicular and axial skeletons of women: Evidence of substantial vertebral bone loss before menopause. J Clin Invest 77:1487–1491, 1986.
23. Rogers J, Sinaki M, Bergstrahl E, et al: The effect of back extensor strength, physical activity, and vertebral bone density on postural change [abstract]. Arthritis Rheum 33(suppl):S124, 1990.

24. Ryan PJ, Evans P, Gibson T, Fogelman I: Osteoporosis and chronic back pain: A study with single-photon emission computed tomography bone scintography. J Bone Miner Res 7:1455–1460, 1992.
25. San Gil A, Sinaki M: Efficacy of rehabilitative interventions on reduction of bone loss and compression fractures in osteoporotic spine: Comparison of two groups [abstract]. In Christiansen C (ed): Fourth International Symposium on Osteoporosis and Consensus Development Conference. Hong Kong, Gardiner-Caldwell Communications, 1993.
26. Sartoris DJ, Clopton P, Nemcek A, et al: Vertebral-body collapse in focal and diffuse disease: Patterns of pathologic processes. Radiology 160:479–483, 1986.
27. Saville PD: The syndrome of spinal osteoporosis. Clin Endocrinol Metab 2:177–185, 1973.
28. Sinaki M: Postmenopausal spinal osteoporosis: Physical therapy and rehabilitation principles. Mayo Clin Proc 57:699–703, 1982.
29. Sinaki M: Exercise and physical therapy. In Riggs BL, Melton LJ III (eds): Osteoporosis: Etiology, Diagnosis, and Management. New York, Raven, 1988, pp 457–479.
30. Sinaki M: Metabolic bone disease. In Sinaki M (ed): Basic Clinical Rehabilitation Medicine. 2nd ed. St. Louis, Mosby-Year Book, 1993, pp 209–236.
31. Sinaki M: Osteoporosis. In DeLisa JA, Gans BM (eds): Rehabilitation Medicine: Principles and Practice. 2nd ed. Philadelphia, JB Lippincott, 1993, pp 1018–1035.
32. Sinaki M, Khosla S, Limburg PJ, et al: Muscle strength in osteoporotic versus normal women. Osteoporosis Int 3:8–12, 1993.
33. Sinaki M, Mikkelsen BA: Postmenopausal spinal osteoporosis: Flexion versus extension exercises. Arch Phys Med Rehabil 65:593–596, 1984.
34. Sinaki M, Wahner HW, Offord KP, Hodgson SF: Efficacy of nonloading exercises in prevention of vertebral bone loss in postmenopausal women: A controlled trial. Mayo Clin Proc 64:762–769, 1989.
35. Stillwell GK: The law of Laplace: Some clinical applications. Mayo Clin Proc 48:863–869, 1973.
36. Urist MR: Orthopaedic management of osteoporosis in postmenopausal women. Clin Endocrinol Metab 2:159–176, 1973.
37. Wahner HW, Riggs BL: Methods and application of bone densitometry in clinical diagnosis. CRC Crit Rev Clin Lab Sci 24:217–233, 1986.

DAVID X. CIFU, MD

REHABILITATION OF FRACTURES OF THE HIP

From the Department of Physical
  Medicine and Rehabilitation
  and
Rehabilitation and Research
  Center
Medical College of Virginia
Richmond, Virginia

Reprint requests to:
David X. Cifu, MD
Box 661, MCV Station
Richmond, VA 23298-0661

A full 95% of hip fractures occur in people age 50 and older, and it is estimated that 250,000 hip fractures occur each year in people older than 65.[28] The incidence of hip fractures in the United States is approximately 80 per 100,000,[10] and it increases with increasing age, doubling with every 5–7 years over age 60.[32] The number of Americans 65 and older increased from 3 million in 1900 to more than 12 million in 1985 and is projected to increase to 28 million by the year 2000. The fastest growing segment of the population is composed of people who are 85 and older, and it is anticipated they will number 5.6 million by the year 2000.[13] Not only is there a greater proportion of people 65 and older, but these people are also tending to stay increasingly active and thus may be more prone to accidents and falls. This increase in the number of "vigorous" older adults, along with advances in medical science that allow the "frail" elderly to live longer and have increased survivability after motor vehicle trauma and falls, has resulted in a greater number of older adults with hip fractures.[5,9,24] Risk factors for hip fracture include increased age,[22] increased incidence of falls (falls account for nearly 90% of hip fractures in older adults),[22] increased osteoporosis,[8,28] female gender,[8,10] Caucasian race,[8] prior hip fractures,[10] Alzheimer's dementia,[4] and low-calcium diet.[15]

Hip fractures account for about half of all inpatient days for fracture care and, when all medical and rehabilitation costs are considered, the annual costs exceed $7 billion in the United States.[14] Morbidity and mortality after hip fracture contribute significantly to this total.[1] The highest risk of mortality after hip fractures occurs in the first 4–6 months, and the estimated current overall mortality rate at 1 year is 14–36%.[6,17,31] Factors that contribute to increased morbidity and mortality after hip fracture include increasing age (although often confounded by concomitant morbidity),[3,18,31] male gender,[6,31] concomitant morbidity,[18,31] cognitive deficits,[25] premorbid institutionalization,[26] and limited premorbid function.[3,16] Reducing the incidence of hip fractures and postfracture morbidity and mortality by using preventive strategies in the face of known risk factors is an important means of reducing health care costs. Additionally, optimizing acute and long-term treatment methods to achieve maximal functional outcome while minimizing morbidity and mortality will assist in limiting expenses.

ANATOMY OF THE HIP

Skeletal Architecture
The hip joint is a "ball and socket" joint composed of the acetabulum of the pelvis and the femoral head portion of the proximal femur. The meshwork of trabecular bone of the femoral head allows for the initial absorption and subsequent distribution of stresses to the dense cortical bone of the femoral neck and proximal femur. The head of the femur and the majority of the femoral neck lie within the hip joint capsule; thus, femoral neck fractures are intracapsular. The intertrochanteric region distal to the femoral neck is extracapsular and includes the greater and lesser trochanters and the calcar femorale. The trochanters provide bony insertions for the gluteal musculature. The calcar femorale, which extends from the posterior portion of the neck to the posteromedial aspect of the shaft, provides a strong conduit for the transfer of stresses through this region. The subtrochanteric region extends from the lesser trochanter to 5 cm distally.[12,32]

Musculature and Nervous Structures
The musculature of the hip may be divided into the adductors (gracilis and adductor longus, brevis, and magnus), abductors (gluteus medius and minimus), flexors (rectus femoris, pectineus, sartorius, and iliopsoas), extensors (gluteus maximus, adductor magnus, semimembranosus, semitendinosus, and long head of the biceps femoris), internal rotators (gluteus minimus and medius and tensor fascia lata) and external rotators (gluteus maximus, piriformis, obturator internus and externus, inferior and superior gemelli, and quadratus femoris). Nervous innervation of the musculature of the hip includes the obturator nerve (adductors), superior gluteal nerve (abductors and internal rotators), femoral nerve (flexors), tibial branch of the sciatic nerve (extensors), inferior gluteal nerve (external rotators and extensors), and small branches directly off the lumbosacral plexus (external rotators). Sensory innervation to the hip joint is provided by the femoral, obturator, superior gluteal nerves, and the nerve to the quadratus femoris.[12] Hip fractures rarely result in neurologic injury; however, posterior hip dislocations and surgical implantation of femoral endoprostheses may result in contusion or traction injuries to the sciatic nerve.[30] Anterior dislocations may cause similar injuries to the femoral nerve.

Ligamentous Structures
The pubofemoral, iliofemoral, and ischiofemoral ligaments are thickenings of the joint capsule that provide stability to the hip. Because the capsule provides

greater anterior than posterior stability, posterior dislocations are more common. Additionally, the capsule is taut with full extension of the hip and slack with full hip flexion. This allows for hip stability in full extension without hip musculature activity, as in quiet standing, and accounts for the majority of dislocations occurring when the hip is in flexion.[12]

Blood Supply

The blood supply to the hip is particularly important with regard to the femoral head, because there is a greater than 20% incidence of osteonecrosis of the head in displaced femoral neck fractures.[21] A branch of the femoral artery, the profunda femoris, divides into the medial and lateral circumflex arteries. The ascending branches of these arteries form an extracapsular arterial ring at the base of the femoral neck. Ascending cervical arteries from this ring then join with the intramedullary nutrient artery of the femur to form an intracapsular arterial ring. Branches from this ring then provide the primary blood supply to the head, with an insignificant secondary supply coming through an artery within the ligamentum teres. In short, the blood supply to the head traverses the neck in a distal to proximal direction, and disruption of the neck may cause disruption of the blood flow and, with it, osteonecrosis of the head.[12]

CLASSIFICATION OF HIP FRACTURES

Dislocations

Hip dislocations occur most commonly in 30- to 40-year-olds as a result of high-speed trauma (motor vehicle accidents) and may occur in conjunction with acetabular, femoral head, and femoral neck fractures. About 10–15% are anterior dislocations, and 85–90% are posterior dislocations. Further classification includes the presence or absence of fracture and whether the fracture is stable or unstable.

Femoral Neck Fractures

Fractures of the femoral neck are most commonly caused by falls or near-falls in the older adult. They occur in the elderly at approximately the same incidence as intertrochanteric fractures,[10,22,23] but may be more likely to affect women and the frail elderly.[22] The most common classification of femoral neck fractures was introduced by Garden in 1961.[11] A type 1 fracture is an incomplete or impacted fracture in which the bony trabeculae of the inferior portion of the femoral neck remain intact. A type 2 fracture is a complete fracture without displacement of the fracture fragments. A type 3 fracture is a complete fracture with partial displacement of the fracture fragments. A type 4 fracture is a complete fracture with total displacement of the fracture fragments, allowing the femoral head to rotate back to an anatomic position. A simpler classification system, which correlates with treatment options and groups fractures according to whether they are nondisplaced (types 1 and 2) or displaced (types 3 and 4), is also used.

Intertrochanteric Fractures

Fractures of the intertrochanteric region of the femur are commonly caused by significant trauma (falls, motor vehicle accidents) and occur more often in males and the vigorous elderly.[22,23] A commonly used classification was refined by Kyle in 1979.[19] Type 1 fractures are two-part fractures that are nondisplaced. Type 2 fractures are displaced into varus, with a smaller lesser trochanteric fragment but an intact posteromedial cortex. Type 3 fractures are displaced into varus with posteromedial cortical comminution and a greater trochanteric fracture (four-part fracture). Type 4 fractures are similar to type 3 fractures with extension into the subtrochanteric region. As with femoral neck fractures, a simpler classification is also used that correlates with treatment options and groups fractures as either stable (type 1 and 2) or unstable (type 3 and 4). Isolated injuries to the greater or lesser trochanters are uncommon.

Subtrochanteric Fractures

Fractures of the subtrochanteric region of the femur are generally caused by falls in older adults and motor vehicle accidents in younger adults. The subtrochanteric region is also a common site of pathologic fractures from neoplastic disease. Fractures may be classified as having either a stable or unstable posteromedial cortical buttress.

ACUTE MANAGEMENT OF HIP FRACTURES

Acute nonoperative or operative management should be instituted as soon as necessary medical evaluation and treatment has been completed. The majority of patients can and should have surgery within 24 hours of the fracture. Rehabilitative efforts are begun as soon as possible, either the first postoperative day or when medically feasible in nonoperative cases.

Dislocations

Because dislocations and fracture-dislocation injuries of the hip are typically caused by high-energy trauma, a comprehensive trauma evaluation must be performed in these patients. Neurologic, vascular, visceral, and additional skeletal injuries are not uncommon.

ANTERIOR DISLOCATIONS

Anterior dislocations without associated fractures that can be successfully closed reduced are treated with 5–7 days of bed rest. Mild skin traction or pillows are used to maintain hip flexion. Range of motion can be initiated when tolerated, and ambulation with full weightbearing is begun by the fifth day. If hip stability or patient compliance are issues, an orthosis that limits extension and abduction may be used for 6–8 weeks. Anterior dislocations without associated fractures that need to be open reduced are treated similarly; however, greater care is taken with range of motion restrictions (i.e., orthoses are always used). Associated fractures

TABLE 1. Practical Classification of Femur Fractures and Dislocations

Injury/Dislocation	Classification
Dislocation	Stable without fracture
	Unstable without fracture
	Unstable with fracture
Femoral neck fracture	Nondisplaced
	Displaced
Intertrochanteric fracture	Stable
	Unstable
Subtrochanteric fracture	Stable
	Unstable

of the femoral head or neck may be excised, if small, and mobilized similarly. Larger fractures may require open reduction and internal fixation (in younger patients), primary prosthetic replacement (in older patients), or total hip arthroplasty (when stability is lost due to acetabular, labral, or capsular injuries). Postoperative management will be determined primarily by the fracture type and fixation. Posttraumatic arthritis (30–50%) and femoral head osteonecrosis (8%) are the most common late complications.[32]

POSTERIOR DISLOCATIONS

Posterior dislocations that are stable and without fracture are closed reduced, managed with 5–7 days of bed rest, and positioned with an abduction pillow. Range of motion is initiated to pain tolerance and full weightbearing ambulation initiated by day 5. In poorly compliant patients, an orthosis that limits hip flexion, adduction, and internal rotation is used for 6–8 weeks. Posterior dislocations with fractures require open reduction and internal fixation, primary prosthetic replacement, or total hip arthroplasty. Postoperative management will be determined primarily by the fracture type and fixation. Unstable posterior dislocations that cannot be stabilized surgically are treated with traction for 6–8 weeks. A continuous passive motion (CPM) machine for hip flexion, initiated on the first postoperative day, is used throughout the day and night to maintain some degree of movement in these patients. Isometric and active assisted exercises are used in bed to maximize range of motion, muscle bulk and strength, and cardiopulmonary endurance. Touch down or foot flat weightbearing (less than 10% weightbearing) may be initiated once stability is achieved, and it is liberalized over 4–6 weeks. An orthosis is used to limit adduction, flexion, and internal rotation when out of traction. Posttraumatic arthritis (30–100%) and femoral head osteonecrosis (10–50%) are the most common late complications.[32]

Femoral Neck Fractures

Fractures of the femoral neck can be difficult to diagnose initially if they are nondisplaced, because groin pain and reluctance to fully bear weight are often the only symptoms. A thorough evaluation is crucial to ascertain diagnosis. All femoral neck fractures are treated initially with bed rest, positioning the leg with slight hip flexion and external rotation. Early aspiration or surgical decompression of hemarthrosis is controversial and not commonly used. Surgical intervention is indicated for all patients, except when severe medical conditions precluding surgery are present or patients are nonambulatory and have dementia. Nonoperative treatment can either involve 6–8 weeks of traction for the displaced fracture, followed by gradual weightbearing and ambulation, or it can involve mobilization from bed to chair when tolerating pain for the nondisplaced fracture.[32]

NONDISPLACED FRACTURES

Impacted, nondisplaced femoral neck fractures (Garden type 1) are often treated with in situ internal fixation using multiple screws or pins. Patients should be mobilized rapidly, out of bed the first postoperative day, and ambulating with weightbearing as tolerated by the second day.[32]

DISPLACED FRACTURES

Displaced fractures may be managed either with reduction (closed or open) and internal fixation (screws and pins) or with primary prosthetic replacement.

The tenuous blood supply to the femoral head may be compromised by the fracture or by the treatment. Reduction and fixation is used primarily, if possible, for the active, healthy patient younger than 70. Postoperative management encourages mobilization out of bed by the day after surgery. Controversy remains about the limits of weightbearing for reduced, fixated femoral neck fractures. Some clinicians have advocated restricted weightbearing (toe touch to foot flat) for 6–8 weeks; others have indicated that, with adequate fixation, there should be no limits except to tolerance; and a third faction believes in a compromise between the two (foot flat for 1–2 weeks, followed by partial weightbearing for 2 weeks).[32] Range of motion restrictions may be dictated by the surgical approach used; however, orthoses or long-term precautions are rarely indicated.

ENDOPROSTHESES

Because older patients have a higher risk for failure of fixation or femoral head osteonecrosis, prosthetic replacement is often used. The first unipolar endoprostheses used in the 1950s through the 1970s (Austin-Moore, Thompson), which articulated directly with the anatomic acetabulum, provided good fixation but often caused acetabular erosion and pain within 5 years. The newer bipolar endoprostheses (Bateman, Gilberty) consist of a smaller femoral head that articulates by a snap-fit with a polyethylene liner of a metal acetabular shell that, in turn, articulates with the anatomic acetabulum. This feature reduces the incidence of acetabular erosion and also allows simple conversion for total hip arthroplasty, if necessary. The surgical approach to the hip will vary by clinical preference; however, each (anterior, lateral, or posterior) results in some degree of joint capsule instability. The lateral approach is used most often. The majority of endoprostheses today are cemented with methylmethacrylate, which offers the advantage of immediate stabilization of the prosthesis in the femoral canal. It also allows for almost immediate full weightbearing. Disadvantages of a cemented endoprosthesis include difficulty with revision to total hip arthroplasty, greater difficulty eradicating hip joint infections, potential restrictions on the use of deep heating modalities such as ultrasound, and difficulty revising for fractures below the prosthesis. Patients are mobilized out of bed by the first postoperative day and then ambulated without weightbearing restrictions. An abduction pillow is used in bed. Range of motion restrictions may be dictated by the surgical approach, but orthoses or long-term precautions are rarely indicated. Uncemented prostheses, which allow a more physiologic fixation by encouraging growth of bone into the porous prosthesis, may be used in younger patients with hip fractures. A longer life span of the prosthesis and more secure fit are advantages, while nonweightbearing status for 4–6 weeks is a major disadvantage.[32]

PRIMARY TOTAL HIP ARTHROPLASTY

Primary total hip arthroplasty following a femoral neck fracture should be reserved for patients with preexisting acetabular disease, including rheumatoid arthritis, osteoarthritis, and Paget's disease. Patients are mobilized out of bed by the first postoperative day and, in the majority of cases, ambulated without weightbearing restrictions. An abduction pillow is used while in bed and with sitting. Range of motion restrictions are strictly enforced for at least the first 3 months and include no hip flexion greater than 90°, no internal rotation past neutral, and no adduction past neutral (the "90-90-90 rule"). Uncemented total hip arthroplasties, which allow a more physiologic fixation by encouraging growth of

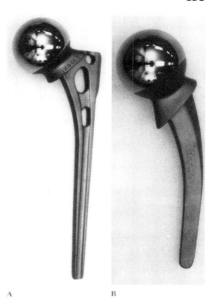

FIGURE 1.   *A,* Austin-Moore endoprosthesis with a fenestrated straight stem. *B,* Thompson endoprosthesis provided a longer neck than the Austin-Moore design. (From Zuckerman JD (ed): Comprehensive Care of Orthopedic Injuries in the Elderly. Baltimore, Urban & Schwarzenberg, 1990; with permission.)

A   B

bone into the porous prosthesis, may be used in younger patients with hip fractures. A longer life span of the prosthesis and more secure fit are advantages, while nonweightbearing status for 4–6 weeks is a major disadvantage.[32]

Intertrochanteric Fractures

Because intertrochanteric fractures occur extracapsularly, the complications of nonunion or osteonecrosis are avoided and the stability of the joint capsule is not

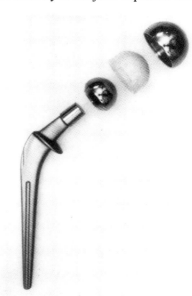

FIGURE 2.   Bipolar endoprosthesis consisting of a modular femoral stem with a femoral head component; the femoral head articulates with the polyethylene liner by a snap-fit that is captured by the metal acetabular shell; the shell articulates with the acetabulum by a suction-fit. (From Zuckerman JD (ed): Comprehensive Care of Orthopedic Injuries in the Elderly. Baltimore, Urban & Schwarzenberg, 1990; with permission.)

affected. Surgical intervention is indicated for all patients, except when severe medical conditions precluding surgery are present or when the patient is nonambulatory and demented. Nonoperative treatment can either involve 6–8 weeks of traction followed by gradual weightbearing and ambulation, or it can involve mobilization from bed to chair when tolerating pain.[32]

INTERNAL FIXATION DEVICES

The first implants used to fixate intertrochanteric fractures were fixed-angle, nail-plate devices (Jewett nail, Holt nail). Although these devices allowed for a static fixation of the fracture, they did not allow for the impaction of the fracture fragments. This often resulted in breakage of the devices or migration of nail into the hip joint. An improvement on these early devices was the sliding hip screw, which provided good static fixation (like the nail-plate devices) in combination with the physiologic healing brought about by the dynamic impaction of the proximal and distal bone fragments. Patients are mobilized out of bed by the first postoperative day. Weightbearing restrictions vary from toe touch for 6–8 weeks to immediate weightbearing as tolerated.[32] No range of motion restrictions are imposed.

INTRAMEDULLARY DEVICES

Intertrochanteric fractures may also be fixated using flexible intramedullary nails or rods (Ender nails), which are inserted distal to the fracture site (at the distal femur) and passed across the fracture site. This approach is advantageous for patients with skin problems in the area of the fracture. Patients are mobilized out of bed by the first postoperative day. Weightbearing restrictions vary from toe touch for 6–8 weeks to immediate weightbearing as tolerated.[32] No range of motion restrictions are imposed.

ENDOPROSTHESES

The uses of a bipolar endoprosthesis following an intertrochanteric fracture are extremely limited. Anchoring the prosthesis becomes difficult due to fracture location. It may be used to allow full weightbearing for a frail or demented older adult.

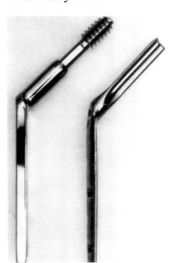

FIGURE 3. The fixed-angle Jewett nail (right) is compared to the sliding hip screw (left). The sliding hip screw allows impaction to occur, and the Jewett nail does not. (From Zuckerman JD (ed): Comprehensive Care of Orthopedic Injuries in the Elderly. Baltimore, Urban & Schwarzenberg, 1990; with permission.)

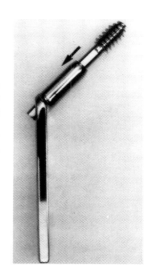

FIGURE 4. The sliding hip screw allows controlled impaction to occur at the fracture site. A screw sliding within the barrel of the plate (arrow) effectively shortens the bending movement and reduces the risk of loss of fixation and implant failure. (From Zuckerman JD (ed): Comprehensive Care of Orthopedic Injuries in the Elderly. Baltimore, Urban & Schwarzenberg, 1990; with permission.)

Subtrochanteric Fractures

Similar to femoral neck and intertrochanteric fractures, subtrochanteric fractures should be surgically fixed, if possible. The same fixation techniques used for intertrochanteric fractures are used for subtrochanteric fractures; however, intramedullary devices are used more frequently. Prosthetic replacement is not an option. Complications of fixation (nonunion, malunion, and implant failure) are more common following subtrochanteric fractures than for intertrochanteric or femoral neck fractures. Pathologic fractures are typically fixated if the patient has a life span of greater than 30 days and is in significant pain. Patients are mobilized out of bed by the first postoperative day. Weightbearing restrictions vary from toe touch for 6–8 weeks to immediate weightbearing as tolerated.[32] No range of motion restrictions are imposed.

REHABILITATIVE MANAGEMENT OF HIP FRACTURES

Physiatric Evaluation

All patients who survive a hip fracture will benefit from some type of rehabilitative services. The primary goal of a rehabilitation program after hip fracture is to reduce disability and maximize function to allow the person to return to his or her prior activity level. The intensity of services and the setting of care are on a continuum, depending on the type and duration of disability. The goal of any rehabilitation program is to develop a home or community-based program that can be performed by the disabled person and his or her caregivers and family. It is imperative that services begin early (typically by the first postoperative day), be interdisciplinary in nature, continue until the person reaches his or her maximal functional level, and be focused on the goals of the patient and his or her family. Functional skills and potential for improvement with rehabilitation can only be assessed if a person's premorbid and present social supports, physical status, and functional level are known. After hip fracture, the majority of patients will return to their premorbid level of basic functions within 4–6 weeks of the fracture.[5] Recovery of more advanced skills (driving, vocation, avocations) may take longer.

TABLE 2.   Rehabilitative Precautions After Hip Fracture and Dislocation

Injury Type	Precautions
Dislocations without fracture	
Anterior	After stabilization, weightbearing as tolerated, with limited extension and abduction
Posterior	After stabilization, weightbearing as tolerated, with limited flexion, adduction and internal rotation
Dislocations with fracture	Same as above; additional limitations based on fracture type
Femoral neck fracture	
Nondisplaced	Weightbearing as tolerated by second postoperative day
Displaced	If internal fixation is used, weightbearing is variable, but usually foot-flat to partial for 4–6 weeks. If cemented endoprosthesis is used, weightbearing as tolerated immediately. No hip flexion, adduction, or internal rotation if endoprosthesis is used.
Inter/subtrochanteric fracture	
Stable	If internal fixation is used, weightbearing is variable, but usually weightbearing as tolerated by the second postoperative day. No range of motion limits.
Unstable	If internal fixation is used, weightbearing is variable, but usually foot-flat to partial for 4–6 weeks. No range of motion limits.

Some activities may need to be modified to permit performance. Driving skills are best delayed until at least 8 weeks following fracture.[5,20]

SOCIAL SUPPORT ASSESSMENT

Evaluations focus on the patient's social structure and supports prior to the change in ability or illness and present status of these supports. Input from family and caregivers is vital and allows them to be involved with the rehabilitation process. The specific areas to be investigated include the physical environment, social supports, and economic factors. The physical environment includes the type of abode, steps to entry and ramps, steps and obstacles within the home, type of flooring, wheelchair and walker accessibility, and location of the bedroom, kitchen, and bathroom. The social supports system includes the role of patient, roles of other persons living in home, roles of persons living in proximity, roles of other significant persons, and the health and functioning of these supports. Economic factors include type and coverage of health insurance, sources and amounts of income and assets, and financial capabilities of significant others.[5]

PHYSICAL ASSSESSMENT

Physical status may be reflected by the history of hospitalizations and medical visits, past medical history, types and amounts of medications, and other physical parameters, such as pulmonary function tests and cardiac stress tests. The physical status should focus on physical findings and parameters that directly affect function and ability to participate in a program to improve function. These include blood pressure and pulse (dynamic), respiration and the need for supplemental oxygen, cardiac limitations (post-myocardial infarction, angina, claudication), nutritional status, skin integrity, chest wall or abdominal pain, limb edema and pain, mentation (ability to follow commands, ability to retain learned information, ability to tolerate mental activity), vision, hearing, sensation, strength, joint range of motion and pain, balance (sitting and standing), visual-perceptual skills (verticality), skeletal weightbearing limitations, medications that may limit abilities (anticoagulants, beta-blockers), and conditions that may limit participation (virulent infections, psychiatric disorders). In the patient with a hip fracture, joint pain and limitation and bony weightbearing considerations are very important and are determined by the type of fracture sustained, type of fixation used, ability of the patient to follow prescribed limitations, and the clinical judgment of the orthopedic surgeon.[5]

FUNCTIONAL ASSESSMENT

Functional status is best quantified by the Functional Independence Measure (FIM), looking at self-care, mobility, communication, psychosocial and cognitive skills.[29] It is particularly important to identify skills that could not be done premorbidly and who was helping the patient to perform them. The assessment should be dynamic in nature and is best accomplished over 2–3 days, at different times during the day. It also should be supplemented by input from other health professionals such as nurses, therapists, and perhaps the family. This allows one to assess consistency, improvement, and diurnal variability. While a static (one-time) assessment is less desirable, it may be become somewhat dynamic if one can note changes over the course of the exam, changes with different examiners or examination style, and the role of the family.[5]

Rehabilitation Programs

ACUTE REHABILITATION SERVICES

In all patients, physical and occupational therapy in the form of a program of bed-level range of motion, strengthening, and conditioning exercises should be initiated immediately postoperatively or after the initiation of traction. This program is taught to the patient, caregivers, and nursing staff so that it may be performed throughout the day. Patients in traction are continued with bed-level activities until released for out-of-bed activity. Patients who are not limited by traction are mobilized out of bed to a chair by the first postoperative day. Chair-level exercises (active quadriceps exercises, ankle pumps) are implemented. On postoperative days 2–4 the program consists of bed-to-chair mobility using a standing pivot transfer, wheelchair skills, pregait (from sit to stand, standing balance, and tolerance) and gait (parallel bars, to walker, to crutches) activities, bathroom skills, activities of daily living (ADL) training, and continued performance of range of motion, strengthening, and conditioning exercises. Advanced skills in transfers (tub, car), mobility (stairs) and ADLs are instituted by days 4–7, and equipment is procured (raised toilet seat, bathtub bench with hand-held shower, bathroom grab bars, long handled dressing and ADL devices, walker and/or rental wheelchair) in preparation for discharge. Outpatient or home health therapy (usually only physical therapy) is typically used for 2–8 weeks after discharge to assist with the transition to home and advance mobility skills (use of crutches or cane) and endurance. These rehabilitative services are typically reimbursed by Medicare, Medicaid, and private insurance carriers.

INTERDISCIPLINARY REHABILITATION SERVICES

Patients who are unable to progress within 4–7 days to a level of functional independence that will allow them to safely return to and remain in the community, and who are willing and able to tolerate a 2–4 week comprehensive rehabilitation program, should be admitted to a rehabilitation unit. Factor that often predispose patients to require such a program include concomitant morbidity that limits rapid mobilization (arthritis, cardiac disease), a complicated stay in acute care, limited social supports, and premorbid disability. The program will focus on similar aspects of function that are addressed in acute care rehabilitation but will do so at a slower pace and with greater repetition. Day rehabilitation that allows for 6–7 hours of intensive and interdisciplinary rehabilitation while still allowing the patient to return to home at night may be a good alternative for patients unwilling or unable to remain in the hospital. Outpatient or home-based rehabilitation services are available to help the patient make the transition back to the community, but they are not used as often when inpatient or day rehabilitation programs are implemented. Medicare reimburses for inpatient and day rehabilitation; Medicaid does so in most states; and private insurance carriers usually reimburse for these services, but specifics will vary by policy.

SUBACUTE REHABILITATION SERVICES

Patients who are unable to return to the community in the acute phase of care, and who do not qualify or wish to undertake comprehensive rehabilitation, can also be managed with a more slowly paced rehabilitation program in a nursing home or other skilled facility. These programs are not typically interdisciplinary and often are primarily based on physical therapy. Medicare will reimburse for limited skilled nursing facility stays if extensive rehabilitation services are necessary; Medicaid will reimburse for skilled nursing facility rehabilitation; but private insurance rarely reimburses for this service.

Complications After Hip Fracture

Hip fractures have a 20% mortality 1 year and a 33% mortality 2 years following injury.[7] Orthopedic complications may include nonunion of fracture, infection of joint or prosthesis, leg length discrepancy (often unavoidable),

TABLE 3.   Rehabilitative Program Following Hip Fractures and Dislocations

Stage	Number of Postoperative Days	Program
Acute	1	Comprehensive evaluation. Bed-level strengthening, range of motion and conditioning exercises. Out of bed to chair, chair-level exercises. Review weightbearing/range of motion limits.
	2–4	Basic transfer skills, wheelchair skills, pre-gait activities, ambulation training, bathroom mobility, basic activities of daily living. Transfer to rehabilitation facility if slow to progress. (See Rehabilitation, below)
	4–7	Advanced transfer skills, stair climbing, advanced activities of daily living. Equipment procurement. Return home if possible.
	5–40	Home or outpatient physical therapy for household mobility, community mobility, endurance training. Return to work/driving by 6–8 weeks postoperatively.
Rehabilitation	5–25	Advanced transfer skills, stair climbing, advanced activities of daily living, community mobility, household mobility with home evaluation. Equipment procurement. Return home. Return to work/driving by 6–8 weeks postoperatively.

heterotopic ossification, and loosening of the prosthetic or internal fixation device. Nonorthopedic complications may include exacerbation of premorbid medical conditions, sciatic (more often the lateral or peroneal division), obturator and femoral nerve injuries secondary to stretch injury at the time of injury or surgery, peroneal nerve injury at the fibula head due to excess pressure, poor wound healing in the debilitated patient, skin breakdown secondary to prolonged pressure (heels, sacrum), atelectasis and pneumonia, constipation secondary to immobilization and use of narcotic pain medication, and deep venous thrombosis.

HETEROTOPIC OSSIFICATION

Heterotopic ossification (HO) is the production of bone in aberrant locations around the hip with resultant loss of motion. It occurs following 5–70% of hip fractures and is most frequent after total hip replacement, followed by endoprosthesis use, and then open reduction and internal fixation. While the cause is unclear, risk factors include a history of hypertrophic osteoarthritis in males, prior heterotopic ossification, ankylosing spondylitis, diffuse idiopathic skeletal hyperostosis, posttraumatic arthritis, or Paget's disease. The diagnosis can be made early (within 1 week) by using a three-phase radionuclide bone imaging and correlated later (in 3–4 weeks) with plain film radiography. Prevention of HO can be attempted with NSAIDs, calcium chelating agents, radiation therapy (600–2000 rad), and controlled range of motion and activity. Treatment is similar to preventative measures, with a goal of maintaining functional mobility. Surgical removal of HO is rarely indicated.[2]

DEEP VENOUS THROMBOSIS

Deep venous thrombosis (DVT) may occur in up to 70% of patients after hip fracture and in up to 16% of patients with concomitant pulmonary embolus. The vast majority of cases will occur in the first week and may occur intraoperatively. Risk factors for DVT following hip fracture include prior thromboembolic disease, prior hip fracture, presence of congestive heart failure, use of estrogen supplements, obesity, immobilization, and increased age. Physical exam is only accurate about half of the time; however, duplex Doppler scanning and venography are accurate greater than 90% of the time. All patients who sustain hip fractures should receive prophylaxis with either adjusted-dose heparin or warfarin for 1–3 months following the fracture. Intermittent pneumatic compression devices and early mobilization are acceptable alternatives in patients who cannot tolerate anticoagulation. Antiembolism stockings (TEDs), subcutaneous heparin, aspirin, or mobilization alone is not sufficient prophylaxis.[27] Treatment of DVTs involves either 3–6 months of anticoagulation or placement of an inferior vena cava filter.

SUMMARY

In conclusion, hip fractures account for about half of all inpatient hospital days for fracture care, with all medical and rehabilitation costs exceeding $7 billion. Although femoral neck and intertrochanteric hip fractures are the most common, subtrochanteric fractures and hip dislocations also contribute to these costs. Acute nonoperative or operative management should be instituted as soon as necessary medical evaluation and treatment have been completed. The majority of patients can and should undergo surgery within 24 hours of the fracture. All patients who survive a hip fracture will benefit from some type of rehabilitative services. Rehabilitative efforts are begun as soon as possible, either the first postoperative day or when medically feasible in nonoperative cases. The intensity of services and the setting of care are on a continuum, depending on the type and duration of disability. The primary goal of a rehabilitation program after hip fracture is to reduce disability and maximize function to allow patients to return to their prior activity level. A knowledge of the anatomy and physiology of the hip, the types and classifications of hip fractures, methods of surgical and nonsurgical fixation, and the mobility and weightbearing restrictions imposed as a result are vital in prescribing appropriate rehabilitative interventions.

REFERENCES

1. Agarwal N, Reyes JD, Westerman DA, Cayten CG: Factors influencing DRG 210 (hip fracture) reimbursement. J Trauma 26:426–431, 1986.
2. Ayes PC, McCollister E, Parkinson JR: The prevention of heterotopic ossification in high-risk patients by low-dose radiation after total hip arthroplasty. J Bone Joint Surg 68A:1423–1429, 1986.
3. Beals RK: Survival following hip fracture: Long follow-up of 607 patients. J Chronic Dis 25:235–244, 1986.
4. Buchner DM, Larson EB: Falls and fractures in patients with Alzheimer-type dementia. JAMA 257:1492–1495, 1987.
5. Cifu DX: Rehabilitation of the elderly crash victim. Clin Geriatr Med 9:473–483, 1993.
6. Dahl E: Mortality and life expectancy after hip fractures. Acta Orthop Scand 51:163–170, 1980.
7. Emerson S, Zetterberg, Andersen GBJ: Ten year survival after fractures of the proximal end of the femur. Gerontology 34:186–191, 1988.
8. Farmer ME, White LR, Brody JA: Race and sex differences in hip fracture incidence. Am J Public Health 74:1374–1380, 1984.
9. Fenton LA: Fractures of the neck of the femur: Changing incidence BMJ 283:1217–1220, 1981.
10. Gallagher JC, Melton LJ, Riggs BC, Bergtrath E: Epidemiology of fractures of the proximal femur in Rochester, Minnesota. Clin Orthop 150:163–167, 1980.
11. Garden RS: Low-angle fixation in fractures of the femoral neck. J Bone Joint Surg 43B:647–661, 1961.
12. Gardner E, Gray DJ, O'Rahilly R: The lower limb. In Gardner E, Gray DJ, O'Rahilly R (eds): Anatomy: A Regional Study of Human Structure. Philadelphia, WB Saunders, 1975, pp 165–180.
13. Gershkoff AM, Cifu DX, Means KM: Geriatric rehabilitation: Social, attitudinal, and economic factors. Arch Phys Med Rehabil 74(suppl):402–405, 1993.
14. Holbrook TL, Grazier K, Kelsey JL, Stauffer RN: The frequency of occurrence, impact and cost of selected musculoskeletal conditions in the United States. Rosemont, IL, American Academy of Orthopaedic Surgeons, 1984.
15. Holbrook TL, Barrett-Connor E, Wingard DL: Dietary calcium and risk of hip fracture: A 14 year prospective population study. Lancet 2:1046–1049, 1988.
16. Jensen JS, Bagger J: Long term social prognosis after hip fractures. Injury 15:411–414, 1984.
17. Ions GK, Stevens J: Prediction of survival in patients with femoral neck fracture. J Bone Joint Surg 69B:384–387, 1987.
18. Kenzora JE, McCarthy R, Lowell JD, Sledge CB: Hip fracture mortality. Clin Orthop 186:45–56, 1984.
19. Kyle RF, Gustilo RB, Premer RF: Analysis of 622 intertrochanteric hip fractures: A retrospective study. J Bone Joint Surg 61A:216–221, 1979.
20. MacDonald W, Owen JW: The effect of total hip replacement on driving reactions. J Bone Joint Surg 70B:202–205, 1988.
21. Massie WK: Treatment of femoral neck fractures emphasizing long-term follow-up observations on aseptic necrosis. Clin Orthop 92:16–62, 1973.
22. Means KM: Falls and fractures. Phys Med Rehabil State Art Rev 4:39–48, 1990.
23. Melton LJ, Ilstrup DM, Riggs BL, Beckenbaugh RD: Fifty year trend in hip fracture incidence. Clin Orthop 162:144–149, 1982.
24. Melton LJ, O'Fallon WM, Riggs BL: Secular trends in the incidence of hip fractures. Calcif Tissue Int 41:57–64, 1987.
25. Miller CW: Survival and ambulation following hip fracture. J Bone Joint Surg 60A:930–934, 1978.
26. Niemann KMW, Markin HJ: Fractures about the hip in institutionalized patient population. J Bone Joint Surg 50A:1327–1340, 1968.

27. Paiemont GD, Beisaw N, Lotke PA, Elia EA, et al: Advances in prevention of venous thromboembolic disease after hip and knee surgery. Orthop Rev 18(suppl):1–16, 1989.
28. Riggs BL, Melton LJ III: Involutional osteoporosis. N Engl J Med 314:1676–1686, 1986.
29. State University of New York at Buffalo, Department of Rehabilitation Medicine, School of Medicine and Biochemical Sciences Center for Functional Assessment Research: Guide for use of the uniform data set for medical rehabilitation including the functional independence measure (FIM). Version 3.1. New York, State University of New York, 1990.
30. Stewart MJ, McCarroll HR, Mulhollan JS: Fracture-dislocation of the hip. Acta Orthop Scand 46:507–525, 1975.
31. White BL, Fisher WD, Laurin CA: Rate of mortality for elderly patients after fracture of the hip in the 1980s. J Bone Joint Surg 69A:1335–1340, 1987.
32. Zuckerman JD, Schon LC: Hip fractures. In Zuckerman JD (ed): Comprehensive Care of Orthopedic Injuries in the Elderly. Baltimore, Urban & Schwarzenberg, 1990, pp 23–111.

ABNA A. OGLE, MD

REHABILITATION OF UPPER EXTREMITY FRACTURES

From the Department of
  Rehabilitation Medicine
The University of Kansas Medical
  Center
Kansas City, Kansas

Reprint requests to:
Abna A. Ogle, MD
Assistant Professor
Department of Rehabilitation
  Medicine
The University of Kansas Medical
  Center
3901 Rainbow Blvd.
Kansas City, KS 66160-7306

The basis of fracture treatment is tripartite, encompassing the goals of reduction, immobilization, and preservation/restoration of function. It is the last goal that is the purview of rehabilitation. Although any fracture can be easily classified, every injured person has his or her own unique personal, social, and vocational sphere to which to return. The initial rehabilitation evaluation of the individual must therefore encompass not only an assessment of the fracture but also the patient's previous level of function.

EVALUATION OF THE PATIENT

Although the evaluation can be structured by any number of functional assessment tools, such as the PULSES profile,[32,34] Barthel,[31] or Functional Independence Measure[21a] system, any history must include the following:

1. General Physical Condition. Any other medical or surgical condition that will affect the performance of the patient in the treatment program, constitutes a contraindication to some forms of treatment, or that will affect ultimate outcome, must be assessed.

2. Mental and Psychological Assessment. The patient's capacity to follow therapy instructions and demonstrate comprehension of the treatment plan, as well as compensatory techniques, must be evaluated. Any deficits affect outcome.

For example, a demented 84-year-old man, previously cared for in his home by 24-hour aides, will need a rehabilitation program heavily geared toward attendant training. Appropriate positioning of the extremity, applying and removing a brace, and performance of passive and/or active assisted exercises by the aide will become critical goals of therapy.

A patient with a long-standing injury who has been unemployed for several weeks or months may be burdened by feelings of poor self esteem, helplessness, or depression.[43] The presence of such psychological ramifications will frequently affect the progress of therapies.

Whenever possible, it is always best to involve the patient and/or family in setting rehabilitation goals. Unique needs that are essential to their lives are usually only determined by direct questioning. A personalized treatment plan encourages patient identification with, and enthusiasm for, therapies and serves to increase compliance.

3. Social History. Determination of a support system is critical. Frequently, older and previously independent patients will have been living alone, with relatives living out of state. Issues such as transportation to and from therapies and assistance with the use of equipment at home will need to be addressed.

4. Premorbid Living Situation. The presence of architectural barriers must be ascertained, the evaluation for adaptive equipment completed, and safety and accessibility recommendations made.

5. Premorbid Function. An adequate history must include evaluation of the patient's level of function prior to the injury. Was this person independently performing basic self-care tasks? Was he or she driving, doing grocery shopping and errands without assistance? If not, the amount and type of help must be noted. The functional assessment scales previously mentioned can provide the framework for gathering data.

Premorbid function affects the expected outcome of any rehabilitation program. Patients with a history of higher level functioning have a better prognosis for a more complete and quicker return to their functional baseline.

6. Vocational/Avocational History. It is imperative to determine the nature of the patient's work. A professional baseball player will have different rehabilitation goals than a retired executive secretary.

Likewise, cherished hobbies should be known so that strength and endurance training specific to those activities can be incorporated into a comprehensive rehabilitation treatment plan.

EVALUATION OF THE INJURED LIMB

Neurologic Evaluation

Soft tissue injury necessarily accompanies any fracture, and damage to peripheral nerves occurs more frequently than injury to major arteries.

Sensory and/or motor deficits found at the time of presentation with fracture are generally assumed to represent incomplete and reversible nerve damage (a neuropraxia).[1,8,21] Neurologic changes that occur after closed manipulation or surgical reduction are of more concern and may be indicative of an axonotmesis (loss of continuity of the nerve axon) and, possibly, irreversible changes. Electrodiagnostic testing that includes electromyography and nerve conduction studies is very useful in the determination of the degree of nerve involvement. This type of examination cannot differentiate between a neuropraxia and axonotmesis until at least 4 days following injury. Serial studies may therefore be indicated to document denervation changes and assist with prognostications for reinnervation.

Discovery of peripheral nerve damage must be recognized early to allow for surgical exploration and reanastomosis, if necessary. A motor neuropraxia may warrant neuromuscular electrical stimulation to denervated muscles to avoid atrophy and permanently decreased strength when and if reinnervation finally occurs. Splinting of the extremity may also be necessary to support weakened muscles and prevent overstretching. Specific fractures are especially prone to an accompanying peripheral nerve injury, and these will be discussed as treatment of individual fractures is reviewed.

Vascular Evaluation

The peripheral circulation must not only be evaluated at the time of presentation of the initial injury, but monitored closely throughout the rehabilitation process. In the upper extremity, documentation must be made of the presence and symmetry of any accessible axial, brachial, and radial pulses.

Pain, particularly on extension of the fingers, asymmetric pallor of the skin, the presence of new onset paresthesias, and/or paralysis should be further assessed immediately to rule out impending circulatory compromise.

Musculoskeletal Evaluation

Both active and passive range of motion of proximal and distal joints must be documented to establish a baseline for a treatment plan and to allow documentation of progress. The presence of pain, fear, or muscle spasm can affect the results of range of motion testing and should be noted. Biarticular muscles, such as the biceps brachii and the finger flexors, will influence joint range depending on the relative degree of muscle stretch at adjacent joints. Range of motion is also influenced by age, sex, general conditioning, and genetics. Preexisting conditions can affect range of motion. These include joint deformities due to arthritic conditions and contractures due to previous injuries and subsequent disuse. For example, an elderly woman with a fractured humerus may also have a "frozen shoulder" with limited shoulder range as a result of an old rotator cuff tear.

In long-bone fractures, development of an intramuscular hematoma can result in secondary fibrosis in the muscle belly and can contribute to shortening of the muscle with subsequent restriction of joint movement.[33] If a hemarthrosis has developed, residual fiber strands present after resolution of blood within the joint may form adhesions between synovial folds, thereby contributing to joint stiffness. A more common cause of joint stiffness is the persistence of edema fluid in subcutaneous tissue. This facilitates adhesions between connective tissue fibers, or even between bones and overlying muscles.[1]

Strength testing of muscles surrounding all joints not covered by an immobilizing cast must be completed. It is important to note that the results of manual muscle testing may also be hampered by pain and fear, and note should be made of those confounding factors. Not infrequently, the patient may misunderstand the instructions for muscle testing. Extra time must be taken to ensure the patient has an absolute grasp of the desired muscle contraction.

PRINCIPLES OF TREATMENT

The achievement of bony union is not equivalent to the achievement of maximum function. Injuries sustained at the time of fracture and, indeed, sequelae from actual fracture treatment (immobilization) may combine to result in persistent loss of physical performance.

Rehabilitation begins during the initial evaluation of the fracture. The members of the rehabilitation team include the orthopedic surgeon, physiatrist, physical and occupational therapists, and, of course, the patient. All team members must collaborate well for optimal outcome; however, at different stages of recovery, one or a few will have primary responsibility for carrying out the treatment plan.

Most fracture treatment can be divided into (1) acute, (2) immobilization, and (3) mobilization stages.

In the initial acute stage, the orthopedic surgeon determines the site and stability of the fracture and the need for reduction. A neurovascular evaluation by the treating surgeon is critical for early determination of the need for further evaluation or treatment. Cast or splint immobilization in a position that allows maximal function also occurs in the acute stage.

In the second stage, the physiatrist and therapists devise a treatment plan that will minimize the deleterious effects of immobilization, within weightbearing and joint range limitations determined by the surgeon. Exercises that preserve joint strength and range of motion proximal and distal to the fracture are initiated. Edema is reduced by active and passive means. Close monitoring to ensure preserved neurovascular function continues. Use of adaptive equipment is introduced to compensate for the impaired extremity. Instruction in one-handed techniques for performance of daily tasks such as tying shoe-laces or fastening buttons is completed.

The mobilization phase follows discontinuation of weightbearing restrictions, casts, or splints. The emphasis of rehabilitation is now placed on full recovery and/ or improvement of premorbid function. Treatment goals include decreasing joint stiffness, improving strength in the face of disuse atrophy or neuropraxia, return to bimanual activities, and supervision of graded return to work or avocational activities.

The goals of upper extremity fracture rehabilitation are (1) maintenance and improvement of muscle strength and endurance, (2) maintenance or improvement of joint range of motion, (3) control of edema, and (4) improvement of the rate of union by increasing activity.

The therapeutic armamentaria applied to achieve the above include superficial and/or deep heat application, massage, orthotic application, and therapeutic exercise.

Heat

The application of local heat before the initiation of an exercise program reduces muscle spasm, joint stiffness, and pain, and can also increase the extensibility of collagen.[3,26,29] However, before using any heat modality, the area must be visually inspected for open areas and examined to rule out sensory deficits. A patient with full or partial sensory impairments should only undergo heat treatment under extremely close supervision and certainly never alone.

Superficial heat modalities are the most common. Although their physical characteristics vary, they are able to effect local temperature elevation of no more than a few degrees at depths of a few centimeters.[3,30]

Hydrocollator packs, or hot packs, are a form of superficial heat frequently used to decrease pain and muscle spasm. The extremity must be placed with the muscle in spasm in a relatively lengthened or extended position and with gravity eliminated. The application of heat to an already swollen limb in a dependent position will result in vasodilatation, which can lead to exacerbation of edema. Therefore, heat application must only be accomplished with the limb elevated.

Whirlpool baths are also helpful for facilitating mobilization of joints after prolonged cast immobilization. The patient should be instructed to perform active range of motion exercises and to avoid a static dependent position in the bath in order to minimize the development of edema. The temperature of the bath may also be lowered to decrease the likelihood of vasodilatation and subsequent swelling.

Paraffin baths (usually consisting of a 1:7 mixture of mineral oil and paraffin at 52–54° C) are useful for the treatment of hand contractures.[3]

Short-wave diathermy is a form of deep heat that uses radio waves to produce temperature elevations in subcutaneous tissue such as muscle and fat. It should never be used in patients with metal implants, since it can induce high temperatures in the metal with subsequent risk of injury to surrounding soft tissues.

Ultrasound can heat tissues to depths of 8 cm. Its application is useful for heating and thereby increasing the extensibility of collagen in the treatment of shortened joint capsules, ligaments, and muscle tendons.[3,29]

Massage

Retrograde massage is useful for reduction of edema,[23,24] particularly in the hand. It is carried out from the distal to proximal portion of the limb with the extremity in a gravity-eliminated position. Compressive elastic garments or tape (for example, Coban) may need to be applied in order to maintain the edema reduction achieved during therapy.

Deep friction massage has been used to decrease tendon and muscle belly adhesions in the hand.[26] Superficial massage parallel to the direction of muscle fibers has been reported to help decrease muscle spasm and to improve joint motion.[15,33] Scar tissue, which can limit skin elasticity and lend to adherence of gliding tendons, is responsive to massage that helps stretch collagen fibers.[11,26,33] Massage is contraindicated in the presence of open wounds, infected tissues, and thrombophlebitis.

Orthotics

The use of static and dynamic splints in upper extremity fractures is often critical to achievement of maximal functional recovery (chapter 2). A protective static splint can be used to maintain the specific joint position and can be sequentially altered to provide slow increases in joint range. Dynamic splints allow application of a low-load, extended-duration force to a joint to improve its range in a desired plane.[14] Dynamic splints also can be used to allow optimal joint positioning while providing for light resistive motion.

The concept of functional fracture bracing was first introduced approximately 20 years ago when Sarmiento showed that early mobilization circumvented many of the complications associated with protracted immobilization.[39,41] Functional bracing of the upper extremity reduces tendencies toward angular deformities and allows unrestricted use of other joints as the need for extensive casting is avoided. These braces are essentially cylindrical and made of a thermal-molded plastic such as polypropylene. They are used for supporting long-bone fractures in the upper extremity and have adjustable anterior and posterior interlocking shells. Velcro straps provide closure.

Sarmiento's work strongly suggests that the callus that forms in the presence of limited movement at fracture sites has superior mechanical characteristics and contributes to more rapid and enhanced fracture stability. Fracture bracing allows small amounts of movement at the fracture line, as compared to the more extensive immobilization of fragments that occurs in a standard cast.

When a functional brace is applied to a fracture, stresses can be applied prior to the achievement of bony union. This is advantageous, since both clinical and laboratory studies have revealed data supporting the hypothesis that controlled motion at the fracture site produces an environment that enhances osteogenesis.[28,38,40] Specific uses of functional bracing are discussed later in this chapter as they relate to particular fractures.

Therapeutic Exercise

An exercise program must focus on activities that are critical for independent function. Generally speaking, movements that reproduce the mechanism of injury and that increase the angle of the fracture deformity should not be emphasized. The exercise regimen will progress from having maximal therapist assistance to patient independence with resisted movement. Although range of motion and strength training necessarily occur concurrently, the initial phases of the exercise program emphasize maintenance and/or improvement of joint range. Later phases emphasize strength and endurance training.

Serial reevaluation of the patient for assessment of progress and adjustment to the exercise prescription must be completed. A prescription should include precautions (e.g., peripheral nerve lesions leading to sensory and/or motor deficits, presence of infection, or delayed union). Specifics regarding weightbearing status of the limb must be a part of the therapy prescription.

Exercise can be defined by the ratio of patient-to-therapist effort. Passive exercise implies no patient effort, with all of the work of joint movement being provided by the therapist. This type of exercise is primarily used to prevent joint stiffness or contractures in very weak or paralyzed limbs. Passive exercise may also be used as a warm-up prior to more active involvement by the patient. The therapist is responsible for adequate proximal stabilization of the limb to ensure that true joint movement is occurring at the joint in question and that there is no substitution by more proximal portions of the limb or at the fracture site.

Continuous passive motion (chapter 5) is a relatively new form of passive exercise that has been shown to decrease joint stiffness and facilitate articular cartilage regeneration.[10] In addition, studies indicate that production of synovial fluid may be increased and edema reduced.[9,35] Continuous passive motion devices are particularly useful in anxious patients, since the joint is consistently ranged through a preset and limited arc of motion that can be slowly increased to patient tolerance and in accordance with the goals of rehabilitation.[42]

Active assisted exercise involves activity from both the patient and therapist. Alternatively, assistance to the patient can be provided by gravity, by buoyancy of water, counterbalancing with weights, or with devices that decrease friction such as powder boards or skateboards.[18,20]

Active exercise is performed only by the patient. The therapist may be present to stabilize the proximal limb in order to minimize inappropriate muscular substitution and to ensure true movement through the joint in question.

Resistive exercise is performed with either the therapist or equipment providing resistance to the patient's independent muscle contraction. It is useful to initiate resistive exercises with the therapist providing manual resistance in order to ensure adequate limb positioning and appropriate muscle group involvement for the desired action. Patients in an independent program will often avoid uncomfortable muscle contractions or joint positions and substitute with pain-free and, frequently, incorrect movements.

Progressive resistance exercise should be initiated only after the patient is independently and correctly performing active exercises. Resistance can be provided isokinetically, isotonically, or isometrically.

SPECIFIC FRACTURES

Fractures of the Clavicle

Frequently caused by a fall on the shoulder, fractures of the clavicle also may be sustained from forces generated by falling on an outstretched hand. The most common site of injury is at the junction of the middle and outer thirds.[1,36]

Complete immobilization is not possible. Fractures that are either mildly displaced or undisplaced are treated with a simple collar and cuff sling applied to the ipsilateral upper extremity, primarily for patient comfort.

Most clavicular fractures are displaced, usually with the lateral fragment displaced medially and downward. Some clinicians recommend application of a figure eight bandage that facilitates shoulder retraction and minimizes the displacement. There are increasing concerns that the figure eight harness rarely achieves the goal of sustained fracture alignment. An incorrectly placed bandage that is too tight may impede venous return to the upper extremity or may even cause axillary nerve damage due to sustained pressure over the peripheral nerve.

Clavicular fractures have a high rate of union. Not infrequently, some bony irregularity is palpable at the fracture site. If cosmesis is a significant concern, surgical reshaping is an option. Occasionally, disruption of the adjacent acromioclavicular joint occurs due to persistent displacement of the fracture site, leading to chronic symptoms in the joint.

A sling should be worn no longer than 2 weeks to avoid secondary complications, in particular, glenohumeral capsule tightness. Active shoulder exercises should be started no later than 1 week after injury, with emphasis on abduction and external rotation. With removal of the sling, encouragement of bimanual performance of self-care tasks begins. Resistive upper extremity exercises should be introduced by 3 weeks, when bony union is well under way. Weights are increased as tolerated by the patient.

Fractures of the Scapula

Unlike fractures of the clavicle, fractures of the scapula are usually the result of a direct force or violence. There are four classifications: fractures of the body, fractures of the neck, fractures of the acromion, and fractures of the coracoid process.

Fractures of the body rarely display any significant displacement, even if comminution occurs, because of the extensive muscular attachment. A sling is frequently prescribed, primarily for the patient's comfort. However, as soon as acute symptoms subside, scapular mobilization and active exercises must be initiated to achieve full shoulder range.

Fractures of the neck may result in some downward displacement of the glenoid portion, but this is rarely significant. If, however, a medially displaced glenoid neck fracture accompanies a displaced clavicular fracture, the result is an unstable segment involving the lateral clavicle, acromion, and glenoid. In this case, plate fixation of the clavicle provides for a speedier functional recovery.[1,4] Rigid immobilization is not indicated and, as the patient's tolerance permits, active shoulder range of motion exercises must be implemented.

Minimally displaced fractures of the acromion process are treated with a sling and passive and active assistive exercises. No resisted deltoid contraction is recommended until after full bony union occurs.[4] If the fracture is significantly comminuted and/or displaced, surgical excision or fixation must be considered. Postoperatively, immobilization in a sling for about 3 weeks allows not only for fracture healing but for adequate muscle reattachment. Following removal of the sling, mobilization is begun to achieve full glenohumeral range and shoulder girdle strength.

Fractures of the coracoid process are of little clinical significance, even in the presence of marked downward and associated conjoined tendon or pectoralis minor muscle avulsion. No specific treatment is warranted for these fractures, and rehabilitation, again, focuses on regaining shoulder range and strength.

Fractures of the Humerus

There are six classes of humeral fractures: fractures of the greater tuberosity, fractures of the neck of the humerus, fractures of the shaft, supracondylar fractures, fractures of the condyles, and fractures of the epicondyles.

Fractures of the Greater Tuberosity of the Humerus

Fractures of the greater tuberosity of the humerus are usually the result of a direct fall on the shoulder. The majority are undisplaced, but some may be comminuted or even widely displaced from the humerus because of the action of the rotator cuff muscles whose common tendon inserts into the greater tuberosity. Treatment is dictated by the degree of displacement. In nondisplaced fractures, splinting is not necessary, and a therapy program progressing from passive to active ranging of the shoulder is all that is necessary.

A widely avulsed bony fragment represents a more challenging clinical problem. Closed reduction is dificult to maintain unless a bulky abduction or "airplane"' splint is devised. Surgical fixation is the usual remedy. Postoperatively, therapies emphasizing abduction and external rotation, along with improving shoulder strength, are provided.

In some patients, residual irregularity of the greater tuberosity can restrict glenohumeral abduction, which is caused by impingement against the acromion process, or coracoacromial ligament. Pain due to impingement occurs between 60–120° of abduction. The symptoms usually subside over time; however, persistent symptoms may warrant referral for surgical excision of the acromion.[1]

Fractures of the Neck of the Humerus

Fractures of the neck of the humerus most often occur after a fall on the limb with the arm in an adducted and internally rotated position. Fortunately, most humeral neck fractures are impacted, allowing for early mobilization and return to functional baseline.

Although radiographs identify the fracture, the clinical examination determines the presence of impaction. The patient should be in the supine position to allow relaxation of the shoulder girdle musculature and reduction of anxiety. The patient's elbow should be flexed. The examiner then palpates the head of the humerus with one hand while gently externally rotating the distal humerus with the other. The humeral head and distal fragment will move simultaneously if the fracture fragments are impacted.[33] Alternatively, the examiner will be able to passively abduct the extremity without significant discomfort to the patient. In nonimpacted fractures, any movement of the distal fragment, no matter how slight, is poorly tolerated.

If fracture fragments are not impacted, early active or even passive exercises are precluded. The arm can be supported in a Velpeau[4] sling or a collar and cuff sling. A swathe or body bandage can provide additional splinting. Active wrist and finger exercises are initiated immediately. Shoulder movement should be deferred for 2–3 weeks, at which time enough union has been initiated to allow active shoulder range without fear of affecting the rate of progression of bony healing.

The approach to treatment of a displaced fracture should acknowledge that even significant displacement is compatible with excellent functional outcome. Extensive immobilization following open or closed reduction is frequently plagued by persistent shoulder and elbow stiffness. The optimal acute treatment always allows the earliest possible shoulder mobilization.

In elderly patients, a considerably greater degree of displacement is tolerable. In younger patients, however, reduction is often accomplished under anesthesia and maintained in a shoulder spica or an abduction frame for 1 month. Surgical repair is indicated when reduction by manipulation is not possible and particularly when a fracture of the greater tuberosity is also present (a three-part fracture). Greater tuberosity fractures are usually displaced superiorly and posteriorly and are generally not amenable to closed reduction.

If the fracture is impacted, immobilization is not indicated and rehabilitation is started immediately. A sling may be provided between therapy sessions for support of the upper extremity.

A three-phase rehabilitation protocol developed by Hughes and Neer[18] for proximal humeral fractures is widely used. The system is highly adaptable and can be adjusted based on the anatomy of the fracture, the stability of the fracture, or presence of surgical repair.

The first phase comprises passive and active assistive exercises. The second phase encompasses active assistive, early resistive, and stretching exercises, and the third phase progresses to advanced stretching and strengthening exercises. Prior to beginning exercises, application of a hot pack may be beneficial to promote muscle relaxation and facilitate stretching.

In minimally displaced fractures, or those demonstrating a stable closed reduction, phase 1 is initiated 7–10 days after injury. This phase comprises passive and active assistive exercises. The first activity is a pendulum (Codman) exercise. The patient stands with the trunk flexed at the hips, with the involved arm hanging perpendicularly and forming a "pendulum." This position facilitates shoulder adductor and scapulothoracic muscle relaxation. The arm is rotated in small circles with the humerus in both internal and external rotation (palm facing inward and outward, respectively).

The second exercise facilitates shoulder external rotation using a stick. The patient lies supine with the involved arm supported and the shoulder abducted 15–20°. The uninvolved arm pushes the stick into the palm of the fractured extremity.

Approximately 3 weeks after injury, therapist-assisted shoulder flexion may be initiated along with pulley exercises. Shoulder extension exercises are introduced later. At 4 weeks, isometric exercises emphasizing internal and external rotation of the shoulder are also recommended.

If a stable surgical repair is achieved, phase 1 exercises may begin 24–48 hours postoperatively. Active assistive shoulder flexion, elbow flexion, and extension are introduced first, as well as instruction in pendulum exercises. Active supine external rotation is also performed. Three to five days after surgery, external rotation with a stick, supine forward flexion, and extension exercises are added. Resistive exercises in the form of isometrics are introduced after 3 weeks.

Phase 2 comprises active, resistive, and stretching exercises. The first exercise is active shoulder flexion (or elevation) performed supine. This position partially eliminates gravity and facilitates completion of the movement by the patient. As patient performance improves, progression to shoulder flexion in an erect position is made. Using a stick grasped in both hands provides some forward momentum for the affected arm. The patient should be cued to keep elbows flexed and pointed forward.

Resistive exercises are added to strengthen internal and external shoulder rotators as well as deltoids. Three sets of 10–15 repetitions are usually prescribed.

Stretching exercises in this phase include forward arm flexion to try to reach the top of a wall, raising arms with hands clasped overhead, and placing the hands behind the head to achieve shoulder abduction and external rotation. Internal rotation is assisted by clasping hands behind the back.

Phase 3 exercises are begun 3 months after injury for all fracture types. The intensity of resistive exercises is increased. Light weights are added, beginning at 1-pound weights and increasing in 1-pound increments up to 5 pounds. Persistent pain following use of weights is an indication for their reduction or discontinuation. Rubber tubing may be substituted for rubber strips to increase resistance for isometric exercises. Stretches in this phase include prone stretching with the shoulder in forward flexion and leaning into a wall or door after shoulder flexion to achieve end flexion range.

Humeral neck fractures may be accompanied by an axillary nerve injury. The patient will demonstrate decreased deltoid muscle contraction and anesthesia over the area of the deltoid. Assessment and treatment of this condition are discussed in chapter 3.

Fractures of the Shaft of the Humerus

Humeral fractures can be the result of direct trauma resulting in transverse, short, oblique, or comminuted fractures. They can also be the result of a twisting force that leads to a spiral fracture. The shaft is most frequently fractured in the middle third. Pathologic fractures due to metastatic disease often occur in the proximal half of the humerus.

The degree of displacement varies; however, fragment contact over at least one quarter of the area is enough for adequate fracture healing.

Closed reduction may be necessary because of significant displacement of fragments. A cyndrical cast from shoulder to just distal to the flexed elbow with a simple sling for extremity support is a common form of immobilization. Active wrist and finger range of motion exercises should be started immediately. Seven to ten days after injury, shoulder mobilization as described by Hughes and Neer[18] can be initiated.

Zagorski et al.[49] at the University of Miami have developed a functional bracing protocol that comprises (1) alignment of the fracture, (2) application of the prefabricated device over cast padding, and (3) application of the sling on the initial injury.

The patient is reevaluated 24 hours after injury for a neurovascular status check. One week later, pendulum exercises, passive flexion of the shoulder, and active elbow, wrist, and finger exercises are begun. They allow removal of the brace for attendance to personal hygiene only. Patients are seen for follow-up 2 weeks after the fracture and then at 3- to 4-week intervals for clinical and radiographic checks. When adequate bony healing is confirmed, use of the brace is discontinued. Because significant distal edema is sometimes associated with functional brace use, scrupulous attention to arm elevation and encouragement of active hand movement is recommended.

In the event of unstable fracture fragments or a pathologic fracture, more rigid immobilization is necessary. If closed reduction is possible, a shoulder spica can be used to maintain adequate alignment.[1] The cast encloses the trunk and entire upper extremity except for the fingers, with the shoulder held semiabducted and the elbow flexed to 90°.

A less cumbersome alternative is internal fixation by means of a metal plate and screws or an intramedullary nail. The latter is generally inserted inferiorly from just above the olecranon fossa. A more superior approach through the greater tuberosity can hamper shoulder movement.

Contaminated, open, or infected humeral shaft fractures are treated with external fixation. Twin threaded pins are inserted percutaneously through each fragment and held externally by a metal bar, clamps, or cement.

Humeral shaft fractures are frequently associated with radial nerve injury. A discrete area of sensory deficit over the dorsal web space between the thumb and index finger, along with weakness or paralysis of the thumb, finger, and wrist extensors is characteristic. Most clinicians recommend observation, because the vast majority of radial palsies resolve.[21] Any deficit noted after the initial injury (for example, symptoms noted only after manipulation or surgery) is of greater concern and warrants closer and more immediate evaluation. If significant paralysis of radial innervated muscles exists, splinting will be necessary to maintain wrist and finger range and to avoid wrist and finger flexion contractures. A wrist cock-up splint may be used alone or in conjunction with an outrigger for providing thumb and finger extension.

Supracondylar Fractures

Supracondylar fractures usually are the result of a fall onto an outstretched hand. They are infrequently seen in adults but represent one of the more common fractures in children. If displacement occurs, it is nearly always with the distal fragment displaced backward.

Brachial artery damage is a prominent complication of this type of fracture. Close monitoring of the circulation of the forearm is critical. Casts should be cut away to allow monitoring of the radial pulse. Signs of impending circulatory compromise, such as pain in the forearm particularly on passive finger extension, or the patient's inability to fully extend fingers is worrisome.

In severe cases of arterial occlusion or injury, gangrene of the digits ensues. When significant ischemia is present, some hand viability is spared because of blood passing into the collateral circulation. Flexor muscles of the forearm and hand are often irreversibly damaged as a result. Muscle fibrosis and shortening occurs, leading to wrist and finger flexion contractures. This condition is known as a Volkmann's contracture.

Treatment in the incipient stage is emergent and aims to alleviate the arterial occlusion. Any immobilization device that may be constricting the extremity is removed and superficial heat applied to promote vasodilatation. If no results are noted in 30 minutes, surgical exploration is indicated. If untreated, a contracted wrist and claw hand will result. Rehabilitative efforts are directed toward passive range of motion and appropriate splinting to counter these deformities. Heat applied to the hand prior to ranging will facilitate improved range of motion but must be used with caution in insensate extremities.

Median and ulnar neuropathies may also be associated with a supracondylar fracture but much less frequently. The development of a claw hand with hyperextended metacarpophalangeal joints and an abducted and extended thumb is characteristic. Passive ranging is critical to avoid shortening of the extrinsic finger flexors and extensors. A dynamic splint may be fabricated to maintain interphalangeal joint extension in the fingers.

Initial treatment of supracondylar fractures is in the form of immobilization for undisplaced fractures and displaced fractures following reduction. Cast placement is usually prescribed for approximately 3 weeks. Active assistive and active range of motion exercises for shoulder, wrist, and fingers begin immediately. After cast removal, active and active assistive exercises emphasizing elbow extension, wrist supination, and pronation are added. Progression to light resistive activity can occur within a week.

Fractures of the Humeral Condyle

Fractures of the humeral condyle are relatively uncommon in the general population but are more frequently seen in children. Condylar fractures are often the result of a fall, and the lateral condyle appears to be more prone to fracture.

Displacement is usually minor but critical, since these fractures involve the joint surface. Undisplaced fractures are treated with immobilization for 3–4 weeks, followed by the rehabilitation protocol described for supracondylar fractures. Displaced fractures must be reduced either by manipulation or with surgical fixation. Persistence of the displacement can result in a significant disability. These fractures have a relatively high incidence of nonunion, which can result in deformity and development of osteoarthritis.

Fractures of the Epicondyle

Like condylar fractures, epicondylar fractures are also more common in children. The medial epicondyle is fractured more often than the others. Displacement is rarely of clinical significance, and treatment is with cast immobilization for 3 weeks followed by elbow exercises as described previously. If the fracture fragment is widely displaced or enters the elbow joint, surgical reattachment is indicated. Ulnar nerve damage may occur, particularly in a displaced medial epicondylar fracture. Surgical transposition of the nerve anterior to the elbow is a consideration.

Fractures of the Olecranon Process

There are three types of olecranon fractures: undisplaced, displaced, and comminuted. Treatment, as always, is decided by fracture type. Undisplaced fractures are simply immobilized, preferably with the elbow flexed to 90°.[1] The surrounding aponeurosis holds the fragments in place and the flexed elbow allows for a more functional hand position.

Displaced fractures are not amenable to closed reduction. Because the action of the triceps maintains angulation of the proximal fracture fragment, fixation is achieved by means of a screw or tension wires. Postoperatively, cast immobilization for up to 3 weeks is considered if there is any question about the stability of the fracture.

Comminuted fractures are usually treated either with attempts at closed surgical fixation or, in the presence of very small fragments, with excision of the fracture fragments. The triceps is sutured to the most proximal portion of the residual ulna. The elbow is subsequently immobilized for 3 weeks.

During the immobilization of the elbow, active shoulder and hand exercises are performed. After cast removal, active assistive elbow exercises emphasizing extension, supination, and pronation are practiced.[17] If recovery of elbow range is delayed, dynamic splinting may be added to the treatment regimen. Continuous passive motion also has been successfully used.[6,44]

Fractures of the Radius

Fractures of the radius usually occur after falling on an outstretched hand and are common upper extremity fractures in young adults. The fracture often is a simple crack without any displacement. Significant comminution and depression of the radial head can occur.

The diagnosis of this type of fracture is often overlooked, since radiographic findings may be easily missed. If the characteristic fall is described and examination reveals a discrete area of pain on palpation of the radial head, or pain at the lateral joint on end supination or pronation, a fracture should be considered. If radiographs are nonconfirmatory, they should be repeated with the radius at varying degrees of rotation.

If a small nondisplaced fracture is present, a cast is applied with the elbow flexed and the forearm in supination, or no more than neutral rotation. Immobilization lasts for at least 3 weeks with an exercise prescription identical to that described for olecranon fractures.

In the presence of a comminuted radial head fracture with implied damage to the articular surface, surgical excision is the treatment of choice. Again, cast immobilization for 2 weeks follows the surgery. Active elbow exercises previously described are initiated after cast removal.

Elbow joint stiffness for a protracted time following the injury is not uncommon. It is important to note that the elbow tolerates manipulation or even forceful passive range of motion poorly. These maneuvers are associated with a high incidence of heterotopic ossification formation and resulting bony ankylosis. The majority of patients improve with persistent adherence to the active exercise regimen.

Fractures of the Shaft of the Radius with Ulnar Dislocation

Fractures of the shaft of the radius with ulnar dislocation are also called Galeazzi fracture dislocations for Ricardo Galeazzi, who first fully described the injury in 1935. As with many other upper extremity fractures, they are frequently caused by a fall onto the outstretched upper extremity. The radius is most frequently fractured at the junction of its middle and distal thirds. The inferior radial ulnar ligament is ruptured and the head of the ulna displaced from its articulation with the radius.

Meticulous reduction is critical for full functional restoration, and this can rarely be achieved and maintained by closed methods. Surgical fixation by means of a metal plate and screws is the preferred intervention. A full-length arm cast extending from the axilla to midpalm is applied postoperatively with the elbow in flexion.

Active movement of proximal and distal joints is also encouraged, with a protocol to improve active elbow flexion added after cast removal.

Fractures of the Distal Radius

Also called a Colles' fracture, fractures of the distal radius are one of the most common fractures of the upper extremity. The fracture characteristically occurs within 2 cm of the articular surface. Most of these fractures are accompanied by significant displacement. The distal fragment is frequently displaced dorsally, resulting in the characteristic "dinner fork" deformity of the wrist.

Treatment usually comprises manipulation under anesthesia with subsequent immobilization in a forearm cast. Since there is a small but sizable risk of loss of reduction after cast placement, it is recommended that radiographs be performed weekly for 2–3 weeks to monitor alignment.

Some surgeons use the standard circumferential cast while others use a dorsal splint that is maintained in position by means of bandages. The theoretical advantage of the latter is ease of removal if significant swelling should occur.

The cast should leave the first metacarpophalangeal joint free and should not extend past the proximal palmar crease. Active range of motion exercises for fingers, elbow, and shoulder should begin immediately. One center[8] uses a "six-pack" of hand exercises that facilitate maintenance of hand range of motion:

1. Maximal active extension of all digits
2. Touch thumb to each fingertip
3. Maximal flexion of all fingers (to the proximal palmar crease if possible
4. Maximal flexion of distal interphalangeal and proximal interphalangeal joints with metacarpophalangeal joints extended
5. Maximal flexion of the metacarpophalangeal joint with the distal interphalangeal joints and proximal interphalangeal joints extended
6. Abduction and adduction of all digits

When the cast is removed, massage for edema reduction and passive and active exercises for all digits are provided. The patient is instructed in a program to improve wrist flexion and extension and forearm supination and pronation. The exercise regimen also must include exercises to maintain shoulder and elbow range of motion and strength.

Rupture of the extensor pollicis longus tendon can accompany distal radial fractures. The muscle tendon courses over the radius, gliding backward and forward with extension of the thumb. There is generally fraying of the tendon that progresses to a complete tear 4–8 weeks after injury. There appears to be no relationship between the severity of the fracture and the incidence of tendon rupture.

The patient may not always be aware of any deficits. Examination reveals weak metacarpophalangeal joint extension and absent interphalangeal extension. Since the tendon ends are usually shredded, tendon transfer (frequently from the extensor indicis) is preferable to attempting end-to-end anastomosis.

Median neuropathy at the wrist also can occur. This may be due to significant tension on the nerve caused by hyperextension of the wrist at the time of injury. It may also represent compression secondary to edema rather than direct trauma. Evaluation and treatment of median neuropraxia are discussed in chapter 3.

Less commonly, the distal fracture fragment is displaced volarly. This presentation is also called a Smith's fracture, Barton's fracture, or reverse Colles' fracture. In this instance, the fracture is prone to displacement after initial manual reduction. If weekly radiograph checks confirm loss of alignment, surgical fixation with metal plate and screws is recommended.[1,8]

Fractures of the Shaft of the Radius and/or Ulna

Fractures of the radius, ulna, or both are prone to significant displacement. Undisplaced fractures can be treated with immobilization in a long-arm cast with good results. Unfortunately, a satisfactory outcome with conservative therapy is unlikely in the presence of displaced fractures.[16,17,22]

If initial closed reduction is successful, check radiographs are performed weekly. If the reduction cannot be maintained, surgical fixation either via plate and screws or intramedullary nailing is pursued.

Zagorski et al.[49] have reported use of functional bracing in isolated ulnar shaft fractures. They recommend closed reduction if the fracture has less than 10° of angulation, followed by placement of a long-arm cast. Check radiographs are performed after 2 weeks. If alignment is satisfactory, a fracture brace similar to that described in the treatment of humeral fractures is applied instead of the cast. Radiographs are followed to monitor maintenance of reduction. The patient is instructed in active range of motion exercises for all proximal and distal joints. The brace is removed only for purposes of hygiene.

The role of functional bracing in isolated radial shaft fractures is much more limited. Most radial fractures occur distally with an associated derangement of the radial ulnar articulation that frequently necessitates surgical intervention.

While the arm is immobilized, the patient must be instructed in appropriate positioning of the extremity. Dependent positions that exacerbate edema must be avoided. Active wrist and finger flexion and extension should be performed several times daily. When immobilization is discontinued, rehabilitation again focuses on increasing forearm rotation and strength. Exercises should be performed on a firm surface and the patient carefully supervised to avoid inappropriate muscle substitution.

Proximal Ulnar Shaft Fractures and Radial Dislocation

Proximal ulnar shaft fractures and radial dislocation are also called Monteggia fracture dislocations. This injury is often sustained when the arm is raised to ward off a blow. Examination will reveal marked tenderness in the elbow region. The patient will usually resist any attempted passive elbow flexion, elbow extension, or forearm pronation or supination. There is frequently an anterior angulation of the ulna and anterior dislocation of the radius. Although there is no uniformity of thinking regarding surgical treatment, many surgeons opt for open reduction of the ulnar fracture and closed reduction of the radial dislocation via wrist supination.[1,8] The arm is then casted postoperatively and the wrist supination maintained for 6–8 weeks. Following cast removal, active elbow and wrist exercises are begun as described above.

Fractures of the Scaphoid

Fractures of the scaphoid represent the most common fractures of the carpal bones.[12,45] They are usually caused by a fall on an outstretched hand with the wrist hyperextended and ulnarly deviated.[7,37] Diagnosis can be difficult since pain and swelling are usually not significant and initial radiographs may be negative.[1,25]

Suspicions should be raised when examination reveals discrete tenderness in the region of the anatomic snuff box, formed by the abductor pollicis longus and extensor pollicis brevis tendons. Radiographic examination should include oblique views. When symptoms are consistent with a scaphoid fracture but x-rays are negative, as is common, the wrist should be casted and films repeated in 2 weeks since a fracture may not become immediately apparent. Technetium bone scans, poly-tomography, and MRI may also be useful for providing confirmatory evidence.[8]

Immediate immobilization is critical, since delayed diagnosis is associated with an increased incidence of nonunion.[13] Fracture fragments are usually not displaced, and the treatment of choice is placement of a cast until radiographic union occurs—usually in 2–3 months. The cast should encompass the first metacarpal and proximal phalanx of the thumb, leaving the distal phalanx free. The portion surrounding the hand should not extend past the proximal palmar crease. Displaced fractures can be treated with immobilization alone if the fragments can be reduced and alignment maintained. Otherwise, surgical fixation via pin fixation or compression screws should be considered.

Scaphoid fractures have a high rate of malunion, progression to avascular necrosis, and development of posttraumatic arthritis.[13,25] Treatment should be guided by the degree of functional impairment present in the face of these complications. In fractures with delayed union (approximately 4 months after the injury), if mobilization does not result in exacerbation of wrist symptoms, no further treatment is generally warranted. Persistent discomfort or decreased wrist function may require compression screw placement and bone grafting.[8,13]

Pulsed electromagnetic stimulation (PEMS) has been suggested for use in undisplaced fractures with delayed union.[2,5] Radioisotope scanning assists with the diagnosis of avascular necrosis. Excision of the dead fragment is usually advised. During immobilization, active range of motion exercises of all proximal and distal joints should be encouraged. The set of six hand exercises previously described is useful.

Following cast removal, the common deficits are usually decreased wrist flexion and extension, although decreased supination may be present. The patient is instructed in rotation exercises of the forearm. The patient sits with the forearm resting on a surface such that the elbow is flexed to 90°. With the upper arm held in an adducted position, the hand is rotated into alternate positions of supination and pronation. Active wrist flexion and extension exercises are performed with the patient's forearm resting on the edge of the table. The wrist hangs free, and the forearm is stabilized by the opposite hand. Active wrist flexion and extension can then be performed.

Fractures of the Metacarpals

Fractures of the metacarpals often result from a dorsal crush injury to the hand and are sustained after direct violence, such as in boxing. The fractures are classified according to site:

1. Fractures through the base at the proximal end
2. Fractures through the shaft, which may be transverse or oblique
3. Fractures through the neck of the metacarpal at the distal end

Undisplaced fractures may require only a dorsal splint for 2–4 weeks. Displaced fractures must be reduced and alignment maintained, either by closed reduction and splinting, or by surgical fixation. Malrotation and shortening of metacarpal fracture fragments can be an associated finding. Shortening can still allow full functional return; however, metacarpal rotation of only 5–10° can result in significant overlapping of the fingers and a less than cosmetic result.

Metacarpophalangeal joints are susceptible to extension contractures, and interphalangeal joints are prone to stiffening quickly in flexion. Immobilization is best accomplished with the metacarpophalangeal joints at approximately 70–90° of flexion and with the interphalangeal joints in close to full extension.

Because these fractures are frequently associated with a dorsal injury involving the soft tissues, significant edema in this area is to be expected. Commonly, adherence of extensor tendons and stiffness of the metacarpophalangeal joints in extension complicate the rehabilitation.

Active hand movement should be started by the third week following injury or as soon as tolerated by the patient. Movements must include specific tendon gliding of the flexor digitorum superficialis, extensor digitorum communis, extensor indicis, and extensor digiti quinti, as well as tendons of the intrinsic muscles.

Goals of therapy are to prevent adhesions between bones, tendons, and skin, increase circulation, decrease swelling, and promote compression at the fracture site.[27]

Wehbe and Hunter[46,47,48] have described three exercises that facilitate this selective tendon gliding:

Claw Fist.   Flexion of the distal interphalangeal (DIP) and proximal interphalangeal (PIP) joints occurs, with the metacarpophalangeal joints (MCP) in extension. This action causes the flexor digitorum profundus tendon to move over bone.

Sublimus Fist.   Flexion of MCP and PIP joints occurs, with DIP joints in extension. This allows the flexor digitorum superficialis to glide over the stationary flexor digitorum profundus tendon.

Full Fist.   Flexion of MCP, PIP, and DIP joints together allow gliding of the flexor digitorum superficialis and flexor digitorum communis tendons over each other.

In addition, extensor digit quinti (EDQ) and extensor indicis tendons glide when the second and fourth digits extend fully. The extensor digitorum communis tendon glides when the MCP joints are extended as the interphalangeal joints are flexed.

Resistance exercises can be introduced 4 weeks following injury in most metacarpal fractures. By this time, there should be some radiographic evidence of bony union. In fractures following surgical fixation, resistive exercises are begun only after removal of pins.

Fractures of the Phalanges

Fractures of the phalanges can result from crush injuries to the finger. Fracture types include: comminuted fractures, transverse fractures of the shaft, spiral fractures of the shaft, and oblique fractures of the base. Since interphalangeal joint fractures are very susceptible to flexion contractures, immobilization should be kept to a minimum.

Undisplaced fractures of the phalangeal shaft can be lightly taped to an adjacent finger for support.[19,42] Displaced fractures should be easily reduced by manipulation and immobilized for no more than 3 weeks in a simple splint. If reduction cannot be maintained, Kirschner wires are used for fixation.

Comminuted distal phalangeal fractures are often associated with significant soft tissue injury. The nail bed and pulp injuries should be primarily addressed since no specific treatment is needed for the bony injury.

Therapy follows the same pattern described for metacarpophalangeal joint fractures. The collateral ligaments of the proximal interphalangeal joints are maximally extended with the joints in extension. Full interphalangeal joint range is facilitated by dragging the involved finger through putty on a flat surface, thereby passively extending the joint.

Continuous passive motion is a useful adjunct to range of motion exercises, and dynamic splinting can also be used to improve passive extension and also light resistive finger flexion.

CONCLUSION

There are myriad modalities, equipment, and exercise regimens that can contribute to improving joint range and extremity strength. However, if successful fracture rehabilitation is to occur, it is imperative that the patient be provided with a treatment plan that allows achievement of maximum function in his or her own environment and throughout every stage of recovery from the initial injury.

REFERENCES

1. Adams JC, Hamblen DL: Outline of Fractures. 10th ed. New York, Churchill Livingstone, 1992.
2. Ahl T, Andersson G, Herberts P, et al: Electrical treatment of non-united fractures. Acta Orthop Scand 55:585–588, 1984.
3. Basford JR: Physical agents and biofeedback. In DeLisa J (ed): Rehabilitation Medicine: Principles and Practice. Philadelphia, JB Lippincott, 1988, pp 257–264.
4. Bigliani LU, Craig EV, Butters KP: Fractures of the shoulder. In Rockwood CA, Green DP, Bucholz R (eds): Rockwood and Green's Fractures in Adults. 3rd ed. Philadelphia, JB Lippincott, 1991.
5. Bora FW, Osterman AL, Brighton CT: The electrical treatment of scaphoid non-union. Clin Orthop 161:33–38, 1981.
6. Breen TF, Gelberman RH, Ackerman GN: Elbow flexion contractures: Treatment by anterior release and continuous passive motion. J Hand Surg 13B:286–287, 1988.
7. Bryan RS, Dobyns JH: Fractures of the carpal bones other than lunate and navicular. Clin Orthop 149:107–111, 1980.
8. Cooney WP, Linscheid RL, Dobyns JH: Fractures and dislocations of the wrist. In Rockwood CA, Green DP, Bucholz R (eds): Rockwood and Green's Fractures in Adults. 3rd ed. Philadelphia, JB Lippincott, 1991, pp 563–678.
9. Coutts RD: Continuous passive motion in the rehabilitation of the total knee patient: Its role and effect. Orthop Rev 15:126–134, 1986.
10. Coutts RD, Kaita JH, Barr R, et al: The role of continuous passive motion in the post operative rehabilitation of the total knee patient. Orthop Trans 6:277–278, 1982.
11. Cyriax J: Textbook of Orthopaedic Medicine. 7th ed. London, Cassell, 1979.
12. Dobyns JH, Beckenbaugh RD, Bryan RS, et al: Fractures of the hand and wrist. In Flynn JE (ed): Hand Surgery. 3rd ed. Baltimore, Williams & Wilkins, 1982, pp 111–180.
13. Eddeland A, Eiken O, Hellgren E, et al: Fractures of the scaphoid. Scand J Plast Reconstr Surg 9:234–239, 1975.
14. Fess EE, Gettle KS, Strickland JW: Hand Splinting: Principles and Methods. St. Louis, Mosby, 1981.
15. Geiringer SR, Kincaid CB, Rechtien JJ: Traction, manipulation and massage. In DeLisa J (ed): Rehabilitation Medicine: Principles and Practice. Philadelphia, JB Lippincott, 1988.
16. Horne G: Supracondylar fractures of the humerus in adults. J Trauma 20:71–74, 1980.
17. Hotchkiss N, Green DP: Fractures and dislocations of the elbow. In Rockwood CA, Green DP, Bucholz R (eds): Rockwood and Green's Fractures in Adults. 3rd ed. Philadelphia, JB Lippincott, 1991.
18. Hughes M, Neer CS: Glenohumeral joint replacement and post operative rehabilitation. Phys Ther 55:850–858, 1975.
19. James JIP: Fractures of the proximal and middle phalanges of the fingers. Acta Orthop Scand 32:401–412, 1962.
20. Joynt RL: Therapeutic exercise. In DeLisa J (ed): Rehabilitation Medicine: Principles and Practice. Philadelphia, JB Lippincott, 1988.
21. Kettlekamp DB, Alexander H: Clinical review of radial nerve injury. J Trauma 7:424–432, 1967.
21a. Keith RA, Granger CV, Hamilton BB, Sherwin FS: The Functional Independence Measure: A new tool for rehabilitation. In Eisenberg MG, Grzesiak RC (eds): Advances in Clinical Rehabilitation. New York, Springer-Verlag, 1987, pp 6–18.

22. King D, Secor C: Bow elbow (cubitus varus). J Bone Joint Surg 33A:572–576, 1951.
23. Knapp ME: Treatment of fracture sequelae. Lancet (79):106–112, 1959.
24. Knapp ME: Aftercare of fractures. In Kottke FJ, Lehmann JF (eds): Krusen's Handbook of Physical Medicine and Rehabilitation Medicine. 4th ed. Philadelphia, WB Saunders, 1990.
25. Koman LA, Mooney JF, Poehling GG: Fractures and ligamentous injuries of the wrist. Hand Clin 6:477–491, 1990.
26. Lane C: Therapy for the occupationally injured hand. Hand Clin 2:593–602, 1986.
27. Lanyon LE, Robin CT: Static versus dynamic loads: An influence on bone remodeling. J Biomech 17:897–905, 1984.
28. Latta LL, Sarmiento A: Periosteal Fracture Callus Mechanics. St. Louis, Mosby, 1981.
29. Lehmann JF, Masock AJ, Warren CG, et al: Effect of therapeutic temperatures on tendon extensibility. Arch Phys Med Rehabil 51:481–487, 1970.
30. Lehmann JF, Silverman DR, Baum BR, et al: Temperature distributions in the human thigh, produced by infrared, hot pack and microwave applications. Arch Phys Med Rehabil 40:510–512, 1959.
31. Mahoney FI, Barthel DW: Functional evaluation: Barthel Index. Md Med J 14:61–65, 1965.
32. Moskowitz E: PULSES profile in retrospect. Arch Phys Med Rehabil 66:647, 1985.
33. Moskowitz E: Rehabilitation in Extremity Fractures. Springfield, IL, Charles C Thomas, 1968.
34. Moskowitz E, McCann CB: Classification of disability in chronically ill and aging. J Chronic Dis 5:342–346, 1957.
35. O'Driscol SW, Kumar A, Salter RB: The effect of continuous passive motion on the clearing of a hemarthrosis. Clin Orthop 176:305–311, 1983.
36. Reid DC: Sports Injury Assessment and Rehabilitation. New York, Churchill Livingstone, 1992.
37. Reister JN, Baker BE, Mosher JF, et al: A review of scaphoid fracture healing in competitive athletes. Am J Sports Med 13:159–161, 1985.
38. Sarmiento A: Functional fracture bracing: An update. Instr Course Lect 36:371–376, 1987.
39. Sarmiento A: A functional below-the-knee brace for tibial fractures. J Bone Joint Surg 49A:855, 1967.
40. Sarmiento A, Mullis DL, Latta LL, et al: A quantitative comparative analysis of fracture bracing under the influence of compression plating versus closed weightbearing treatment. Clin Orthop 149:232–239, 1980.
41. Sarmiento A, Schaeffer JF, Beckerman L, et al: Fracture healing in rat femora as affected by functional weightbearing. J Bone Joint Surg 59A:369–375, 1977.
42. Saunders SR: Physical therapy management of hand fractures. Phys Ther 69:1065–1076, 1989.
43. Sternbach RA: Psychological aspects of chronic pain. Clin Orthop 129:150–155, 1977.
44. Urbaniak JF, Hansen PE, Beissinger SF, et al: Correction of post traumatic flexion contracture of the elbow by anterior capsulotomy. J Bone Joint Surg 67A:1160–1164, 1985.
45. Verdan C: Fractures of the scaphoid. Surg Clin North Am 40:461–464, 1960.
46. Wehbe MA: Tendon gliding exercises. Am J Occup Ther 41:164–167, 1987.
47. Wehbe MA, Hunter JM: Flexor tendon gliding in the hand: Part I. In vivo excursions. J Hand Surg 10A:570–574, 1985.
48. Wehbe MA, Hunter JM: Flexor tendon gliding in the hand: Part II. Differential gliding. J Hand Surg 10A:575–579, 1985.
49. Zagorski JB, Zych GA, Latta LL, et al: Modern concepts in functional fracture bracing: The upper limb. Instr Course Lect 36:377–401, 1987.

ROBERT S. ZUCKER, MD, MPH

REHABILITATION OF FRACTURES OF THE LOWER EXTREMITY

From the Physical Medicine
and Rehabilitation Service
Department of Veterans Affairs
Outpatient Clinic
and
Department of Physical Medicine
and Rehabilitation
The Ohio State University
Columbus, Ohio

The comprehensive rehabilitation program for specific lower extremity fractures should include those aspects pertinent to fracture rehabilitation in general, such as reduction of the fracture to near-anatomic alignment, stabilization, active motion of uninvolved and nonimmobilized joints, restoration of range of motion and strength after remobilization,[39] and gait training with progressive weightbearing (WB). Muscle strengthening is important not only for functional restoration, but the stresses it provides also stimulate healing at the fracture site. Early joint mobilization has been shown experimentally to produce more efficient repair of soft tissue.[17] Gait training with an appropriate assistive device helps to prevent the problems of recumbency, particularly in the elderly. WB stress increases both the rate and quality of fracture healing.[28] It also helps to maintain bone mass in the remainder of the injured extremity.[13]

WB should only be allowed to the extent that the stability of the fracture is able to withstand it. Nonweightbearing (NWB) is usually advised initially for intraarticular fractures such as tibial plateau and femoral condylar fractures, because WB may displace articular surfaces resulting in joint incongruity. NWB is also recommended initially for unstable fractures. It should be kept in mind, however, that NWB status is essentially impossible for elderly patients to maintain.[69]

In practice, "full" WB is the same as WB "as tolerated." It is used later in the rehabilitation of unstable fractures as stability is achieved. Stability can be judged by evidence of fracture callus on radiography, or it may be judged arbitrarily based on the anticipated healing rate for the bone involved, in cases of fracture treatment with internal fixation where there may be no external callus. Partial WB (also termed *protected* WB) is recommended for fractures somewhere along the continuum from unstable to stable. *Partial* is preferred as a designation of WB status (rather than the percent) because in practice no injured individual can actually adhere to any specific recommendation. In deciding whether non, partial, or full weightbearing is to be recommended in a particular case, the quality of the preinjury bone stock, the stage of healing (as assessed by both time since injury and radiographic appearance), the weight of the patient, the site of the fracture, and the type of fixation all should be taken into account.

FEMORAL SHAFT FRACTURES

Since the femur is the longest, strongest bone in the body, the force required for fracture is of high energy, such as auto-pedestrian accidents and gunshot wounds. Femoral shaft fractures can rarely be held in reduction by plaster casting. The large powerful muscles surrounding the femur exert angulatory forces on the fragments that lead to displacement and malposition. The muscle envelope also provides an ideally vascular environment for fracture healing; delayed union is rarely a problem. Internal fixation with medullary nailing in an open procedure is the most common surgical treatment for these fractures.[59] Quadriceps- and hamstring-setting exercises should be practiced as soon as possible postoperatively.[44] These exercises maintain muscle tone and strength, thereby compressing the fracture, preventing distraction, and possibly stimulating local vascularity and subsequently union. Active range of motion exercises are also encouraged so that normal ROM can be regained in 4–6 weeks. Gait training with "touch-down" (just barely greater than non-) WB is begun as the patient obtains muscular control of the limb. After about 4–6 weeks, early callus is seen on radiography. Partial WB is then begun, with progression to full WB as early as after 12 weeks. The nail is surgically removed after 1–2 years.

DISTAL FEMORAL FRACTURES

Distal femoral fractures may be treated operatively or nonoperatively. Nonoperative treatment typically consists of skeletal traction for days to 2–3 weeks to obtain and maintain reduction and allow early callus formation. A cast brace is then applied. The classification scheme of Muller et al.[3] is useful. Type A fractures are supracondylar, type B are fractures of one condyle or the other, and type C are intercondylar, with at least three fracture fragments. The recommendations for operative treatment appear to be strongest for type C fractures and the least strong for type A fractures.[19,38,57,65] One retrospective series of operatively treated supracondylar fractures showed significant complications in a majority of the patients; only a minority achieved preinjury ambulatory status.[40] However, a comparative retrospective study showed much better functional outcomes, in general, for open fixation versus closed.[24] Because the surgeries for type C fractures are significantly more difficult and prone to complications, closed treatment may be favored in cases in which anatomic reduction may not be obtained or in which fixation may not be sufficient to allow early ROM of the knee. Open fixation typically involves the use of screws for type B fractures, plate and screws for type C, and, for supracondylar fractures, the Zickel supracondylar device,[69] consisting of two curved medullary rods. The rods are flexible proximally and more rigid at the condylar ends, with tunnels for screw insertion at the condylar ends (Fig. 1).

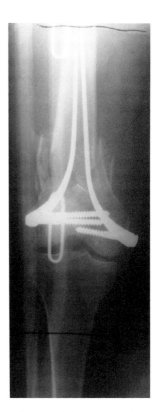

FIGURE 1. The Zickel supracondylar internal fixation device. A third compression screw is used to secure a condylar fracture. (From Zickel RE, Hobeika P, Robbins DS: Zickel supracondylar nails for fractures of the distal end of femur. Clin Orthop 212:79–88, 1986; with permission.)

Following operative treatment of condylar fractures, isometric knee exercises and use of a continuous passive motion (CPM) machine are begun immediately after surgery. The effectiveness of CPM in reducing posttraumatic joint stiffness following stabilization of intraarticular fractures has been demonstrated in animals.[43,51] Active and active-assisted ROM exercises are begun after 3–10 days, depending on soft tissue healing and reduction of swelling. A posterior splint is applied postoperatively and worn for 2 weeks. NWB gait training is begun at 4–10 days. The rapidity of progression of WB is determined by the stability of the fixation intraoperatively. Generally, progression to partial WB is accomplished at 8–10 weeks, then WB as tolerated at about 12 weeks. After operative fixation of intercondylar fractures, the lower limb is initially immobilized for 4–5 days at 90° flexion at the hip and knee before active motion is allowed. NWB gait training is begun at 2 weeks, with an increase to partial WB at 10–12 weeks. Following supracondylar fixation, ROM exercises are begun within a few days of surgery. If angulatory and rotatory forces are adequately controlled, gait training with touchdown WB is begun with progressive WB to pain tolerance and as radiographic evidence of healing is apparent.

PATELLAR FRACTURES

Patellar fractures may be classified as displaced or nondisplaced and as transverse, vertical, oblique, or comminuted. Transverse fractures, which represent the largest category, result from indirect force exerted violently through the patella-quadriceps mechanism. Comminuted fractures are more likely from direct trauma such as the knee striking an automobile dashboard. Nonoperative treatment has been recommended when there is less than 3 mm of displacement of fragments and less than 2 mm of articular surface incongruity.[4] The arguments against patellectomy are numerous: The mechanical advantage of the increased effective radius from the center of rotation of the knee is lost, resulting in less power in knee extension; quadriceps atrophy is more permanent; and the anatomic protection of the knee by the patella is lost. A comparative study of results following patellectomy versus internal fixation clearly favored internal fixation.[35] If the fracture is comminuted, the fragments are removed, but the largest fragment is preserved. Various methods of internal fixation of transverse patellar fractures have been described.[64]

Following circumferential wire loop fixation, rigid fixation is not achieved, so knee motion must be delayed for 3–4 weeks. The knee is immobilized by posterior splint or cylindrical cast. Quad-sets and straight-leg raises are encouraged as soon as possible after surgery. Gait training is begun when the patient can control the limb. WB may begin after cast removal.

Tension band wire fixation allows immediate knee motion (e.g., CPM), because the placement of wires converts distracting forces into compressive forces across the fracture site (Fig. 2). On the third postoperative day, the patient is placed in a hinged removable brace and begins gait training WB as tolerated with the knee locked in extension. The hinges are loosened for active ROM exercise, and the amount of knee flexion allowed during ambulation is gradually increased.[53] If there are significant associated tears in the medial or lateral retinacular expansions, a modified tension band wiring technique is used that allows gait training just as early but requires immobilization with a posterior splint for 1–3 weeks.

Following partial patellectomy for a comminuted fracture, treatment is similar to that following wire loop fixation.

TIBIAL PLATEAU FRACTURES

Tibial plateau fractures result from violent compression forces usually in combination with valgus forces, the classic "bumper fracture."[56] There are several classification schemes for these fractures and fracture-dislocations.[27,55] For non-displaced fractures with intact collateral ligaments, initial treatment is CPM, or a few days of immobilization by splint if CPM is unavailable, followed by active ROM and NWB ambulation for 8–10 weeks. Fracture-dislocations more commonly are associated with ligamentous disruption (the medial collateral ligament most commonly) and meniscal injuries. Treatment options vary from arthrotomy with reconstruction of the joint surface with plate and screw fixation, and repair of ligamentous and meniscal injuries, to closed manipulation and cast bracing. For displaced fractures, the size of the depression of the articular surface and the age and activity level of the patient are considered in the choice of treatment approach. For unicondylar fractures, the knee generally is splinted in extension for 3–4 days, and CPM is then employed, in conjunction with active ROM exercises, quadriceps setting exercises, and NWB ambulation for 12–16 weeks.

If the medial collateral ligament is repaired, 2 weeks of cast immobilization of the knee at 45° flexion, followed by 4 weeks of cast bracing with extension stopping short of full extension, is required. For bicondylar fractures, ambulation

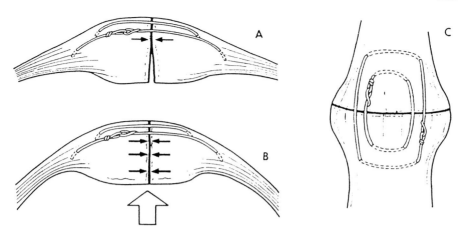

FIGURE 2. Tension band wiring for the patella. *A,* wire that has been passed around insertion of patellar tendon and quadriceps tendon is tightened until the fracture is slightly overcorrected or opened on the articular surface. A second wire is then passed more superficially but through bone fragments. *B,* on flexing the knee or contracting the quadriceps, pressure of the condyles against the patella compresses the bony fragments together. *C,* anterior view of both wires. (From Crenshaw AH (ed): Campbell's Operative Orthopaedics. 8th ed. St. Louis, Mosby, 1992. Redrawn from Müller ME, Allgower M, Willenegger H: Manual of Internal Fixation. New York, Springer-Verlag, 1970; with permission.)

is delayed for 3 weeks, the knee is placed in a cast brace, and WB is delayed for 10–12 weeks. For severely depresesd comminuted fractures, a bone graft may be used to restore the articular surface, and WB is delayed for 4–6 months.

TIBIAL SHAFT FRACTURES

Because the tibia is subcutaneous throughout much of its length and not enclosed by muscles, open fractures are more common in the tibia than in any other long bone. The blood supply for healing is also more precarious. The knee joint at the proximal end of the tibia does not allow rotary movement as the shoulder joint allows rotation of the humerus or as the hip joint allows rotation of the femur. Therefore, complications are relatively frequent and include infection, delayed union, and nonunion. Because each fracture is a unique problem with numerous possible surgical approaches, few generalizations can be made in reference to rehabilitation. The time required for healing may be quite long and variable. Maintenance of ROM and strength about the nonimmobilized uninvolved joints of the extremity may be all that can be done during this extended time. Tibial shaft fractures have been classified as caused by high-energy (motor vehicle accidents and industrial crush injuries) or low-energy (falls on ice, skiing injuries) trauma.[26]

High-energy fractures take longer to heal and have poorer prognosis. Associated factors include the amount of displacement, degree of comminution, and the severity of the soft tissue injury.

Closed reduction, cast bracing, and early WB are recommended only for closed and/or stable, low-energy fractures.[54] Other common treatments for tibial shaft fractures are plate and screw fixation, medullary fixation, and external fixation.

Fixation of short oblique or transverse fractures may be by plate and screws. Postoperatively the limb is placed in a long leg cast and kept NWB for 3–4 weeks. Progressive WB is allowed subsequently through a long-leg walking cast for 8–10 weeks, followed by short-leg cast bracing until bony union at 3–4 months. In a reliable patient with stable fixation, a brace is not needed.[7]

Generally following medullary fixation, the rigidity of fixation and control of angulatory and rotary forces determine whether plaster immobilization or bracing is needed and when WB is allowed. Immediate full WB may be possible in many cases. Following use of interlocking nails, some suggest that cast immobilization be used until there are radiographic signs of fracture healing at about 12 weeks.[59] Others advise early WB without external protection in the case of dynamically locked rods.[7] *Dynamic locking* refers to an intramedullary nail that is crossfixed to the bone cortex, usually by a bolt that is either proximal or distal to the fracture site, but not both (Fig. 3). This has been thought to provide a more physiologic environment for fracture healing. A *static-locked* nail is crossfixed both proximally and distally to the fracture, thus more securely controlling rotation at the fracture site.

For static-locked nails, WB is not allowed until the fracture heals. For axially stable fractures, dynamization (removal of either the proximal or distal locking screws, depending on which is least critical) allows progressive WB according to stability, with or without an orthosis.

External fixation has been used increasingly for open, high-energy fractures, facilitating soft tissue care and providing stabilization of fractures with bone loss for delayed autogenous bone grafting. If the fixator has been placed in compression, partial WB gait training is usually possible. Difficult nonunions with extensive bone loss have been managed with the Ilizarov device[61] (Fig. 4).

ANKLE FRACTURES

Following reduction of ankle fractures, only slight variation from normal is compatible with good joint function. Normal relations of the ankle mortise must

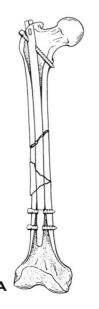

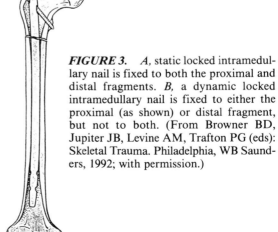

FIGURE 3. *A*, static locked intramedullary nail is fixed to both the proximal and distal fragments. *B*, a dynamic locked intramedullary nail is fixed to either the proximal (as shown) or distal fragment, but not to both. (From Browner BD, Jupiter JB, Levine AM, Trafton PG (eds): Skeletal Trauma. Philadelphia, WB Saunders, 1992; with permission.)

A   B

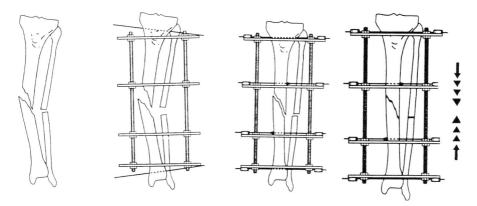

FIGURE 4. Difficult displaced fractures of tibial and fibular shafts treated with an Ilizarov fixator, demonstrating elimination of fragment distraction with tensioned wires. (From Crenshaw AH (ed): Campbell's Operative Orthopaedics, 8th ed. St. Louis, Mosby, 1992; with permission.)

be restored. Small alterations in the position of the malleoli can markedly distort the talotibial WB area and lead to rapid degenerative arthritic changes within the ankle joint.[59] Ankle fractures may be classified along anatomic lines as unimalleolar, bimalleolar, trimalleolar, and pilon fractures. The most common mechanism of ankle fracture is supination-external rotation, producing an oblique fracture of the distal fibula and a rupture of the deltoid ligament or fracture of the medial malleolus.

Operative treatment of ankle fractures may be early or late. Open reduction and internal fixation (ORIF) may be possible within the first day after injury or may be delayed for 2–3 weeks due to excessive swelling. Following unimalleolar (lateral malleolar) fractures, the deltoid ligament must be repaired with suture first, before the fibular fracture is reduced and internally fixed. If the deltoid ligament is not repaired, it may become caught between the medial malleolus and the talus, preventing accurate reduction. The fibular fracture is fixed with one or two lag screws or with pinning if the fracture has a small distal fragment or is transverse. After surgical repair, the limb is placed in a long-leg cast with the ankle in neutral position for 4 weeks. This is changed to a short-leg walking cast for another 4 weeks. Although this protocol has been widely used, controversy exists as to whether it is acutally better than others. A randomized prospective trial compared NWB without immobilization after 3 days postoperatively, versus NWB with cast immobilization, versus immediate WB on a walking cast, for a period of 6 weeks following surgical fixation.[14] There were no important differences in clinical outcomes in serial follow-up for 2 years. Another randomized trial comparing WB versus NWB with orthoses showed better loaded dorsiflexion capacity in the WB group.[1] Others have recommended early ROM and WB without orthoses.[66]

For bimalleolar fractures, ORIF of both malleoli and anatomic restoration of the distal tibiofibular syndesmosis is recommended. Depending on the quality of the fixation, either a long-leg cast or a short-leg cast with the anterior half cut away in front to allow ankle motion is applied for 4–6 weeks. The long-leg cast is changed to a short-leg cast for 4 weeks and then a walking cast until union occurs. With more secure fixation, the short-leg cast is removed after the 4–6 weeks, and progressive partial WB is continued until union.

Trimalleolar, or Cotton, fractures include fracture and displacement of the posterior lip of the articular surface of the tibia. If this fracture is not reduced and stabilized, the irregularity in the articular surface of the tibia is brought into contact with the surface of the talus, in which case WB and motion may cause severe traumatic arthritis. For small fracture fragments, often reduction and fixation of the fibula results in reduction of the posterior tibial fragment. When the posterior fragment is one third or more of the articular surface, separate internal fixation of the fragment is recommended.[63] When the fragment is one fourth or less of the articular surface, no difference was observed between clinical outcomes of fractures that were fixed or not fixed.[22] Following surgery, treatment is the same as for bimalleolar fractures.

Pilon fractures are comminuted fractures resulting from axial compressive force applied to the joint surface of the distal tibia. The fractures may involve bone loss, gaps from compaction of metaphyseal cancellous bone cavities, soft tissue swelling, and compromised circulation. The complications of ORIF are frequent, including further surgery for arthrodesis or amputation, and reflex sympathetic dystrophy. WB is generally delayed for 3–4 months. One series reported zero good results.[48]

TALAR FRACTURES

The talus is the only tarsal bone without muscular attachments. Because most of its surface is articular cartilage, most fractures involving the talus are intraarticular. All of the articulations of the talus are WB, and more weight per unit surface area is borne by the surface of the talus than by any other bone. If traumatic arthritis is to be prevented, exact anatomic reduction is necessary following fractures. Talar neck fractures are the most common talar fractures and are particularly susceptible to avascular necrosis. They usually occur as a result of forceful dorsiflexion of the foot in which the anterior margin of the tibia acts as a wedge. Hawkins classified talar neck fractures into three groups.[23] Type 1 fractures are nondisplaced and are treated conservatively by plaster immobilization in a short-leg cast for 6–8 weeks. These are initially NWB, then advanced in WB as union is demonstrated radiographically. In Hawkins' series, none of the type 1 fractures developed avascular necrosis; however, Canale later showed a 15% occurrence of avascular necrosis,[6] and Lorentzen showed a 30% occurrence of degenerative arthritis.[33] In type 2 talar neck fractures, the talus is dislocated with respect to the subtalar joint, but the tibiotalar joint is normally aligned. In type 3 fractures, the body of the talus is completely dislocated from both the ankle and the subtalar joint. Types 2 and 3 talar neck fractures require ORIF, usually with a cancellous lag screw.[32] Following surgery, the ankle is immobilized in a short-leg cast and maintained NWB 6–8 weeks, after which a cast boot is worn. The cast may be removed after 3 months, and an orthopedic shoe is worn for another 3 months. An alternative to casting is the use of a patellar tendon bearing brace.

Avascular necrosis occurs almost inevitably after type 3 fractures but does not necessarily preclude a satisfactory result.[32] When disability develops, the results of talectomy are poor unless done in conjunction with calcaneotibial arthrodesis either in a combined procedure[49] or in two stages.[47] Postoperatively, the limb is placed in a long-leg cast incorporating external fixation devices and maintained

NWB for 6 weeks, followed by a short-leg walking cast for another 6 weeks, followed by an ankle-foot orthosis for 2–3 months.[50]

Transchondral fractures of the talar dome are caused by inversion of the ankle with force transmitted from the articular surface of the tibia, across the joint, through the articular cartilage, to the subchondral trabeculae of the fractured bone. They have been classified by Berndt and Harty[3] into stages 1–4, corresponding to compression fracture, partial detachment of an osteochondral fragment, complete detachment of the fragment remaining in anatomic position, and completely displaced osteochondral fragment (loose body). These fractures are more common in men, as caused by landing on the toes associated with a torsional inversion in basketball, than in women, usually caused by inversion injuries from wearing high heels.[9,67] These lesions are frequently missed because routine radiographs are negative and because the more obvious sprain of lateral ligaments obscures their detection. CT scanning is the definitive study.

If the injury is recognized early and the fracture is nondisplaced, NWB cast immobilization for at least 6 weeks may result in adequate healing. If closed reduction is unsatisfactory, ORIF is employed. The foot is kept elevated and may not be casted for 2 weeks due to severe swelling and possible development of a compartment syndrome. After 6 weeks of NWB, a walking cast is applied for 4–6 weeks. Plantar forces may result in fracture dislocation of Chopart's joint, with displacement of the cuboid and navicular bones. Again, closed reduction with 6–8 weeks of NWB plaster immobilization is sufficient.

Results of one long-term follow-up study suggest that any displaced talar fracture should be excised.[5] Others recommend that if the displacement is recognized early and the fracture fragments are relatively large, the fracture should be surgically reduced and internally fixed.[15] An anterolateral or anteromedial approach is used depending on the location of the fragment. Adequate exposure may require osteotomy of the medial malleolus, which is reattached with a screw.[45] Postoperatively, a soft, bulky dressing is applied and active ROM is begun immediately. Full WB is delayed for 6 weeks. Ankle arthroscopy is now widely used for these lesions and may allow earlier WB at 2 weeks.[2,46]

CALCANEAL FRACTURES

Of the tarsal bones, the calcaneus is fractured the most frequently. Falls or jumps from ladders or roofs onto the heel are common mechanisms of injury. Calcaneal fractures may be classified most simply into intraarticular fractures causing disruption of the subtalar joint (the majority of cases) and extraarticular fractures not involving the subtalar joint (only about one fourth of cases). Extraarticular fractures are generally treated with plaster immobilization and early WB with two exceptions: ORIF is indicated for posterosuperior tuberosity fractures when a large fragment extends inferiorly to include avulsion of the Achilles tendon and also is indicated for displaced fractures of the anterior process of the calcaneus if it extends into the calcaneocuboid joint.

In intraarticular fractures, the sharp posterolateral edge of the talus carries vertical compressive and shearing forces into Gissane's angle of the calcaneus, splitting it obliquely.[12] There is a fairly constant pattern known as the *primary fracture*, with several variants and degrees of comminution. There are several methods of treating these fractures, but there is no consensus on indications for surgery or on postoperative management when surgery is performed. There is a high rate of severe permanent disability regardless of approach.[18] There does seem to be general agreement that nonoperative treatment is of little benefit and that traumatic arthritis of the subtalar joint may be inevitable. However, later arthrodesis may be technically easier if the joint has previously been surgically restored to a more anatomic configuration.[50] Whatever the operative technique, it appears that early (as soon as pain allows, 1–3 days postoperatively) subtalar active movement results in significantly better function subsequently.[58] One author recommends that a short-leg cast be applied postoperatively, with NWB ambulation for the first 2–3 weeks, followed by touch-down WB for another 3 weeks, followed by partial WB with cast removal at 8 weeks, and progression to full WB at 12 weeks.[21]

MIDFOOT FRACTURES

Fractures of the cuneiforms, cuboid, or navicular bones are likely to be associated with subluxation or dislocation at the proximal (Chopart) or distal (Lisfranc) articulations. When isolated, these fractures may be treated nonoperatively unless significantly displaced. The largest proportion of these fractures is caused by longitudinal forces such as landing from a jump when the plantar-flexed foot impacts on the metatarsal (MT) heads and compresses the navicular between the cuneiforms and the talus.[34]

Plaster NWB immobilization in a short-leg cast for 6 weeks is usually adequate. If bony union is not achieved, percutaneous fixation may be needed. If the fracture fragments are separated, bone grafting may be required. NWB is maintained postoperatively until union. Most Lisfranc injuries can be treated by closed reduction and stabilization with a percutaneous Kirschner wire or a Steinmann pin. Six weeks of NWB in a short-leg cast followed by 3 weeks in a walking cast are recommended.

METATARSAL FRACTURES

Displacement of simple fractures of the MT shafts is limited due to rigid attachments of the MTs to each other by the deep transverse MT ligaments distally and the interossei and other intrinsic muscles. Fractures of the first four MTs usually result from a heavy object falling on the dorsum of the foot. Because the skin and soft tissue are fragile and swelling may further compromise the neurocirculatory status, these injuries should never be treated with a constrictive dressing or cast. Minimal displacement of these fractures may be reduced manually. A plaster splint is applied to the plantar surface of the foot, and the leg is covered with a bulky cotton dressing to protect it from further soft tissue injury. Reduction is generally maintained with the splint, as irregular fracture edges interdigitate.

The dressing and splint are removed after a few days, and full WB ambulation is encouraged as soon as possible. Padded postoperative shoes can be worn for comfort. As the skin's condition permits, the forefoot should be circumferentially tape wrapped. Nondisplaced fractures of the first MT should be treated more carefully because they are less stable; a short-leg cast is used after swelling is resolved, and NWB status is maintained for 2 weeks.[10]

Surgical fixation is indicated if manual reduction of displaced fractures or maintenance of reduction is not possible. Internal fixation using a small plate and screws or Kirschner wire is employed. Postoperatively, a short-leg cast is used for 2–4 weeks, the first 2 weeks of which are NWB. Wire, if used, is removed at 3–4 weeks.

Fractures of the fifth MT involving the middle and distal diaphysis are typically caused by a fall on the plantar-flexed and inverted forefoot, usually after a leap. These occur so commonly in ballet that the injury has been referred to as the "dancer's fracture."[20] These are usually long-oblique or spiral fractures with minimal displacement. For nondisplaced and minimally displaced fractures of this type, treatment may be merely symptomatic, with a well-padded shoe. Displaced fractures may be manually reduced and fixed percutaneously with Kirschner wire, or ORIF is performed if closed reduction was not possible. The fractures usually heal rapidly, WB is begun immediately in a postoperative shoe, and the wires are removed at 4 weeks.

Fractures of the proximal fifth MT are distinctly different from middle and distal fractures, with great risk for delayed union and nonunion.[31,60,68] Fractures of the tuberosity of the base of the fifth MT are caused by indirect forces and represent an avulsion produced by strong contraction of the peroneus brevis tendon (which attaches there).[8] These fractures generally unite within 6–8 weeks or are asymptomatic by then; even those that heal by fibrous union are rarely symptomatic. A few weeks of cast immobilization may be used, but symptomatic treatment and a firm shoe are generally sufficient. WB may begin when swelling subsides, and unrestricted mobility is allowed when the fracture is asymptomatic, even if radiographic union is not complete.

However, fractures distal to the tuberosity may not heal with immobilization, even when combined with many weeks of NWB. These fractures, known as Jones fractures,[30] are also classically caused in dancing, with elevation of the heel, braking at the MTP joints, and vertical loading over the lateral aspect of the foot, which is unable to invert. These fractures are now more commonly seen in competitive athletes. It is of critical importance to differentiate a true acute fracture from those associated with prior injuries, prodromal symptoms, or stress reactions, because the prognosis and treatment are distinctly different. Acute Jones fractures are initially treated for 6 weeks in a NWB short-leg cast; most will heal within that time. However, in one series of Jones fractures, about 40% of patients were found in retrospect to have had a prior history of discomfort, and none of these fractures in athletes healed nonoperatively.[31]

Even after acute fractures are healed, refracture is not uncommon. At 6 weeks, a decision is made regarding further treatment. Many will heal with another 4–6 weeks of NWB cast immobilization. However, if there is radiographic evidence of chronicity, marked sclerosis at the fracture margins or obliteration of the medullary canal, surgical treatment should be strongly considered. Another series demonstrated that if an acute fracture does not heal within 12 weeks, it will still eventually heal but will take an average of nearly 15 months.[60] By contrast, a delayed union managed surgically by internal fixation with a malleolar cancellous screw[31] or by corticocancellous inlay bone grafting[60] should heal within 12 weeks of surgery. Following either screw fixaton or bone graft, the original authors[60] recommend a short-leg NWB cast for 6 weeks, followed by a short-leg walking cast for another 4–6 weeks. It has been demonstrated more recently[42] that intramedullary fixation may allow an earlier return to activity, with only 2 weeks of required NWB, followed by 4 weeks of progressive WB in a postoperative shoe, and then light jogging.

Stress fractures result from cumulative repetitive forces insufficient to cause an acute fracture but which eventually lead to failure of the involved bone. These were classically known as "march" fractures as a result of their occurrence in military recruits.[36] In both athletes and military recruits, these injuries tend to occur with a change in the amount or type of training, typically with a latency of about 3 months. Stress fractures also have been reported after bunionectomy, usually in the second MT, apparently caused by weight redistribution to the adjacent MTs.[16,37] Pain first begins diffusely and then becomes localized. It can take longer than 2 months for a stress fracture to become radiologically visible, long after a bone scan is positive. However, serial radiographs should still be obtained in order to demonstrate the exact fracture pattern. Typically, stress fractures of the first MT occur proximally along the medial border, whereas those of the second through fourth MTs occur distally in the neck along the plantar aspect, and stress fractures of the fifth MT occur proximally just distal to the metaphysis on the lateral margin. Stress fractures of the first four MTs are treated primarily with restriction of activity. A MT pad placed under fractures of the MT neck of the second through fourth MTs may prevent malunion by transferring WB away from involved MT head to the shaft.[42] Internal fixation should be considered if these fractures are displaced. Fifth MT stress fractures are notorious for nonunion and must be immobilized with NWB for at least 6 weeks.[68] Internal fixation with an axial medullary screw is the preferred treatment in athletes, because it decreases the healing time and allows return to sports activities more quickly.[11]

The sesamoid bones, located directly under the first MT head, are susceptible to fracture from direct trauma, such as a fall from a height. The tibial sesamoid is particularly prone to fracture and is another injury commonly observed in ballet dancers.[52] Acute sesamoid fractures may be managed conservatively; however, stress fractures of the sesamoid do not heal even with months of immobilization and inactivity.[62] Excision of the involved sesamoid has been recommended to allow asymptomatic return to prefracture activities.

PHALANGEAL FRACTURES

Toe fractures occur frequently, usually as the result of a direct blow or, in the case of the hallux phalanges, stubbing injuries.[29] Nondisplaced phalangeal fractures are treated by buddy-tape splinting to adjacent toes and the use of a stiff-soled shoe for 2–3 weeks. Displaced fractures should be reduced by longitudinal traction with woven wire traps. Reduction usually can be maintained by taping, but on rare occasions when not sufficiently stable the fracture may be stabilized with an axial Kirschner wire for 3–4 weeks. Furthermore, intraarticular fractures involving the interphalangeal joint of the great toe should be internally fixed to prevent joint incongruity and arthritic changes.[25] Twenty degrees of motion of the first interphalangeal joint are needed for normal function, whereas no motion is needed in either the proximal or distal interphalangeal joints of the lesser toes. Postoperatively, foot casting with the great toe in neutral position has been advised.[21] Following ORIF of other phalangeal fractures, protected WB in a postoperative shoe can begin as soon as soft tissue healing permits.

REFERENCES

1. Ahl T, Dalen N, Selvik G: Mobilization after operation of ankle fractures: Good results of early motion and weight bearing. Acta Orthop Scand 59:302–306, 1988.
2. Baker CL, Andrews JR, Ryan JB: Arthroscopic treatment of transchondral talar dome fractures. Arthroscopy 2:82–87, 1986.
3. Berndt AL, Harty M: Transchondral fractures (osteochondritis dissecans) of the talus. J Bone Joint Surg 41A:988–1020, 1959.
4. Bostrom A: Fracture of the patella: A study of 422 patellar fractures. Acta Orthop Scand (suppl) 143:1–80, 1972.
5. Canale ST, Belding RH: Osteochondral lesions of the talus. J Bone Joint Surg 62A:97–102, 1980.

6. Canale ST, Kelly FB: Fractures of the neck of the talus: Longterm evaluation of 71 cases. J Bone Joint Surg 60A:143–156, 1978.
7. Chapman MW: Fractures of the tibial and fibular shafts. In Evarts CM (ed): Surgery of the Musculoskeletal System. New York, Churchill Livingstone, 1990, pp 3741–3799.
8. Dameron TB: Fractures and anatomical variations of the proximal portion of the fifth metatarsal. J Bone Joint Surg 57A:788–792, 1975.
9. Davidson CD, Steele HD, et al: A review of twenty-one cases of transchondral fractures of the talus. J Trauma 7:378–415, 1967.
10. DeLee JC: Fractures and dislocations of the foot. In Mann RA (ed): Surgery of the Foot. St. Louis, Mosby, 1986, pp 592–808.
11. Delee JC, Evans P, Julian J: Stress fracture of the fifth metatarsal. Am J Sports Med 11:349–353, 1983.
12. Essex-Lopresti P: The mechanism, reduction, technique, and results in fractures of the os calcis. Br J Surg 39:395–419, 1952.
13. Finsen V, Benum P: Osteopenia after ankle fractures: The influence of early weight bearing and muscle activity. Clin Orthop 245:261–268, 1989.
14. Finsen V, Saetermo R, Kibsgaard L, et al: Early postoperative weight-bearing and muscle activity in patients who have a fracture of the ankle. J Bone Joint Surg 71A:23–27, 1989.
15. Flick AB, Gould N: Osteochondritis dissecans of the talus (transchondral fractures of the talus). Foot Ankle 5:165–185, 1985.
16. Ford LT, Gilula LA: Stress fractures of the middle metatarsals following the Keller operation. J Bone Joint Surg 59A:117–118, 1977.
17. Gelberman RH, Botte MJ, Spiegelman JJ, Akeson WH: The excursion and deformation of repaired flexor tendons treated with protected early motion. J Hand Surg 11A:106–110, 1986.
18. Giachino AA, Unthoff HK: Intraarticular fractures of the calcaneus. J Bone Joint Surg 71A:784–787, 1989.
19. Halpenny J, Rorabeck CH: Supracondylar fractures of the femur: Results of treatment of 61 patients. Can J Surg 27:606–609, 1984.
20. Hamilton WG: Injuries in ballet dancers. Sports Med Digest 8:1, 1986.
21. Hansen ST: Foot injuries. In Browner BD, Jupiter JB, Levine AM, Trafton PG (eds): Skeletal Trauma. Philadelphia, WB Saunders, 1992, pp 1959–1991.
22. Harper MC, Handin G: Posterior malleolar fractures of the ankle associated with external rotation-abduction injuries: Results with and without internal fixation. J Bone Joint Surg 70A:1348–1356, 1988.
23. Hawkins LG: Fractures of the neck of the talus. J Bone Joint Surg 52A:991–1002, 1970.
24. Healy WL, Brooker AF: Distal femoral fractures: Comparison of open and closed methods of treatment. Clin Orthop 174:166–171, 1983.
25. Heckman JD: Fractures and dislocations of the midpart and forepart of the foot. In Evarts CM (ed): Surgery of the Musculoskeletal System. 2nd ed. New York, Churchill Livingstone, 1990, pp 4269–4296.
26. Hoagland FT, States JD: Factors influencing the rate of healing in tibial shaft fractures. Surg Gynecol Obstet 124:71–76, 1967.
27. Hohl M, Moore TM: Articular fractures of the proximal tibia. In Evarts CM (ed): Surgery of the Musculoskeletal System. 2nd ed. New York, Churchill Livingstone, 1990, pp 3471–3497.
28. Hulth A: Curent concepts of fracture healing. Clin Orthop 249:265–284, 1989.
29. Jahss MH: Stubbing injuries to the hallux. Foot Ankle 1:327–332, 1981.
30. Jones R: Fractures of the base of the fifth metatarsal by indirect violence. Ann Surg 35:697–700, 1902.
31. Kavanagh JH, Brower TD, Mann RV: The Jones fracture revisited. J Bone Joint Surg 60A:776–782, 1978.
32. King RE, Powell DF: Injury to the talus. In Jahss MH (ed): Disorders of the Foot and Ankle. 2nd ed. Philadelphia, WB Saunders, 1991, pp 2293–2325.
33. Lorentzen JE, Christensen SB, et al: Fractures of the neck of the talus. Acta Orthop Scand 48:115–120, 1977.
34. Main BL, Jowett RL: Injuries of the midtarsal joint. J Bone Joint Surg 57B:89–97, 1975.
35. Marya SK, Bhan S, Dave PK: Comparative study of knee function after patellectomy and osteosynthesis with a tension band wire following patellar fractures. Int Surg 72:211–213, 1987.
36. Meyerding HW, Pollock GA: March fracture. Surg Gynecol Obstet 67:234, 1938.
37. Michetti ML: March fracture following a McBride bunionectomy: A case report. J Am Podiatr Assoc 60:286–287, 1970.
38. Mize RD, Bucholz RW, Grogan DP: Surgical treatment of displaced, comminuted fractures of the distal end of the femur: An extensile approach. J Bone Joint Surg 64A:871–879, 1982.

39. Mooney V, Becker S: Major fractures. In Nickel VL, Botte MJ (eds): Orthopaedic Rehabilitation. New York, Churchill Livingstone, 1992, pp 601–610.
40. Moore TJ, Watson T, Green SA, et al: Complications of surgically treated supracondylar fractures of the femur. J Trauma 27:402–406, 1987.
41. Muller ME, Nazarian S, Koch P: The Comprehensive Classification of Fractures of Long Bones. Berlin, Springer Verlag, 1988.
42. Myerson MS: Injuries to the forefoot and toes. In Jahss MH (ed): Disorders of the Foot and Ankle. 2nd ed. Philadelphia, WB Saunders, 1991, pp 2233–2273.
43. Namba RS, Kabo JM, Dorey FJ, Meals RA: Continuous passive motion versus immobilization: The effect of posttraumatic joint stiffness. Clin Orthop 267:218–223, 1991.
44. Nichols PJR: Rehabilitation after fractures of the shaft of the femur. J Bone Joint Surg 45B:96–102, 1963.
45. Ove PN, Bosse MJ, Reinert CM: Excision of posterolateral talar dome lesions through a medial transmalleolar approach. Foot Ankle 9:171–175, 1989.
46. Parisien JS: Arthroscopic treatment of osteochondral lesions of the talus. Am J Sports Med 14:211–217, 1986.
47. Penny JN, Davis LA: Fractures and fracture dislocations of the neck of the talus. J Trauma 20:1029–1037, 1980.
48. Pierce RO, Heinrich JH: Comminuted intra-articular fractures of the distal tibia. J Trauma 19:828–832, 1979.
49. Reckling FW: Early tibiocalcaneal fusion in the treatment of severe injuries of the talus. J Trauma 12:390–396, 1972.
50. Richardson EG, Graves SC: Fractures and dislocations of foot. In Crenshaw AH (ed): Campbell's Operative Orthopaedics. 8th ed. St. Louis, Mosby, 1992, pp 2875–2922.
51. Salter RB, Simmonds DF, Malcolm BW, et al: The biologic effect of continuous passive motion on the healing of full thickness defects in articular cartilage: An experimental investigation in the rabbit. J Bone Joint Surg 62A:1232–1251, 1980.
52. Sammarco GJ: Forefoot conditions in dancers. Part II. Foot Ankle 3:85–92, 1982.
53. Sanders R: Patella fractures and extensor mechanism injuries. In Browner BD, Jupiter JB, Levine AM, Trafton PG (eds): Skeletal Trauma. Philadelphia, WB Saunders, 1992, pp 1685–1716.
54. Sarmiento A: Functional bracing of tibial fractures. Clin Orthop 105:202–219, 1974.
55. Schatzker J, McBroom R, Bruce D: The tibial plateau fracture: The Toronto Experience 1968–75. Clin Orthop 138:94–104, 1979.
56. Schulak DJ, Gunn DR: Fractures of the tibial plateau: A review of the literature. Clin Orthop 109:166–177, 1975.
57. Seinsheimer F: Fractures of the distal femur. Clin Orthop 153:169–179, 1980.
58. Stephenson JR: Treatment of displaced intra-articular fractures of the calcaneus using medial and lateral approaches, internal fixation, and early motion. J Bone Joint Surg 69A:115–130, 1987.
59. Taylor JC: Fractures of the lower extremity. In Crenshaw AH (ed): Campbell's Operative Orthopaedics. 8th ed. St. Louis, Mosby, 1992, pp 785–893.
60. Torg JS, Balduini FC, Zelko RR, et al: Fractures of the base of the fifth metatarsal distal to the tuberosity: Classification and guidelines for surgical and non-surgical management. J Bone Joint Surg 66A:209–214, 1984.
61. Tucker H: Management of unstable tibial fractures using the method of Ilizarov. Florida Orthop Soc J 2:36, 1989.
62. Van Hal ME, Keene JS, Lange TA, Clancy WG: Stress fractures of the great toe sesamoids. Am J Sports Med 10:122–128, 1982.
63. Warner WC, Farber LA: Trimalleolar fractures. South Med J 58:1292, 1965.
64. Weber MJ, Janecki CJ, McLeod P, et al: Efficacy of various forms of fixation of transverse fractures of the patella. J Bone Joint Surg 62A:215–220, 1980.
65. Winters C, Dabezies EJ: Supracondylar fractures of the femur. Orthopedics 7:1051, 1984.
66. Yablon IG, Segal D: Ankle fractures. In Evarts CM (ed): Surgery of the Musculoskeletal System. New York, Churchill Livingstone, 1990, pp 3827–3860.
67. Yvars MF: Osteochondral fractures of the dome of the talus. Clin Orthop 114:185–191, 1976.
68. Zelko RR, Torg JS, Rachun A: Proximal diaphyseal fractures of the fifth metatarsal: Treatment of the fractures and their complications in athletes. Am J Sports Med 7:95–101, 1979.
69. Zickel RE, Hobeika P, Robbins DS: Zickel supracondylar nails for fractures of the distal end of the femur. Clin Orthop 212:79–88, 1986.
70. Zuckerman JD, Newport ML: Rehabilitation of fractures in adults. In Goodgold J (ed): Rehabilitation Medicine. St. Louis, Mosby, 1988, pp 441–456.

LYNNE M. STEMPIEN, MD
GERARD L. GLANCY, MD

SPECIAL CONSIDERATIONS IN THE REHABILITATION OF FRACTURES IN CHILDREN

From the Rehabilitation Center
(LMS)
and
Department of Orthopaedics (GG)
The Children's Hospital
Denver, Colorado

Reprint requests to:
Lynne M. Stempien, MD
Assistant Medical Director
Rehabilitation Center
The Children's Hospital
1056 East 19th Ave.
Denver, CO 80218

It is axiomatic that childrens' fractures are common, heal rapidly, and, in most cases, present little in the way of residual sequelae. This statement, however, can lead the unwary practitioner into a false sense of security when treating a child's fracture. Certain fractures must be handled with great expertise at the onset of treatment to obtain an optimal outcome. Furthermore, the existence of other injuries or other disease states may require considerable modification in the treatment of what might otherwise be considered a routine pediatric fracture. It is the purpose of this chapter to highlight those conditions and discuss the alteration in fracture care that is required.

UNIQUE FEATURES OF FRACTURES IN CHILDREN

Childrens' bones are considered biologically "plastic." Therefore, frequent long-bone fractures are of the greenstick or buckle variety; they are minimally angulated, heal rapidly, often require no reduction, and immobilization is primarily for comfort and protection. In treating displaced fractures of long bones in girls younger than 10 and boys younger than 12, it is often sufficient to simply realign the bone. Anatomic reduction is not absolutely essential, especially if the fracture is near the physis of maximal growth for that bone (proximal humerus, distal radius, distal femur).

There are, however, exceptions to this generalization for childrens' long-bone fractures.

Supracondylar elbow fractures present a special challenge, as cubitus varus or valgus is a frequent outcome resulting from failure to obtain an adequate reduction. Treatment often requires percutaneous pin fixation under image control with a general anesthetic. Monteggia fractures (fractured ulna with radial head dislocation) also require special attention. The radial head dislocation must first be recognized and a prompt reduction obtained. Any intraarticular fracture, while unusual in a child, requires precise reduction, often by operative means.

Childrens' long bones possess a physis, or growth plate, at either end. Fractures that traverse through this area present special problems. The Salter-Harris classification of these fractures is in general use[33a] and will not be reiterated here. Suffice it to say that any injury through the physis has the potential to alter subsequent growth of that bone. A partial physeal arrest will result in a progressive angular deformity. The younger the age of the patient in which this occurs, of course, the greater the resulting deformity. If the area of shutdown comprises less than 50% of the total area of the physis, it is possible to resect this area of injury and thereby restore growth potential. If the physeal injury results in complete premature closure, limb length discrepancy will result. Age of occurrence will determine the resultant discrepancy at maturity. Limb length inequalities of less than 1 inch frequently need no treatment, between 1 and 2 inches are treated by epiphysiodesis at the appropriate time, and discrepancies of greater than 2 inches are managed with either shortening of the long side or lengthening of the short side.

SPECIAL CIRCUMSTANCES

Multiple System Trauma

Multiple system trauma in a child presents the same problems and challenges as similar injuries to the adult. The concomitant presence of closed head injury and visceral injury may require more than one trip to the operating room and frequent moves from the intensive care unit to the radiology department for special studies such as computed tomography and magnetic resonance imaging. Pulmonary support, especially in an upright position, is critical. Nursing care must be intense, meticulous, and provide frequent changes in the child's position to avoid pressure sores. Early stabilization of fractures greatly facilitates all of the foregoing. Therefore, suitable modifications in fracture care must be made in the polytraumatized child. For example, a mid shaft humerus fracture when treated as an isolated injury requires only a sling or cuff and collar. This, however, is totally inadequate in patients who are comatose or combative or have multiple system injury; stabilization with either external fixator or Rush rods is entirely appropriate (Fig. 1). A mid shaft femur fracture is often managed with either a spica cast or skeletal traction. Again, both methods are difficult when the child has other injuries requiring specialized care. In these cases, use of an external fixator greatly facilitates overall patient management (Fig. 2). The use of such a device thoroughly immobilizes the fracture, permits motion of the joint above and the joint below, leaves the entire extremity exposed for observation, and allows the child to be placed in any position in bed. As overall recovery takes place, it is possible to ambulate with the fixator in place (Fig. 3).

Fractures may go unrecognized in the multiply traumatized child. The absence of deformity and attention directed solely to the major injuries result in delay of diagnosis. Unrecognized fractures can be discovered with spontaneous

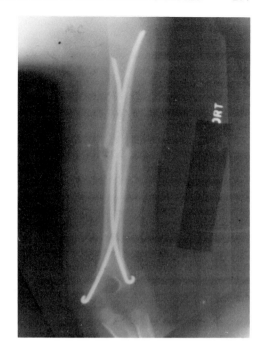

FIGURE 1.   Rush intramedullary rod in a humerus (right).

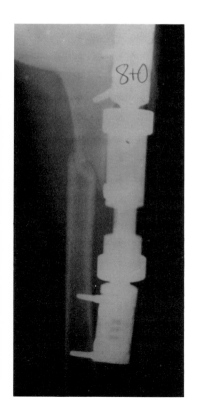

FIGURE 2.   Femoral external fixation (left).

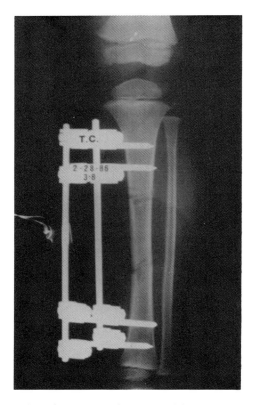

FIGURE 3. External fixator in a patient with polytrauma.

callus in a malaligned position, necessitating complex fixation, often with resection. Also, the change in function with neurologic recovery often includes spasticity, which can promote unwanted angulation.[11,12]

Soft tissue calcification discovered later in the course of treatment has several potential causes. The two major forms are heterotopic ossification (HO) and myositis ossificans. HO is organized bone that occurs in the periarticular soft tissue. HO can cause increased uptake on triple phase bone scan and elevated serum alkaline phosphatase. Clinically it can cause localized soft tissue irritation and eventual joint ankylosis.[11,12,17,28] Myositis ossificans is calcification of traumatized soft tissue. It can occur in other areas besides periarticular ones and does not organize into trabecular bone like HO.

Traumatic Brain Injury

Children suffering traumatic brain injury generally have a rapidly changing neurologic picture that includes swift changes in level of consciousness, with most of the children experiencing a significantly agitated phase. There is often progressive return of motor function, with spasticity and posturing as a prominent feature. Patients can recover mobility prior to complete fracture healing and return of cognitive skills that allow them adequate safety and judgment. As with multisystem trauma the early mobilization allowed by internal or external fixation is essential to allow these children to maximize their functional recovery.

Spinal Cord Injury

The same principles that apply to long-bone fixation also apply to fractures of the spine. As with adults, the emphasis will be on rapid rehabilitation, especially if there is an associated spinal cord injury. To this end, early stabilization of unstable spine fractures or fracture dislocations will facilitate the efforts of the rehabilitation team.

Cerebral Palsy

Fractures in children with cerebral palsy are often complicated by preexisting osteopenia. Poor bone quality can be caused by disuse, with decreased mobility from weakness, spasticity, posturing, and poor motor control. Nutritional compromise and altered bone mineral metabolism from drugs such as anticonvulsants can contribute to bone fragility.[22,23] Postsurgical spica cast immobilization superimposed on these factors can exacerbate this osteopenia. Therefore, techniques of casting that allow the earliest weightbearing and remobilization are preferable. For example, patients with proximal femoral varus osteotomy have their casts bivalved 3 weeks postoperatively to allow physical therapy to begin for gentle mobilization prior to completion of union at the actual site of osteotomy. This reduces the incidence of buckle fractures in the distal femur after the cast is removed.

The risk for malunion or nonunion is also increased in children with cerebral palsy, especially as the amount of neuromuscular dysfunction increases. The occurrence and severity of malunion are related to the amount of soft tissue contracture, joint deformity, and activity level of the patient.[27] Therefore, the greatest risk for poor fracture healing is in children with spastic quadriplegic cerebral palsy and multiple deformities.

Myelomeningocele

Children with myelomeningocele have an increased risk of fractures secondary to immobilization osteopenia from their paralysis and decreased weightbearing. Because this risk increases with the level of neurologic compromise, the majority of fractures occur in patients with thoracic and upper lumbar neurologic dysfunction.[27] This pattern is also seen in the neonatal period.[2]

The most frequent injuries are in the anatomic areas of neurologic dysfunction and in the lower extremities. Fractures occur most commonly in the femur of patients with thoracic dysfunction and the tibia of those with lumbar dysfunction.[24] Regardless of the level of impairment, there is a protective effect from weightbearing. Children who are encouraged to ambulate with equipment for mobility or exercise, rather than exclusively use a wheelchair for mobility, have fewer fractures.[26]

Osteopenia again necessitates the principles of early mobilization in the treatment of fractures in patients with spina bifida. A concern for prevention of pressure sores comes with the combination of sensory loss, deformity, impaired mobility, and cognitive dysfunction. Treatment techniques vary with fracture location. Diaphyseal and metaphyseal injuries heal well with splinting. Physeal injuries have a higher risk of malunion and require immobilization by casting.[20] Unfortunately, there is also an increased risk of refracture after treatment. This frequently occurs in close proximity to the former cast.

NEUROMUSCULAR DISEASE

Children with muscle disease such as muscular dystrophy or spinal muscular atrophy experience hypotonia, often with progressive muscle weakness. Most of these conditions allow the children some independent mobility early in the course of disease, but frequently with impaired balance reactions and increased risk of falls. The most common fractures are of the humerus and femur as patients attempt to protect themselves during a fall.[14] With significant weakness in chronic conditions, such as the congenital myopathies, or more slowly progressive conditions, such as intermediate type spinal muscular atrophy, there is also the increased risk of fractures secondary to disuse osteopenia.

Brevity of immobilization for fracture treatment has special impact in neuromuscular disease. Any period of immobilization hastens the progression of weakness. Even slight worsening of contractures in patients with marginal functioning due to weakness can adversely affect the patients' functional level.[18] Therefore, the use of techniques that allow early weightbearing in ambulatory patients and shorter immobilization in nonambulatory patients is beneficial.

Metabolic Bone Disease

A variety of disease conditions result in bone that is osteopenic and thereby subject to frequent fracture with less than the usual trauma. Paramount among these conditions is osteogenesis imperfecta (OI). While a thorough discussion of this condition is beyond the scope of this chapter, a few general comments are pertinent. Diagnosis of the milder forms of osteogenesis imperfecta may, at times, be difficult. Nonaccidental trauma must always be considered as a possible alternative explanation for multiple fractures. A skin biopsy with fibroblast culture can, at times, confirm the diagnosis of OI.[2a] In the moderate to severe forms of osteogenesis imperfecta, the problem is twofold: recurrent fractures and progressive deformity (Fig. 4). Use of intramedullary fixation is frequently effective in controlling the deformity. In children younger than 2, the double Rush rod technique is effective (Fig. 5). In older children, the Bailey-Dubow rod is a

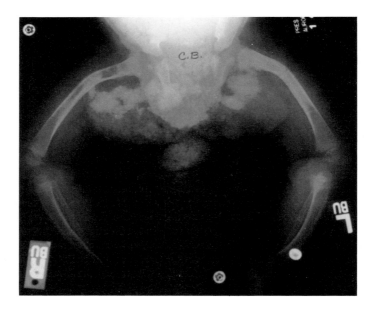

FIGURE 4. Osteogenesis imperfecta.

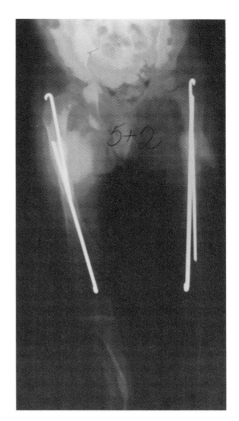

FIGURE 5. Early intramedullary rods in a patient with osteogenesis imperfecta.

suitable alternative and may have a distinct advantage in the bone with a very narrow intramedullary canal. Frequent rod changes to accommodate long-bone growth are often necessary (Fig. 6). Indeed, these should be planned and anticipated in advance, prior to the occurrence of deformity and/or fracture. There is, in fact, some evidence to suggest that early intramedullary rodding, with continued maintenance of long bone alignment, may reduce the actual incidence of fractures. The services of a physical therapist are important in the postoperative period to minimize muscle atrophy. External immobilization either for postoperative recovery or fracture union should be minimal in extent and of as short a duration as possible. This will diminish the extent of secondary disuse osteopenia.

The same general principles of early stabilization with minimal "down time" should be applied to any child with an underlying metabolic bone disease. An example of this is cystinosis with resulting secondary osteomalacia. Treatment of a mid shaft femur fracture in a spica cast would only promote demineralization. Therefore, use of an external fixator and encouragement of early motion and weightbearing minimizes these effects. The use of external fixators for fracture fixation in children is not without hazard. Selection of device, appropriate size, and meticulous attention to detail in pin placement are all critical factors that are required for success.

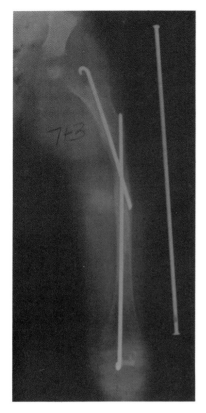

FIGURE 6. These dual Rush rods will be replaced with a Bailey-Dubow rod, which is being sized adjacent to the thigh, in the same patient shown in Figure 5.

Children taking chronic corticosteroids also have osteopenia. The prime example is steroid-dependent asthmatics. Fortunately, long-bone fractures seem to be unusual in this age group. However, compression fractures of vertebral bodies are disturbingly common. They rarely result in neurologic compromise but can be significantly disabling. Most require little more than external support, either a lumbosacral corset or a thoracolumbar spinal orthosis until healing takes place.

Tumors

Pathologic fracture may be the presenting symptom for either a benign or malignant pediatric bone tumor. If the lesion is clearly benign on radiographic criteria (unicameral bone cyst), it can often be ignored and the fracture treated as one would treat the nonpathologic equivalent. On occasion, the healing process of the fracture is sufficient to trigger a resolution of the lesion. Other times, however, the radiographic appearance of the lesion may be worrisome, or the location and size of the lesion may dictate operative intervention. In addition to the obvious need for adequate biopsy, appropriate stabilization and/or bone grafting of the lesion is appropriate. Even benign bone tumors such as aneurysmal bone cysts often are quite sizable, and available autograft is inadequate to adequately fill the lesion. Allografts are nearly as efficacious and have considerably less morbidity to the child.[12a]

Obvious malignant lesions still need biopsy for confirmation. If possible, an adequate specimen should be obtained without violating the bone itself. A postbiopsy stress fracture greatly compromises management, both from the standpoint of chemotherapy and subsequent limb salvage. There may be some evidence, in addition, that it affects prognosis. Fractures through a limb salvage or irradiated extremity present special problems that are beyond the scope of this discussion. The skills and efforts of a physical therapist are critical in the management of the child who has undergone limb salvage.

In summary, the bones of children possess remarkable healing and remodeling potential. The inherent enthusiasm and ingenuousness of children makes rehabilitation a pleasure and a delight. However, special circumstances dictate alternative strategies in the management of children's fractures. These circumstances include multiple system trauma, cerebral palsy, myelomeningocele, neuromuscular disease, metabolic bone disease, and bone tumors. When confronted with a fracture under these circumstances, it is important that the caregivers coordinate their efforts and that the fracture be managed in a way that facilitates and optimizes the ultimate rehabilitation of the child.

REFERENCES

1. Anschuetz RH, Freehafer AA, Shaffer JW, Dixon MS: Severe fracture complications in myelodysplasia. J Pediatr Orthop 4:22–24, 1984.
2. Boytim MJ, Davidson RS, Charney E, Melchionni JB: Neonatal fractures in myelomeningocele patients. J Pediatr Orthop 11:28–30, 1991.
2a. Cetta G, Ramirez F, Tsipouras P (eds): Third international conference on osteogenesis imperfecta. Ann N Y Acad Sci 543:1–185, 1988.
3. Conrad EU, Rang MC: Fractures and sprains: Common orthopedic problems. Ped Clin North Am 33:1523–1540, 1986.
4. Drummond DS, Moreau M, Cruess RL: Post-operative neuropathic fractures in patients with myelomeningocele. Dev Med Child Neurol 23:147–150, 1981.
5. Drummond DS, Moreau M, Cruess R: The results and complications of surgery for the paralytic hip and spine in myelomeningocele. J Bone Joint Surg 62B:49–53, 1980.
6. Edwards CC: Management of multisegment injuries in the polytrauma patient. In Johnston RM (ed): Advances in External Fixation. Miami, Symposia Specialists, 1980, pp 43–59.
7. Eichenholtz SN: Management of long-bone fractures in paraplegic patients. J Bone Joint Surg 45:299–310, 1963.
8. Fulford GE: Surgical management of ankle and foot deformities in cerebral palsy. Clin Orthop 253:55–61, 1990.
9. Fry K, Hoffer MM, Brink J: Femoral shaft fractures in brain-injured children. J Trauma 16:371–373, 1976.
10. Gamble JG, Strudwick WJ, Rinsky LA, Bleck EE: Complications of intramedullary rods in osteogenesis imperfecta: Bailey-Dubow rods versus non-elongating rods. J Pediatr Orthop 8:645–649, 1988.
11. Garland DE: Clinical observations on fractures and heterotopic ossification in the spinal cord and traumatic brain injured populations. Clin Orthop 233:86–101, 1988.
12. Garland DE: Spinal cord insults and heterotopic ossification in the pediatric population. Clin Orthop 245:303–319, 1989.
12a. Glancy GL, Brugioni DJ, Eilert RB, Chang FM: Autograft versus allograft for benign lesions in children. Clin Orthop 262:28–33, 1991.
13. Goldman AB, Lane JM, Salvati E: Slipped capital femoral epiphyses complicating renal osteodystrophy: A report of three cases. Radiology 126:333–339, 1978.
14. Gray B, Hsu JD, Furumasu J: Fractures caused by falling from a wheelchair in patients with neuromuscular disease. Dev Med Child Neurol 34:589–592, 1992.
15. Groswasser Z, Cohen M, Blankstein E: Polytrauma associated with traumatic brain injury: Incidence, nature and impact on rehabilitation outcome. Brain Inj 4:161–166, 1990.
16. Hoffer MM, Garrett A, Brink J, Perry J, Hale W, Nickel V: The orthopaedic management of brain-injured children. J Bone Joint Surg 53A:567–577, 1971.

17. Hurvitz EA, Mandac BR, Davidoff G, et al: Risk factors for heterotopic ossification in children and adolescents with severe traumatic brain injury. Arch Phys Med Rehabil 73:459–462, 1992.

18. Hsu JD: Extremity fractures in children with neuromuscular disease. Johns Hopkins Med J 145:89–93, 1979.

19. Hsu JD, Garcia-Ariz M: Fracture of the femur in the Duchenne muscular dystrophy patient. J Pediatr Orthop 1:203–207, 1981.

20. Kumar SJ, Cowell HR, Townsend P: Physeal, metaphyseal, and diaphyseal injuries of the lower extremities in children with myelomeningocele. J Pediatr Orthop 4:25–27, 1984.

21. Lang-Stevenson AI, Sharrard WJW: Intramedullary rodding with Bailey-Dubow extensible rods in osteogenesis imperfecta. An interim report of results and complications. J Bone Joint Surg 66B:227–232, 1984.

22. Lee JJK, Lyne ED: Pathologic fractures in severely handicapped children and young adults. J Pediatr Orthop 10:497–500, 1990.

23. Lee JJK, Lyne ED, Kleerekoper M, et al: Disorders of bone metabolism in severely handicapped children and young adults. Clin Orthop 245:297–302, 1989.

24. Lock TR, Aronson D: Fractures in patients who have myelomeningocele. J Bone Joint Surg 71A:1153–1157, 1989.

25. Mayfield JK, Erkkila JC, Winter RB: Spine deformity subsequent to acquired childhood spinal cord injury. J Bone Joint Surg 63A:1401–1411, 1981.

26. Mazur JM, Shurtleff D, Menelaus M, Colliver J: Orthopedic management of high-level spina bifida: Early walking compared with early use of a wheelchair. J Bone Joint Surg 71A:56–61, 1989.

27. McIvor WC, Samilson RL: Fractures in patients with cerebral palsy. J Bone Joint Surg 48A:858–866, 1966.

28. Mital MA, Garber JE, Stinson JT: Ectopic bone formation in children and adolescents with head injuries: Its management. J Pediatr Orthop 7:83–90, 1987.

29. Navarro A, Peiro A: Healing in denervated bones. Acta Orthop Scand 45:820, 1974.

30. Ogden JA: Skeletal Injury in the Child. Philadelphia, Lea & Febiger, 1982.

31. Rang M (ed): Children's Fractures. 2nd ed. Philadelphia, JB Lippincott, 1983.

32. Reff RB: The use of external fixation devices in the management of severe lower-extremity trauma and pelvic injuries in children. Clin Orthop 188:21–33, 1984.

33. Rockwood CA, Wilkins KE, King RE (eds): Fractures, Vol 3. Philadelphia, JB Lippincott, 1991.

33a. Salter RB, Harris WR: Injuries involving the epiphyseal plate. J Bone Joint Surg 45A:587–622, 1963.

34. Shapiro F: Consequences of an osteogenesis imperfecta diagnosis for survival and ambulation. J Pediatr Orthop 5:456–462, 1985.

35. Tolo VT: External skeletal fixation in children's fractures. J Pediatr Orthop 3:435–442, 1983.

36. Ziv I, Blackburn N, Rang M: Femoral intramedullary nailing in the growing child. J Trauma 24:432–434, 1984.

MARK A. YOUNG, MD
BRYAN J. O'YOUNG, MD
EDWARD G. McFARLAND, MD

REHABILITATION OF THE ORTHOPEDIC TRAUMA PATIENT: GENERAL PRINCIPLES

From the Department of Physical
  Medicine and Rehabilitation
  (MAY, BJO)
  and
Section of Sports Medicine and
  Shoulder Surgery
Department of Orthopaedic
  Surgery (EGM)
The Johns Hopkins University
  School of Medicine
Baltimore, Maryland

Reprint requests to:
Mark A. Young, MD
Department of Physical Medicine
  and Rehabilitation
Good Samaritan Professional
  Building
5601 Loch Raven Blvd.,
  Room 403/406
Baltimore, MD 21239

A growing role for the physical medicine and rehabilitation specialist in the aftercare of the trauma patient has evolved during the last decade. The rising incidence of trauma-associated morbidity[10,37] and the burgeoning number of trauma centers account for this trend. Ongoing improvements in medical, orthopedic, and resuscitative techniques have enhanced treatment of trauma patients, permitting earlier transfer to rehabilitation centers.[7]

Care of the trauma patient demands a coordinated, multidisciplinary team approach.[37] Members of the "trauma rehabilitation team" often include the physiatrist, surgeon, internist, and other allied health professionals (Fig. 1). Since functional deficits are a frequent sequela, the physiatrist orchestrates the rehabilitative aspects of the patient's treatment.[55]

Physiatry's task is to render early assessment, advise, and assist in acute preventive and maintenance strategies and provide education and counseling to family members. Objectives include contracture avoidance, decubitus prevention, thromboembolic prevention, splinting and positioning protocols, and bowel and bladder preservation. The rehabilitation specialist must also work to avert long-term musculoskeletal and cardiovascular effects of immobility. As with other aspects of physical medicine and rehabilitation, formulation of an effective therapy prescription must be based on a thorough review of the chart with emphasis on the underlying

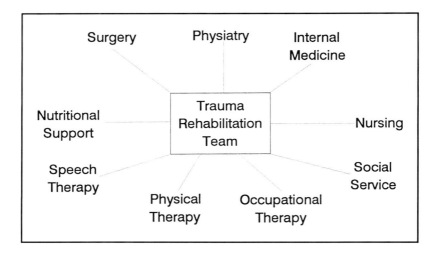

FIGURE 1.   Members of the trauma rehabilitation team.

medical, socioeconomic, and psychologic needs of the patient. Individualization of the therapy plan is always imperative.

Once medical stability of the trauma patient is established, the rehabilitation specialist screens for deficits in functional ability and oversees the implementation of physical therapy and occupational therapy services. For an increasing number of polytrauma patients requiring mechanical ventilation, the rehabilitation team, under physiatric direction, can play a dynamic role in fostering communication ability and swallowing function.[29,50] The advent of a perfected tracheostomy speaking valve has further optimized communication for tracheotomized patients[17,51] (Fig. 2).

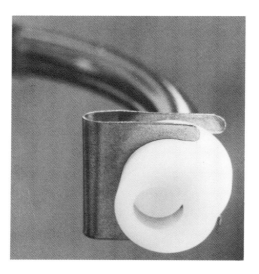

FIGURE 2.   The Hopkins tracheostomy speaking valve.

This chapter will review general principles of rehabilitation in the multiple trauma patient. It will commence with a discussion of the epidemiology of multitrauma, followed by a review of emergency resuscitative techniques used by the surgical team in the care of the polytrauma patient. A dialogue on the evaluation of lower extremity and pelvic orthopedic trauma will follow. Information on acute trauma treatment is included because of the critical implication that early "battlefront" management often has on the later rehabilitative aftercare of patients. After presenting an overview of immobility-related disorders in the trauma patient, the chapter will conclude with a brief discussion on the future of trauma rehabilitation. An example of the entire medical and rehabilitation process[47] is schematized in Figure 3.

Trauma: A Look at Epidemiology

Within the United States, trauma is recognized as the major cause of death in people younger than 40.[37] Irrespective of age, trauma is the third most common cause of mortality, accounting for approximately 150,000 deaths annually. Trauma is a leading cause of disability in American society and presently is responsible for 400,000 cases of permanent disability. The economic effect that trauma imposes is astronomic, with current estimates of loss of goods and services exceeding $50 billion annually.[52] As many as one third of all trauma-related deaths in the U.S. are preventable.[7] With the proper emergency, resuscitative, and rehabilitative intervention, the dramatic impact of trauma can be significantly lessened.

Early Emergency, Resuscitative, and Rehabilitative Measures

Rehabilitation can be viewed as a restorative process that *begins* at the scene of an accident! Although the physiatrist is seldom present moments after injury, he or she must be cognizant of the important "trauma rehab" measures carried out by the resuscitation team. In the state of Maryland, well known for its Shock Trauma system, a significant number of trauma patients are surveyed "in the field."[47] The perfection of an expeditious helicopter transport system has optimized emergency treatment.[9,11] Preliminary emphasis is on assessment and timely identification of life-compromising injuries. Airway preservation, stoppage of bleeding, shock reversal, and multisystem organ issues are all priorities.

Preservation of airway patency is essential during the early moments after traumatic injury. Prolonged anoxia can lead to anoxic encephalopathy, a diagnostic entity commonly encountered in rehabilitation.[42] To assure airway maintenance, the oral cavity and posterior pharyngeal region is freed of vomitus and blood, and a determination about ventilatory sufficiency is made. General indications for endotracheal intubation include protracted unconscious status with an absent gag reflex, open thoracic injuries, flail chest, and a hypoxic state.

Since cervical spine injury can occur in the context of polytrauma, patients complaining of neck discomfort and those with loss of consciousness, facial fractures, and lacerations must be carefully evaluated. Persons thought to have compromise of the cervical spine and who require mechanical ventilation should preferentially undergo nasotracheal intubation.

HYPOVOLEMIA AND SHOCK: IMPLICATIONS FOR REHABILITATION

Patients with multiple trauma who have experienced injury-related blood loss and hypovolemic shock have a heightened need for postacute inpatient

Cause and Effect Diagram of a Patient's Medical and Rehabilitation Process

Baseline: 75-year-old married man, retired engineer (restores antique clocks)

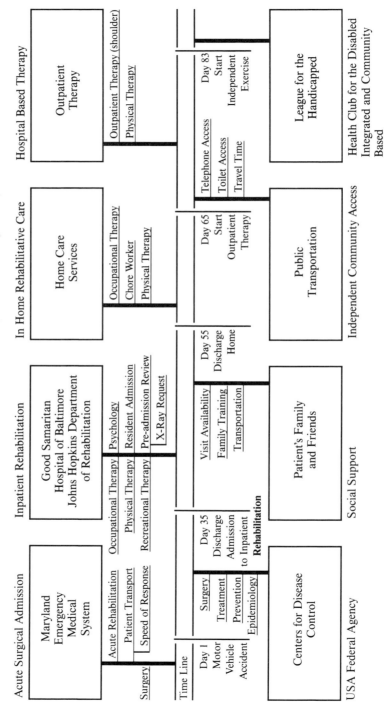

FIGURE 3. An example of the medical and rehabilitation process.

rehabilitation.[46] Bleeding associated with open orthopedic injuries is effectively controlled with simple compression dressings. Compromise to soft tissue structures, nerves, and vessels can sometimes occur with aggressive compressive techniques and vessel clamping. With these interventions, the superficial femoral and brachial artery and veins are the most commonly injured vessels.[16] Occasionally, peripheral nerve injury will become evident during rehabilitation.

Shock is classified according to severity (mild, moderate, severe) depending on the volume of lost blood. Clinical signs of shock include reduction in urinary output, hypotension, and resting tachycardia. The latter are not always present since blood volume must be reduced by 20% (moderate shock) before these clinical indicators are evident. Severe shock is characterized by 40% or greater blood loss and is commonly accompanied by tachycardia, tachypnea, severe hypotension, and metabolic acidosis.

Hypovolemic shock is best treated with volume repletion via large-caliber intravenous catheters. Although the rapid infusion of 2 L of saline solution can be safely accomplished in the hypovolemic patient, a total of 4 L of fluid is needed to compensate for the loss of a single liter of exsanguinated blood. Some centers therefore begin repletion with fresh whole blood or packed red blood cells. Hemodynamic adjustment is carefully monitored by measurement of urinary output and monitoring of hematocrit.

Organ System Assessment: General Approach

Early treatment of the trauma victim with spinal injury and multiple organ involvement has been hampered by the physicians' emphasis on restoring hemovascular integrity.[1] After optimal stabilization of a patient's cardiopulmonary status, a careful systemic assessment of all organ systems must be made. Radiographic survey should include, at the very least, a lateral x-ray of the crevical spine and an upright anteroposterior view of the chest, pelvis, and abdomen.

HEAD AND NECK TRAUMA

Orthopedic polytrauma seldom leaves the spinal region unharmed. Impact injury to the spinal column often results in an unstable, fractured, or malaligned vertebral segment with potential for permanent neurologic damage to spinal cord elements. Motor, sensory, and proprioceptive deficits resulting from insult to the cervical spine are readily detectable in the conscious trauma victim, although immediate recognition of such symptoms are frequently obscured in the obtunded patient.

Vital cranial structures can similarly be adversely affected. Vector forces imposed on the skull in the presence of a flexed neck, a common mechanism in motor vehicle injury, can inflict irreversible damage to cranial structures.[38] Davidoff and his group demonstrated a strong association between closed head injury and spinal cord damage in patients involved in traffic accidents.

The need for timely diagnosis and management of coexisting cervical spine and cranial injury is imperative. Enderson and Maull have characterized "undetected" multiple trauma injuries a "surgeon's nemesis"[15] since hemodynamic instability and altered consciousness tend to obscure underlying injury. Missed injuries are sometimes discovered after transfer to rehabilitation. Occasionally, therapeutic measures implemented during the surgical stabilization of the patient with cervical spine trauma will lead to complications during hospitalization and necessitate close monitoring by the physiatrist.[59]

Brain Injury

After severe head injury, immediate intubation is often necessary to minimize hypoxia and avert added damage to the brain. A thorough neurologic examination is conducted with a view toward pupillary asymmetry, dysconjugate or laterally fixed gaze, and hemiparesis. Often, a patient with lateralizing signs may have an underlying subdural hematoma, cerebral edema, or extradural hematoma. These can increase intracranial pressure and occasionally cause decorticate or decerebrate posturing. When increased intracranial pressure occurs, it may manifest itself subtly, with drowsiness slowly progressing to coma. Patients with extradural hematoma often have temporary unconsciousness followed by an interval of lucidity. In as many as 20% of cases, patients with severe head injury demonstrate the Cushing response, with slowing of pulse and a rise in blood pressure.[3] Computed tomography can aid in the diagnosis of intracranial injuries and has supplanted arteriography. Extradural hematoma typically originates with compromise to the middle meningeal artery. An extradural hematoma is treated as a surgical urgency since expansion of the hematoma, cerebral displacement, and compression can occur at arterial pressure, often resulting in permanent brain damage. Subdural hematomas are characteristically venous in origin and also frequently require evacuation. Frequently, diffuse cerebral edema increases intracranial pressure in the multitrauma patient, necessitating the administration of hyperosmolar agents such as 20% mannitol and corticosteroids, which remain controversial.[3] Ongoing monitoring of these patients is achieved by insertion of a percutaneous catheter into the lateral ventricle. The rehabilitative fate of patients with brain trauma is strongly correlated to neurobehavioral consequences of damage to the central nervous system.[22]

ORTHOPEDIC TRAUMA CONSIDERATIONS

Management of orthopedic injuries in the polytrauma patient has significant implications for morbidity and mortality. Comprehensive early screening is imperative. Head to toe palpation of the appendicular and axial skeleton should be performed. Any areas with abrasion, lacerations, crepitus, or pain with motion should be evaluated with radiographs. This is especially important in the comatose or neurologically impaired patient. Every joint, especially ones with swelling, should be examined for potential bony or ligamentous injury. All lacerations should be explored, preferably with sterile gloves and radiographs obtained to ascertain whether the injury is an open fracture. Any grossly angulated extremity should be carefully assessed and monitored for neurovascular compromise. Correction of a grossly deformed limb with splinting may decrease blood loss and pain. Angiography should be considered when there is suggestion of arterial insufficiency. A thorough examination facilitates triage of the patient and should prevent discovery of injuries later. Once the patient is hospitalized and stable, this examination should be repeated. Adequate delineation of the injuries allows better formulation of a plan for surgical and rehabilitative treatment.

The timing of surgical correction of orthopedic injuries has significance for patient management and rehabilitation. Obviously, surgical treatment of orthopedic injuries in the polytrauma patient can occur only after life-saving procedures such as airway, internal organ, and hemodynamic integrity are safeguarded. Once the patient has been medically stabilized, there is evidence that immediate early fixation of long-bone fractures lowers the incidence of adult respiratory distress syndrome (ARDS), pulmonary sepsis, and mortality.[28] Early fixation of fractures permits better mobilization of the patient, easier pulmonary care, and more timely rehabilitation of the extremity. In one study, the incidence of ARDS was 7% in patients who underwent early fixation and 39% in those with late fixation.[28] Early fixation of fractures also has been shown to decrease the incidence of fat embolism, the need for ventilatory support, the number of days in the intensive care unit, and cost of hosptitalization.[44]

Pelvic Fractures

Assessment of orthopedic injuries includes survey of the pelvis and neighboring anatomic structures. Pelvic fracturs are frequently associated with injuries to the head, chest, abdomen, urogenital structures, rectum, and the vascular tree.[31] Severity of the injury can sometimes be ascertained prior to x-ray by observing pelvic rotation or shortening or rotation of the intact extremity. When pelvic disruption is suspected, urinary catheterization should not be performed until a urethrogram is obtained. A digital exam for concomitant rectal laceration should be performed. Fluid resuscitation and vigilant monitoring of hemodynamic status are essential in patients with suspected pelvic disruption. Hypovolemic shock arising in pelvic injury should be evaluated for other bleeding sources. With severe pelvic fracture, bleeding occurs from venous plexus and occasionally from internal and external iliac vessel laceration. In such situations, angiography may be indicated to define the injury and to embolize the bleeding source. Application of external fixation to an unstable pelvis may decrease bleeding. A cardinal advantage of early stabilization of pelvic ring fractures relates to early mobilization for rehabilitation.

PHYSIATRIC INTERVENTION IN TRAUMA

With adequate stabilization of the acute multitrauma patient, a major challenge confronting the physiatrist is the need to address the insidious effects of deconditioning and immobilization. A variety of organ systems are adversely affected by immobilization, including the integumentary system, muscular system, skeletal system, cardiovascular system, genitourinary system, and gastrointestinal system (Fig. 4).

The Integumentary System

Pressure ulcers are a serious complication of prolonged immobility when soft tissue is compressed between a bony prominence, such as the ischium, sacrum, or trochanter, and a supporting structure such as a bed or wheelchair. Localized areas of necrosis typically result from compression. In early stages, pressure ulcers involve only superficial tissues. Left untreated, the damage extends through fat and muscle and possibly into underlying bone. In extreme cases, bacterial infection of the ulcer may be life-threatening.

According to a recent survey involving 148 acute care hospitals, there was a 9.2% incidence of pressure ulceration among hospitalized patients.[36] An even greater prevalence is known to exist in patients with urinary incontinence.[30]

Skin ulcers are attributable to pressure-induced vascular ischemia, which leads to oxygen and nutrient deprivation of the tissue.[41] Local and systemic factors also contribute to ulceration. Local factors tend to be mechanical, affecting the skin and its superficial layers. These factors include shear forces, skin maceration, edema, and temperature. Animal studies have shown that pressures of 20 mm Hg and upward are necessary to produce skin breakdown.[32] In the presence of shear

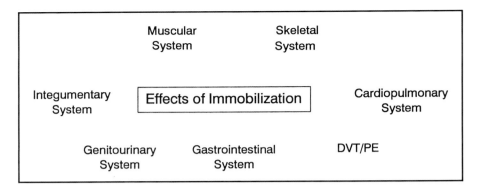

FIGURE 4.   Sytems that are affected by immobilization.

force, the amount of pressure necessary to disrupt the blood flow can be reduced by half.[40] Moisture leads to skin maceration and tissue necrosis by hindering delivery of oxygen and nutrients to the cell.[8] Increased temperature accelerates the metabolic rate of cells. In the absence of adequate blood supply to a cell, ischemia sets in.

Systemic factors critical to the development of pressure ulcers include anemia, malnutrition, and endocrine disorders. Anemia is a significant contributing catalyst that induces cellular hypoxia and necrosis. Malnutrition can amplify this effect by leading to protein insufficiency, which further hinders the healing of pressure ulcers. Hormonal abnormalities such as diabetes can impair metabolism and delay healing. Careful insulin regulation is essential for prevention of ischemic ulcers. Adrenal cortical imbalance also interferes with protein cellular metabolism. Patients with abnormal, insensate, or aging skin are at risk for breakdown since sensory feedback systems are deactivated, resulting in insufficient blood supply.

A classification of skin ulcers is listed in Table 1, and the depth of involvement of pressure ulcers is depicted in Figure 5.

TREATMENT

Prevention is the simplest and most economical method of controlling ulcer formation.[34] For the physiatrist providing consultative service to the acute trauma patient, the essential elements of a prevention program include an integrated team approach emphasizing good medical, nutritional and nursing care, proper patient and family education, timely prescription of pressure relief devices, and a turning-positioning protocol.

TABLE 1.   Classification of Skin Ulcers

Stage	Description
1	Skin area with erythema overlying a bony prominence
2	A superficial ulceration that extends into the dermis
3	An ulcer extending into the subcutaneous tissue but not into muscle
4	Deep ulceration that extends through muscle tissue down to the underlying bony prominence
5	An extensive ulcer with widespread extension along bursae into joints or body cavities

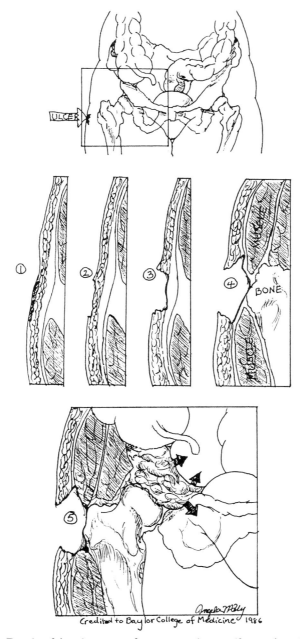

FIGURE 5. Depth of involvement of pressure ulcers. *Above,* site of ulcer. *1,* skin erythema. *2,* superficial ulcer advancing into dermis. *3,* the ulcer penetrates subcutaneously but not into muscle. *4,* the ulcer extends through muscle into bone. *5,* the ulcer encompasses large bursae, involving the joint capsule or penetrating cavities such as the rectum, vagina, or bladder.

Turning is particularly difficult in a patient with multiple trauma. Ideally, turning schedules should consist of 2 hours on the side, 2 hours on the back, and 2 hours on the opposite side.[14] In the supine position, the sacrum and heels are most vulnerable to breakdown. In order to decrease pressure from the sacrum, one should avoid elevation of the head of bed. To protect the heels, the calves are elevated 15° with the calves resting on a pillow. Heel boots also can be worn. For patients who lie on their sides for a long time, the trochanter is the most vulnerable region for breakdown. Preferred posture is a side-lying position in which the inferior leg is flexed 20° at the hip and knee and the superior leg is extended at the hip and flexed 35° at the knee to ensure that the foot and the leg is placed behind the midline of the body. The prone position is most often used following surgery to repair pressure ulcers of the ischium, sacrum, or trochanters. The skin over the knees is the most vulnerable to breakdown in this position. The knees are relieved of pressure by placing a pillow at the shin, hips, chest, and side of the head[13] (Fig. 6).

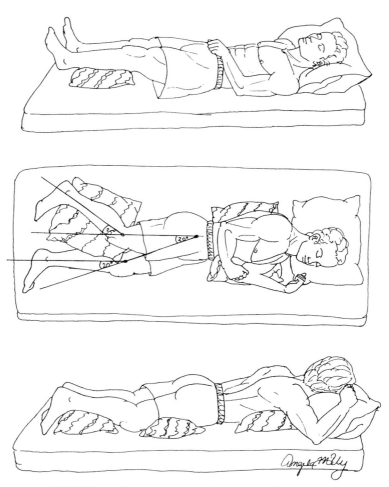

FIGURE 6.   Optimal knee positioning to relieve pressure.

Several types of therapeutic mattresses designed to reduce pressure are available, including the pressure air mattress, air fluidized bed, and the kinetic bed. Ensuring that the skin is neither too dry nor wet helps to foster skin resistance to pressure and bacterial invasion. Optimal mounting of Foley catheterization and other body tubes can help to maintain skin integrity.[57] Maintaining proper nutrition is also essential in maintaining proper oxygenation of the skin.

Conservative Management

The treatment of pressure ulcers is based on a systemic and local approach. The systemic approach has been discussed. The local approach involves grading pressure ulcers based on the local wound characteristics described in the previous grading system and separating the ulcers into conservative (topical therapy with closure by second intention) and surgical treatment groups.[13]

For grade 1 ulcers, a thorough evaluation of extrinsic and intrinsic factors should occur. In particular, measures such as repositioning and turning, proper skin care, and correction of underlying medical risk factors should be instituted.

For grade 2 ulcers, similar measures need to be enforced. In addition, aggressive topical therapy is required to promote wound contraction and reepithelization and thus promote healing by secondary intention. The immediate goal is aggressive debridement of necrotic tissue, suppression of infection, and frequent dressing changes. Many topical agents are available to treat the superficial/deep wounds; however, there is no objective evidence that any of these agents are superior to normal saline wet to dry dressings. Local wound care often depends more on personal preference than on scientific evidence of therapeutic efficacy.[43]

When infection occurs, antibiotics may occasionally play a role. A variety of agents have been applied topically to pressure ulcers for controlling infection. Unfortunately, their use is limited since they often are bacteriostatic and may irritate contiguous tissue. With indiscriminate application, dense fibrosis in the ulcer bed may occur, causing inhibition of capillary budding and suppression of epidermal cells growth. When these events occur, ulcer healing is adversely affected.

Surgical Intervention

Grades 3–5 ulcers will generally require surgical intervention. The goal is to remove necrotic tissue as well as any source of infection and to provide myocutaneous coverage that tolerates pressure, shear, and heat challenges to the tissue's integrity. After the wound heals superficially, deep wound healing can be anticipated in 4–8 weeks.

The Muscular System

Immobility adversely affects muscle strength and size. Additionally, cardiovascular deconditioning predisposes to perceived muscle weakness. In the recumbent position, muscle activity is minimal. With complete bedrest, a muscle will lose 10–15% of its strength per week and 50% in 3–5 weeks.[39] In 2 months, the muscle bulk may shrink to half its original volume. The histologic changes seen in electron microscopy in immobilized muscles after 4–6 weeks include fiber degeneration and an increased proportion of fat and fibrous tissue.[6] Atrophy is due to a decrease in fiber size and not fiber quantity. The first muscles to become weak are those of the lower extremities and the trunk, which resist gravity. Weakness of the quadriceps, gluteus maximus, and back extensors lead to difficulty climbing stairs.

Endurance decreases at a similar rate as muscle strength, and the decrease is attributable to a reduction in metabolic activity related to reduced muscle activity. Decreased oxidative capacity and lowered tolerance to lactic acid and oxygen debt are partially responsible for poor endurance.[25]

Strength gain is best achieved through a regimented progressive resistive exercise program. For a more detailed discussion, the reader is referred elsewhere.[12] Electrical stimulation may be used in isolated muscles or muscle groups to prevent loss of strength or bulk. Quadriceps sets and ankle pumps can be performed in a recumbent position and not only maintain strength but decrease venous stasis by a muscular pumping action. Upright positioning by means of a tilt table helps to strengthen antigravity muscles, as well as improve cardiovascular condition.

The Skeletal System

Bone morphology and density depend on the forces that act on the bone, according to Wolff's law.[53] With immobilization and nonweightbearing situations, normal forces are disrupted. Animals and humans subjected to a weightless state or enforced immobilization are at risk for osteopenia. Intensification of osteoclastic activity and inhibition of osteoblastic activity is thought to occur with immobilization. Several evolutionary stages of bone loss exist.[27] The rate of bone loss is higher in younger individuals and in weightbearing bones. Hormonal abnormalities in geriatric patients may heighten the risk for osteopenia and fracture.[48]

Immobilization leads to osteopenia, which is characterized by the loss of calcium and hydroxyproline from the cancellous bone of long bone epiphyses and metaphyses. Increased resorption of the bone is thought to be a leading mechanism in disuse osteoporosis. Ambulation or partial standing on a tilt table may retard the loss of calcium.[44] Disuse osteoporosis can be prevented by the regular use of isometric and isotonic exercises. Abnormal calcium metabolism can occasionally result in the syndrome of immobilization hypercalcemia. Seen in adolescent boys after spinal cord injury, symptoms include anorexia, abdominal pain, nausea, vomiting, constipation, confusion, and coma. Treatment involves normal saline hydration and furosemide diuresis to promote calcium excretion.

Contractures: Prevention and Therapeutic Intervention

A contracture is defined as a loss of active or passive range of motion due to decreased elasticity in subcutaneous tissue, ligament, muscle, joint capsule, or synovium. Both intrinsic and extrinsic factors are responsible. Intrinsic factors include shortening of collagen fibers in unstretched muscles. Extrinsic factors include imbalance of agonists and antagonists as a consequence of spastic, paralytic or biomechanical conditions. When normal range is not maintained, two joint muscles are the first to shorten. These commonly include the hamstrings, rectus femoris, tensor fasciae latae, erector spinae, and gastrocnemius muscles.[24] The position of maximal comfort in bed, i.e., supine with pillows behind the head, flexed hips, flexed knees, and ankles plantar-flexed, predisposes to contractures.

Cessation of bedrest, proper positioning, and early joint mobilization are of critical importance. If the patient's condition requires more prolonged bed confinement, specific techniques of positioning and stetching are essential. A uniformly firm mattress prevents adverse bed positioning that promotes hip flexion contractures and hinders bed mobility. The use of a trochanteric roll maintains neutral position and prevents hip external rotation and abduction. A foot board or posterior ankle splints limit plantar flexion. The upper extermity is also prone to contracture. The weight of the arm in the recumbent position promotes tightness of the arm adductors and internal rotators. A properly placed pillow can maintain the arm in neutral rotation and abduction. A palmar roll or hand splint can be used to maintain hand, thumb, and finger joints in optimal positions.

Once a contracture has occurred, the primary means of treatment is active and passive range of motion with a sustained terminal stretch. For mild contracture, a short sustained stretch lasting 20–30 minutes twice a day may be effective.[33] The stretch is even more effective with the use of heat application to the musculotendinous junction or joint capsule. Ultrasound as a heat source is the most popular for large joints. Its properties allow therapeutic heating of 40–43°C, which increases the elasticity of the connective tissue, maximizing its tendency to stretch.[24] For more severe contractures that require sustained stretch of at least 2 hours, serial casting or dynamic splinting can be very helpful. Serial casting is the application of plaster or polymer bandages with careful padding over bony prominences. The cast is applied immediately after heat and manual stretch have been applied to obtain maximal range of motion. After the initial cast has been applied for 2–3 days, it should be removed and skin should be checked for pressure areas. The cast can be reapplied every 2–5 days. Serial casting is particularly effective for plantar flexion and knee contractures.

Dynamic splinting is an intervention that allows for repeated stretch with a spring or elastic band providing tension in the desired direction. This type of splinting is often used in the hand and the arm. The continuous passive mobilization device has become relatively routine for knee postoperative range of motion and has recently been applied to other joints. Continuous passive motion is recommended for the early mobilization of hip and knee fractures, synovectomized joints, ligamentous repairs, total knee joint replacement, any arthrogenic contractures, or infected joints.[4] Early passive ranging with continuous passive motion has been shown to promote the exchange of joint fluid, prevent contractures, and reduce the need for pain medication after surgery.

The Genitourinary System

Indwelling urethral catheterization is often unavoidable immediately postoperatively. However, the catheter should be discontinued as soon as possible to reduce the risk of urinary infection, injury to the urethra, and deconditioning of the detrussor. Postvoid residuals are helpful to determine the adequacy of emptying.

With prolonged immobilization there is an increased incidence of bladder/renal stones and urinary tract infections. This is related to hypercalciuria, phosphaturia, and urinary stasis. Patients often find it difficult to initiate voiding in the supine position. This results from reduced intraabdominal pressure secondary to abdominal muscle weakness, restricted diaphragmatic movement, and incomplete relaxation of the pelvic floor. Incomplete bladder emptying results in an ideal situation for stone formation. Bladder stones provide a nidus for bacterial growth and infection.[35]

Important treatment principles include adequate fluid intake, voiding in the upright or sitting position, and avoidance of bladder contamination during instrumentation. Other treatment approaches include acidification of urine and urinary antiseptics.

TABLE 2.   Factors Contributing to Nutritonal Deficiencies
in the Trauma Rehabilitation Patient

Loss of mobility and secretory function of digestive glands as a result of increased adrenergic activity
Loss of appetite resulting from anxiety and depression
Distaste for protein-rich foods
Constipation due to reduction of peristalsis, aggravated by poor fluid intake and lack of ingestion of high-fiber residue[24]

The Gastrointestinal System

Prolonged immobilization can lead to nutritional hypoproteinemia. The four main factors that contribute to nutritional deficiency are outlined in Table 2.

To prevent constipation due to inactivity, it is important to implement a bowel training program that includes a fiber-rich diet and adequate fluids, scheduled bowel movement, and the use of stool softeners, glycerin, or peristaltic stimulating suppositories.[26]

The Cardiovascular System

With bedrest, a progressive rise in the resting heart rate by 0.5 beats per minute per day occurs. The result is immobilization tachycardia and an abnormal pulse with submaximal exertion. After 2 weeks of bedrest, there is a 15% reduction in stroke volume, which is linked to blood volume reduction and lower extremity pooling of blood. Maximal oxygen consumption or VO_2 max declines dramatically with bedrest. Postural hypotension can result from prolonged bedrest and is due to the circulatory system's inability to adjust to the upright position. Orthostatic hypotension can manifest itself with dizziness, lightheadedness, vertigo, tachycardia, and decreased systolic pressure. Early mobilization and conditioning exercises should be initiated when medically and orthopedically feasible. Other measures to be used in patients with orthostatic hypotension include fluid and salt intake, reclining backs, elevating leg rests, tilt table tolerance building, abdominal binders, and compression stockings. Occasionally, sympathomimetic agents such as ephedrine and phenylephrine are used in the multitrauma patient. The presence of sustained cardiovascular aberrations including rhythm abnormalities, angina, and erratic blood pressure and pulse response to exercise mandate an intensive cardiac work-up.

Venous Thromboembolism Prevention in the Trauma Patient

Deep vein thrombosis and pulmonary embolism are major causes of mortality in hospitalized trauma rehabilitation patients. One autopsy study[45] revealed a deep venous thrombosis incidence of 65% in the multiple trauma patient. Increased age and length of immobilization were found to be highly correlated. Virchow's triad of stasis, intimal injury, and hypercoagulability are thought to be the major factors underlying the high incidence of thromboembolic event.

The most common way to prevent thromboembolic complications in the trauma rehabilitation patient is with subcutaneous heparin and support stockings. A regimen of 5,000 units subcutaneously twice daily is customary, although thrombocytopenia and thrombosis syndrome (HATT) can rarely occur.[58] Since patients with generalized weakness, deconditioning, incoordination, and poor balance are often at risk for falls and other exercise-induced mishaps during therapy, treatment modalities that diminish risk of bleeding may be advantageous.[56]

The recent introduction of low-molecular-weight heparin may hold promise because of its lower incidence of bleeding.

Since trauma patients often have associated injuries that are an absolute contraindication for anticoagulation, nonpharmacologic treatment options are often needed. Although intermittent pneumatic compression has proven helpful, its use is limited to patients without lower extermity casts, fractures, or occlusive bandages. For patients with extensive trauma who are ineligible for other forms of prophylaxis, vena cava filter insertion should be considered. Since pulmonary embolism is a significant cause of mortality among asymptomatic rehabilitation patients and often results in thousands of preventable deaths annually, the effect of sudden alterations in intrathoracic and intraabdominal pressure associated with the Valsalva maneuver as a cause for clot propagation should be further investigated.[5]

TRAUMA REHABILITATION: A LOOK AT THE FUTURE

With the dramatic rise in the incidence of trauma and the ongoing perfection of resuscitative techniques, there is likely to be an increased number of multitrauma patients requiring rehabilitation medicine services. As a result of this trend, the specialist in physical medicine and rehabilitation will play a dynamic role in the rehabilitation after care of this challenging population. Maximizing function and minimizing dependence through intensive physiatric intervention will enable the patient to enjoy an enhanced quality of life in the aftermath of major trauma.

ACKNOWLEDGMENT

The authors would like to acknowledge the contribution of Samantha Langer, who assisted in the editing of this chapter.

REFERENCES

1. Albuquerque F, Wolf A, Dunham CM, et al: Frequency of intra-abdominal injury in cases of blunt trauma to cervical spinal cord injury. J Spinal Disord 5:476–480, 1992.
2. Arnold JS, Bartley MH: Skeletal changes in aging and disease. Clin Orthop 49:17–38, 1966.
3. Bakay L: Brain injuries in polytrauma. World J Surg 7:42–48, 1993.
4. Bentham JS, Brereton WDS, Cochrane IW, Lyttle D: Continuous passive motion device for hand rehabilitation. Arch Phys Med Rehabil 68:248–250, 1987.
5. Berkin D, Young MA, Johnston JR: Valsalva maneuver: A risk factor for pulmonary embolism? [abstract]. Arch Phys Med Rehabil 74:669, 1993.
6. Booth FW, Gollnick PD: Effects of disuse on the structure and function of skeletal muscle. Med Sci Sports Exerc 15:415–420, 1983.
7. Bone L, Bucholz R: The management of fractures in the patient with multiple trauma. J Bone Joint Surg 68A:945–949, 1986.
8. Caly CH, Chimoskey JE, Holloway GA, et al: The effect of pressure leading on the blood flow rate in human skin. In Kenedi RM (ed): Bedsore Biomechanics. Baltimore, University Park Press, 1976, pp 69–77.
9. Cooper C, Militello P: The multi-injured patient: The Maryland Shock Trauma protocol approach. Semin Thorac Cardiovasc Surg 4:163–167, 1992.
10. Cowley RA, Dunham CM: Shock Trauma/Critical Care Manual. Initial Assessment and Management. Baltimore, University Park Press, 1982.
11. Davies S: Trauma treatment in Maryland. Nursing Times 86(33):58–62, 1990.
12. deLateur BJ (ed): Exercise. Phys Med Rehabil Clin North Am 5:243–395, 1994.
13. Donovan WH, Garber SL, Hamilton SM, et al: Pressure ulcers. In DeLisa JA (ed): Rehabilitation Medicine: Principles and Practice. Philadelphia, JB Lippincott, 1988, pp 476–491.
14. Dowling AS: Presure sores: Their cause, prevention and treatment. Maryland State Med J 6:131–134, 1970.
15. Enderson BL, Maull KI: Missed injuries. The Trauma Surgeon's Nemesis. Surg Clin North Am 71:399–418, 1991.

16. Feliciani DV: Peripheral vascular injuries in early care of the injured patient. pp 235–240.
17. French JJ, Kummell J, Siebens AA: Adapting the "Hopkins speaking valve" for use with a Shiley cannula. Proceedings of the 14th annual conference of RESNA, Kansas City, MO, June 1991, pp 376–378.
18. Garber SL, Campion LJ, Krouskop TA: Trochanteric pressure in spinal cord injury. Arch Phys Med Rehabil 63:549–552, 1982.
19. Gersten JW: Effect of ultrasound on tendon extensibility. Am J Phys Med 34:360–362, 1955.
20. Gertner RJ Jr, Baker SP, Rutherford RB, Spitz WU: Evaluation of the management of vehicular fatalities secondary to abdominal injury. J Trauma 12:425–431, 1972.
21. Goris RJ: Early osteosynthesis and prophylactic mechanical ventilation in the multitrauma patient.
22. Groswasser Z, Cohen M, Blankstein E: Polytrauma associated with TBI: Incidence, nature and impact on rehabilitation outcome. Brain Injury 4:161–166, 1990.
23. Halar EM, Bell KR: Contracture and other deleterious effects of immobility. In DeLisa JA (ed): Rehabilitation Medicine: Principles and Practice. Philadelphia, JB Lippincott, 1988, pp 448–462.
24. Halar EM, Bell KR: Rehabilitation's relationship to inactivity. In Kottke FJ, Lehmann JF (eds): Krusen's Handbook of Physical Medicine and Rehabilitation. 4th ed. Philadelphia, WB Saunders, 1990, p 1113.
25. Henriksson R, Reitman JS: Time courses of change in human skeletal muscle succinate dehydrogenase and cytochrome oxidase activity and maximal uptake with physical activity and inactivity. Acta Physiol Scand 99:91–97, 1977.
26. Ivy AC, Grossman MI: Gastrointestinal function in convalescence. In Symposium on Physiological Aspects of Convalescence and Rehabilitation. Fed Proc 3:236–239.
27. Jaworski ZFG (ed): Proceedings of the First Workshop on Bone Histomorphometry. Ottawa, University of Ottawa Press, 1976.
28. Johnson KD, Cadambi A, Seibert GB: Incidence of ARDS in patients with multiple musculoskeletal injury: Effect of early operative stabilization of fractures. J Trauma 25:375–384, 1985.
29. Johnston J, Linden P, Kashima H, et al: Management of upper airway complications following head and spinal trauma [abstract]. Arch Phys Med Rehabil 61:484, 1980.
30. Jordan MM, Clark MO: Report of Incidence of Pressure Sores in the Patient Community of the Greater Glasgow Health Board Area. Strathclyde, Scotland, University of Strathclyde, January 21, 1977.
31. Kellam JF, Browner BD: Fractures of the Pelvic Ring. In Browner BD, Jupiter JJ, Levine AM, Tafton PF (eds): Skeletal Trauma. Philadelphia, WB Saunders, 1992, pp 849–922.
32. Kosiak M: Etiology and pathology of ischemic ulcers. Arch Phys Med Rehabil 40:62–69, 1959.
33. Kottke FJ, Pauley DL, Ptka RA: The rationale for prolonged stretching for correction for shortening of connective tissue. Arch Phys Rehabil Med 47:345–352, 1966.
34. Krouskop TA, Noble P, Garber SL, Spencer WA: The effectiveness of preventive management in reducing the occurrence of pressure sores. J Rehabil Res Dev 20:73–83, 1983.
35. Leadbetter WF, Engster HE: Problems of renal lithiasis in convalescent patients. J Urol 53:269, 1957.
36. Meehan M: Multisite Pressure Ulcer Prevalence Survey. Decubitus 3(4):14–17, 1990.
37. Merli GJ: Medical consultation in the patient with multiple trauma. Med Clin North Am 77:493–507, 1993.
38. Miller JG, Pentland B, Berrol S: Early evaluation and management. In Rosenthal M, Griffith ER, Bond MR, Miler JD (eds): Rehabilitation of the Adult and Child with Traumatic Brain Injury. 2nd ed. Philadelphia, FA Davis, 1990, pp 21–51.
39. Mueller EA: Influence of training and inactivity on muscle strength. Arch Phys Med Rehabil 51:449–462, 1970.
40. Murphy E: Transferring load to flesh: I. Concept. Bull Prosthet Res 10(Fall):38–44, 1971.
41. Nichol J, Girling F, Jerrard W, et al: Fundamental instability of small blood vessels and critical closing pressures in vascular beds. Am J Physiol 164:330–344, 1951.
42. Parkin AJ, Miller J, Vincent R: Multiple neuropsychological deficits due to anoxic encephalopathy: A case study. Cortex 23:655–665, 1987.
43. Petro JA: Ethical dilemmas of pressure ulcers. Decubitus 3(2):28–31, 1990.
44. Riska EB: Fat embolism in patients with multiple injury. J Trauma 22:891–894, 1982.
45. Sevitt S, Gallagher N: Venous thromboembolism and pulmonary embolism: A clinico-pathological study in injured and burned patients. Br J Surg 48:475–489, 1961.
46. Siegel JH, Gens DR, Mamantov T, et al: Effect of associated injuries and blood volume replacement on death, rehabilitation needs, and disability in blunt traumatic brain injury. Crit Care Med 19:1251–1265, 1991.

47. Stiens SA, Young MA, O'Young BJ: Trauma rehabilitation in the USA: A local, state and national systems perspective. Presented at the 1994 International Rehabilitation Medicine Association World Congress.
48. Swartz CM, Young MA: Male hypogonadism and bone fracture [letter]. N Engl J Med 318:996, 1988.
49. Sweeney JF, Rosemurgy AS, Gill S, Albrink MH: Is the cervical spine clear? Undetected cervical fractures diagnosed only at autopsy. Ann Emerg Med 21:1288–1290, 1992.
50. Tippett DC, Siebens AA: Using ventilators for speaking and swallowing. Dysphagia 6920:94–99, 1991.
51. Tippett DC, Siebens AA, Lynch CQ, French J: Oral communication in tracheotomized and ventilator-dependent individuals. Arch Phys Med Rehabil 71:789, 1990.
52. Tortella BJ: Trunkey trauma care system. Trauma Q 1:17, 1984.
53. Uhthoff HK, Jaworski ZFG: Bone loss in response to long term immobilization. J Bone Joint Surg 60B:420–429, 1978.
54. Young MA: Rehabilitation makes dysphagia easier to swallow [letter]. J Clin Gastroenterol 17:179, 1993.
55. Young MA: Where all diseases meet: At physiatry. Med Trib August 21, 1993.
56. Young MA: Subcutaneous compared with intravenous heparin for deep vein thrombosis [letter]. Ann Intern Med 117:265, 1992.
57. Young MA, Ehrenpreis ED: Transparent dressing: A new technique for securing nasogastric tubes in CV patients [abstract]. Arch Phys Med Rehabil 69:787, 1988.
58. Young MA, Ehrenpreis ED, Ehrenpreis M, Kirschblum S: Heparin associated thrombocytopenia and thrombosis syndrome in a rehabilitation patient. Arch Phys Med Rehabil 70:468–470, 1989.
59. Young MA, Walko E: The halo orthosis in TBI rehabilitation: A simple technique for assessing migration. Proceedings of the Postgraduate Course on Rehabilitation of the Brain Injured Adult and Child. Williamsburg, VA.

SULABHA MASIH, MD
RAJNIKANT BAKHDA, MD

IMAGING MODALITIES IN DIAGNOSIS AND MANAGEMENT OF FRACTURES

From the West L.A. Veterans
 Affairs Medical Center
Los Angeles, California

Reprint requests to:
Sulabha Masih, MD
West L.A. Veterans Affairs
 Medical Center
Department of Radiology
Los Angeles, CA 90073

The diagnosis and treatment of skeletal trauma was revolutionized by the discovery of x-rays in 1896. Radiology plays a vital role in the evaluation of trauma by providing adequate diagnosis. Plain films are still the primary imaging technique. Serial films are usually taken to document the progress of healing and diagnose any complications. Technical advances in the field of diagnostic imaging assist in the diagnosis of fractures, surgical management, and rehabilitation.

The vastly expanding and newer imaging modalities often make it difficult to choose the right imaging modality. The choices confronting the clinician include the following:[13a,25]

1. Plain films, including initial and follow-up films
2. Conventional tomograms
3. Fluoroscopy
4. Computed tomography (CT) scan
5. Magnetic resonance imaging (MRI)
6. Radionuclide bone scan
7. Arthrography
8. Angiography
9. Myelography

Plain films generally are sufficient to make a diagnosis. As a rule, films are taken in two planes, perpendicular to each other: anteroposterior (AP) and lateral views. At times, oblique views are necessary to make the diagnosis. At least one joint above and one joint below the suspected site of fracture should be included in the films to evaluate a possible subluxation or dislocation (Fig. 1). Comparison films of the opposite extremity greatly assist in making a

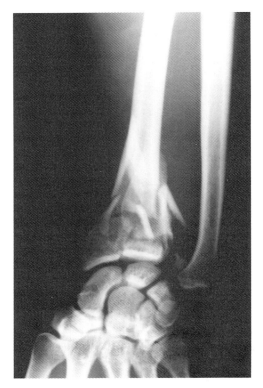

FIGURE 1. AP view of the wrist shows Galleazzi fracture, a comminuted fracture of distal radius with extension into the distal radio-ulnar joint with loose bony fragments. Note the fracture of the distal ulna and dislocation of the distal radio-ulnar joint.

diagnosis of subtle fractures in children. However, to reduce unnecessary radiation to children, comparison views should not be requested routinely.[9]

Follow-up films are valuable in undisplaced fractures, especially when the fractures are undetected on initial films. After a few days following the trauma there is bone resorption along the fracture margins, making it easier to make the diagnosis. Callus begins to form 2–3 weeks after trauma, and in some cases it may be the first time the presence of a fracture is appreciated.

Follow-up films are also required immediately after reduction or postoperatively to check on the satisfactory position of fractures and reduction of any subluxation or dislocation. These films occasionally are done with a portable machine and with a plaster cast, but the details are poor, and conventional tomograms may be necessary. After the initial post-therapy films are done, follow-up x-rays should be done after 2–3 weeks. These films will help to ensure that the alignment of the fragments is satisfactory and there is evidence of callus formation. Fracture healing is seen as early as 2–3 weeks after trauma by the presence of endosteal and periosteal callus formation. At times periosteal reaction develops before callus forms. At this stage the orthopedist may institute further measures as needed or decide to continue without any change in therapy. Assuming all is well, the patient is x-rayed again at 2- to 3-week intervals until there is reabsorption of callus and bony union. The fracture line remains visible for quite some time after clinical union. Any complications will be picked up on serial films. Comparison with previous films is absolutely essential to detect any complications.[19]

In difficult cases conventional tomograms may assist in making the diagnosis. Tomograms are particularly helpful in spinal and pelvic fractures and stress fractures undiagnosed on plain films.

A CT scan is more accurate in diagnosing intraarticular loose bony fragments and fractures of skull, facial bones, pelvis, spine, and ankle (Fig. 2).[5,13,16] If there is overlying hardware, the plain tomograms may show artifacts. Unfortunately, the metallic devices used in treatment of fractures produce similar problems in CT scans. Since CT scans are three-dimensional, they provide better contrast resolution than plain tomograms. CT scans with axial and reconstructed sagittal and coronal views give additional information and help in diagnosing associated injuries to the soft tissues and vascular structures.

MRI is more sensitive to soft tissue definition than CT scanning. MRI is especially good in the assessment of ligamentous injuries, articular injuries, and occult trauma with bone bruise.[1,7,8] Currently, CT scanning is more readily available and cheaper than MRI. As our experience with MRI increases and more scanners are available, it is possible that MRI may replace CT scanning in the evaluation of trauma (Figs. 3, 4, and 5).

COMMON TERMS USED IN MRI

With MRI, images are produced by interactions among the homogenous external magnetic fields, radiofrequency waves, and hydrogen nuclei. The magnetic field is produced by using a magnet with a field strength of 0.3–1.5 T; 1 T is equal to 10,000 G. The earth's magnetic field is approximately 0.6 G. Hydrogen is the

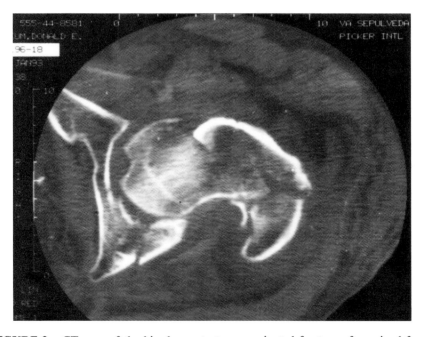

FIGURE 2.   CT scan of the hip demonstrates comminuted fracture of proximal femur with multiple loose bony fragments. The fracture of inferior acetabular rim extends into the hip joint, which was not evident on plain films.

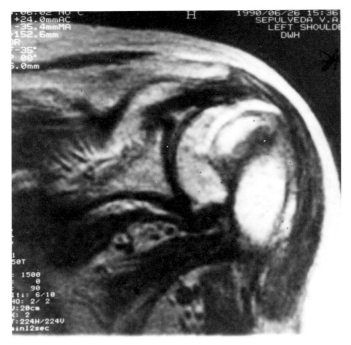

FIGURE 3.   MRI of the shoulder, T2-weighted coronal oblique image, shows comminuted fracture of the head of the humerus with atrophy of the supraspinatus muscle and chronic tear at the musculotendinous junction.

ideal atom for medical imaging, because the hydrogen nucleus has only one proton and it is abundant in human body, making up to two-thirds of all the atoms.

Under normal circumstances, protons in the human body have random orientation. Their small magnetic fields cancel each other with no net magnetization. When the protons in the body are exposed to an external magnetic field, some will align in the direction of the applied field and some in the opposite direction. This creates net magnetization, which is used in MR imaging. T1- and T2-weighted images are usually obtained.

T1 is characterized by a short TR/TE < 1000 msec/50. T2 has longer TR/TE (TR = repetition time; TE = echo time). Proton density images have short TE and longer TR.

Signal intensities of different tissues are as follows: T1, high-signal intensity (white) is seen in fat and bone marrow. Intermediate-signal intensity (gray) is noted in muscles, infection, and tumor. Low-signal intensity (black) is noted in cortical bone, ligaments, tendons, and fluid.

FIGURE 4 (Facing page, top).   MRI of the knee, T1-weighted sagittal image, demonstrates an inhomogeneous increased signal (white) in the medial femoral condyle consistent with bone bruise. No fracture is seen. The plain films were unremarkable. (See Figure 5.)

FIGURE 5 (Facing page, bottom).   MRI of the knee, T2-weighted sagittal image (same patient as in Figure 4) shows nonvisualization of anterior cruciate ligament, indicating a tear. Note the normal posterior cruciate ligament.

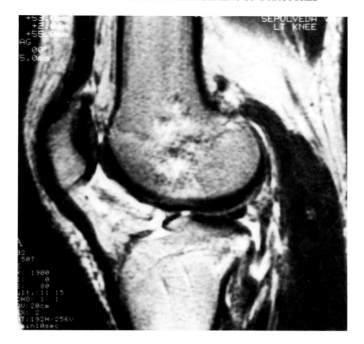

FIGURE 4

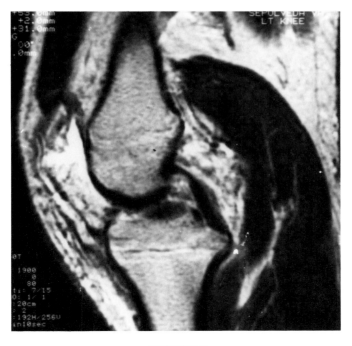

FIGURE 5

TABLE 1.   Signal Characteristics of Different Tissues on MRI

Tissue	T1	T2
Fat	White (Increased signal)	White
Marrow	White	White
Muscle	Gray (Intermediate signal)	Gray
Tumor	Gray	White
Infection	Gray	White
Normal fluid, CSF	Black (Decreased signal)	White
Ligaments	Black	Black
Tendons	Black	Black
Cortical bone	Black	Black
Fibrous tissue	Black	Black

On T2, high-signal intensity (white) is seen in fat, bone marrow, tumor, infection, and fluids. Intermediate-signal (gray) is noted in muscles, and low-signal (black) is seen in cortical bone, ligaments, and tendons (Table 1).

In certain cases when the plain films do not show a fracture and there is a strong suspicion of a fracture, a radionuclide bone scan will confirm the presence of a fracture by demonstrating increased uptake of the radioisotope. In selected cases of suspected vascular or spinal cord injury, an angiogram or a myelogram may be required to demonstrate injury to the neighboring vascular structures or the spinal cord or the spinal nerves. An arthrogram can be done to diagnose damage to the articular cartilage and ligaments (Fig. 6). Currently, the same information is obtained noninvasively with MRI.

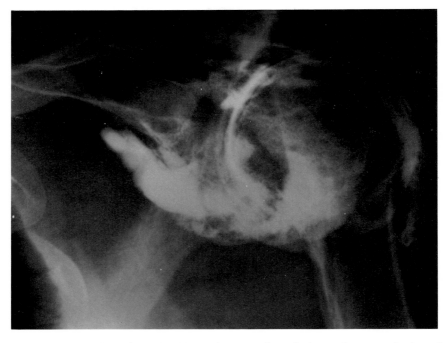

FIGURE 6.   AP view of the shoulder arthrogram shows leakage of contrast in the sub-acromial and subdeltoid bursa, indicating a rotator cuff tear.

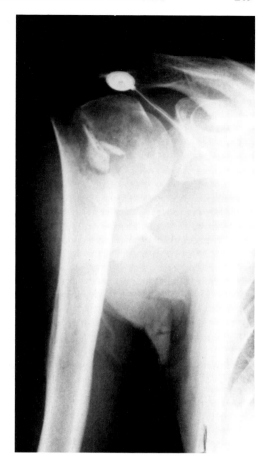

FIGURE 7. AP view of the shoulder demonstrates a comminuted fracture of the head and neck of humerus with loose bony fragments. There is poor alignment with an angulation deformity.

RADIOGRAPHIC FINDINGS IN FRACTURES

On plain films one should check the cortex, trabeculae, and the soft tissues. A subtle fracture may be diagnosed by disruption of the cortex or trabeculae, as in the case of fracture of the neck of femur. When evaluating films in a case of trauma, one should look for the following features:[13a]

1. Degree of apposition of fractures. Look for displacement of bony fragments.
2. Alignment of fragments with respect to lines of weightbearing (Fig. 7).
3. Degree of torsion of fragments, with respect to one another.
4. Degree of shortening of the bone. Compare with the opposite side. Check for angulation between the fragments.
5. Assessment of surrounding soft tissues for displacement of fat and normal soft tissue planes. This is particularly useful around the joints, including the knee, elbow, wrist, shoulder, and the pelvis. Displacement of normal structures such as liver, spleen, urinary bladder, or bowel indicates associated trauma.
6. Involvement of adjacent joints for dislocation, subluxation, or diastasis (Fig. 8).

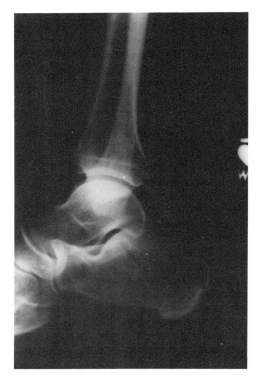

FIGURE 8. Lateral view of the ankle shows a comminuted fracture of calcaneum with extension into the subtalar joint.

7. Check for both intra- and extraarticular loose bony fragments (Fig. 9). In cases of spinal trauma one needs to assess the proximity of the bony fragment to the spinal cord and whether there is any compression of the spinal cord. This is best seen on a CT scan.
8. Determine whether the fracture is simple or comminuted (*see* Fig. 7). A fracture is called simple when there is no break in skin and compound when there is a break.
9. In children, look for the displacement and separation of epiphyses. Comparison with opposite side is quite useful.

The presence of an abnormal fat pad, such as in the elbow, indicates a fracture even if a fracture is not obvious (Fig. 10). A fracture of the head of radius is often difficult to see. A posterior fat pad, or elevation of the anterior fat pad, indicates an effusion in an intact joint and is suggestive of a fracture. The patient is treated for a fracture on the basis of a positive fat pad sign. Normally the posterior fat pad is absent and the anterior fat pad is closely applied to the anterior surface of the distal humerus.[14]

In some instances, a film taken with a horizontal beam, like a decubitus film, may show a fat-fluid level indicating a fracture. This is caused by fat floating on blood. This sign is particularly useful in the sinuses and sometimes in the shoulder and the knee.[9]

A periosteal reaction in a trauma case indicates an occult fracture. Soft tissue swelling is usually present in cases of fracture or dislocation. An absence of soft tissue swelling goes against the diagnosis of a fracture or dislocation.[9]

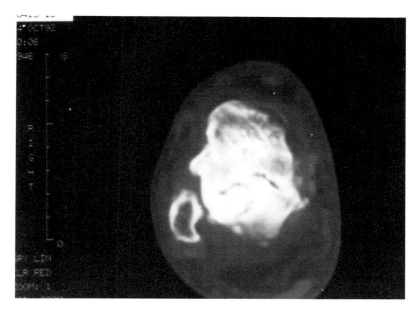

FIGURE 9. CT scan of the calcaneum shows a comminuted fracture with loose bony fragments.

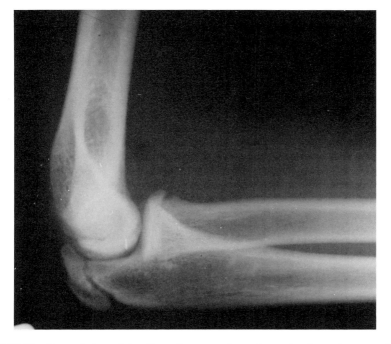

FIGURE 10. Lateral view of the elbow shows an elevated anterior fat pad, a posterior fat pad (difficult to see on reproduction), and a fracture of the olecranon process.

TYPES OF FRACTURES

To manage the patient's injuries, a thorough description of a fracture is important in communicating with the orthopedist and other health professionals. There are many different types of fractures. The main types are discussed below.

Oblique, Spiral and Transverse Fractures. These fractures are named according to the direction of the fracture line in relation to the long axis of the involved bones. There may be interposition of soft tissues between the fragments, which is difficult to visualize on plain films. Oblique and spiral fractures are common in the shafts of long bones. Transverse fractures are less common and are seen when a bending force is responsible for the injury. A fracture line extends at a right angle to the long axis of the bone.

Comminuted Fracture. A fracture that creates two or more fragments is called a comminuted fracture (*see* Figs. 1, 8, and 9).

Pathologic Fracture. Radiographic distinction between pathologic and regular fractures is not always easy. In some of these cases, history of the injury may be absent. The fracture appears in an area of preexisting bony abnormality. There are usually areas of decreased bone density as in metastases. Sometimes there is increased bone density, as in cases of Paget's disease. Other radiologic features are altered trabeculae or density and deformity. The common causes of a pathologic fracture are primary or metastatic tumors and infection (Figs. 11 and 12).

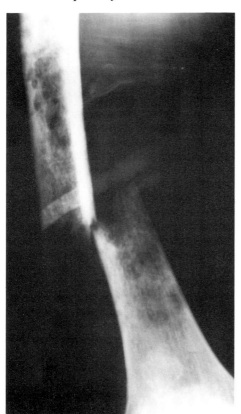

FIGURE 11. AP view of the femur with lytic metastases from a carcinoma of the lung. Note the pathologic fracture of mid shaft of the femur with displacement and poor alignment.

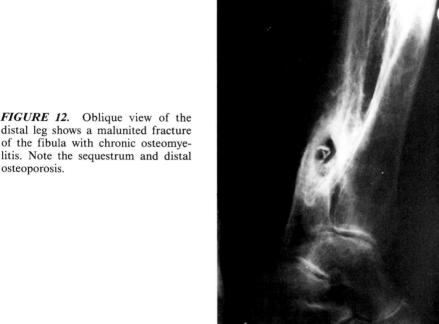

FIGURE 12. Oblique view of the distal leg shows a malunited fracture of the fibula with chronic osteomyelitis. Note the sequestrum and distal osteoporosis.

Stress Fracture. Stress fractures can occur in normal or in abnormal bone and commonly involve the lower extremity. There are two types of stress fractures. In *fatigue fracture*, there is abnormal stress with normal elastic resistance—for instance, the so-called "march fracture" in the metatarsals. *Insufficiency fracture* is associated with normal stress but deficient elastic resistance, as in rheumatoid arthritis or Paget's disease. In the upper extremity or the spine, stress fractures are less frequent.[3]

In the diaphysis there is a linear radiolucent line in the cortex with or without periosteal or endosteal thickening. Epiphyses and cancellous bones mainly show sclerosis. Neural arch of the vertebra shows a spondylolysis or a break in pars interarticularis (Fig. 13) that may be associated with a spondylolisthesis. Lumbar vertebra are usually involved. The fifth lumbar vertebra is involved in 67% and the fourth lumbar vertebra is involved in 25–30% of cases. Males are three times more commonly affected than females. Oblique views show the "Scotty dog" appearance. A break in pars interarticularis shows as a radiolucent line (collar) across the neck of the Scotty dog.

Incomplete Fractures. Incomplete fractures affect only one cortex and do not involve the medullary cavity. The proximal metaphysis and diaphysis of tibia and middle thirds of the radius and ulna are common sites for incomplete fractures. Greenstick fractures and bowing of bones in children are incomplete fractures (Fig. 14).

Salter Harris Fracture. There are many variants of this type of fracture, which occurs in children and may involve the growth plate. These fractures

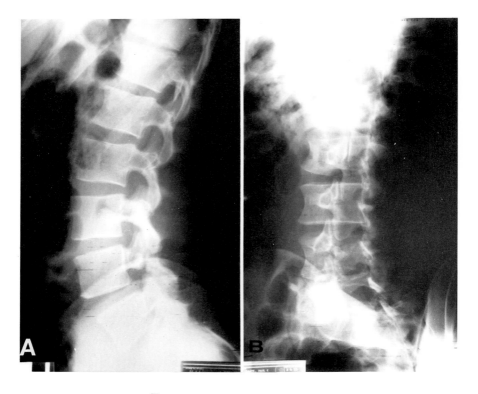

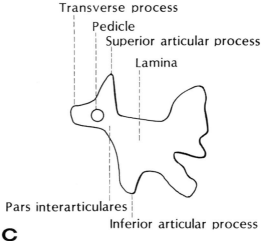

FIGURE 13. *A,* lateral view of the lumbar spine. *B,* oblique view of the lumbar spine. *C,* line drawing of the oblique view. There is a break in pars interarticularis at L4 seen as a radiolucent line (collar) across the neck of the "Scotty dog." There is no evidence of spondylolisthesis.

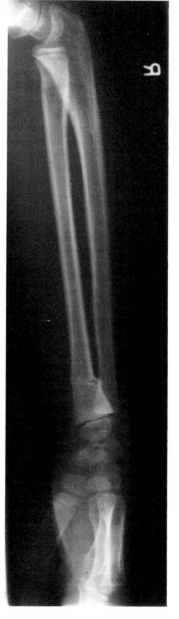

FIGURE 14.   Lateral view of the forearm showing an incomplete (greenstick) fracture of the distal radius.

can be difficult to detect, because the only findings may be widening or narrowing of the growth plate. Films of the opposite side for comparison are invaluable.

   Avulsion or Chip Fractures.   These are associated with forcible injury of ligaments, tendons, and muscle attachments (Fig. 15).

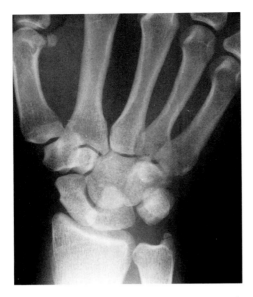

FIGURE 15. AP view of the wrist shows a chip fracture of the ulnar styloid process. Note lunate dislocation shown by the triangular shape of lunate. (Lateral film of this case is seen in Figure 20).

Compression Fracture.   Compression fractures are common in the spine. The diagnosis is evident on plain films. If there is a question of associated involvement of spinal cord or spinal nerves, a myelogram or MRI will help make the diagnosis. MRI is superior because it lacks ionizing radiation and is noninvasive. In cases of spinal trauma, one should always look for loss of alignment. At the level of the upper cervical spine, atlanto-axial subluxation is judged on the lateral film. The distance between the anterior arch of atlas and the odontoid process should be less than 3 mm. If it measures more than 3 mm, a diagnosis of atlanto-axial subluxation is made. In children up to the age of 8 this measurement can be 4 mm under normal circumstances. Lateral films in flexion and extension help in evaluating abnormal motion and loss of alignment.

Transchondral Fractures.   Also called osteochondritis dissecans, transchondral fractures are caused by a fragmentation of a portion of articular surface with or without separation (Fig. 16). They can either be familial or caused by trauma. The diagnosis is made either on plain films or conventional tomograms. Double contrast arthrograms or MRI may also be used for diagnosis. The common sites are the distal femur, patella, talus, elbow, and wrist. Roentgenographic characteristics are linear radiolucent fracture line in the subchondral bone with or without fragmentation.

Depressed Fracture.   They show as a single or double cortical lines. The skull is a common site for depressed fractures (Fig. 17).

Other Common Fractures of Interest

Bennett's fracture is a fracture at the base of the first metacarpal extending into the intraarticular region. This type of fracture may be associated with a carpo-metacarpal dislocation.[26]

Colles' fracture is a fracture of the distal radius with dorsal displacement of the distal fragment, causing a "dinner fork" deformity. This is usually associated with a chip fracture of the ulnar styloid process.[18]

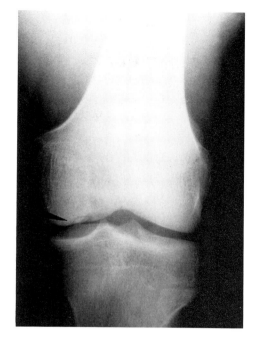

FIGURE 16. AP view of the knee demonstrates osteochondritis dissecans. There is a radiolucent ring surrounding an undisplaced elliptical bony fragment in the medial femoral condyle.

Smith fracture, which is relatively less common than Colles' fracture, is a fracture of the distal radius with a ventral displacement of the distal fragment.[18]

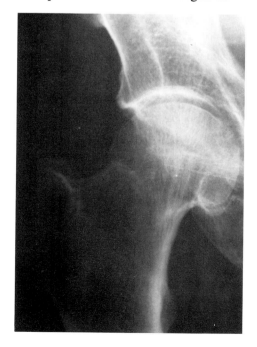

FIGURE 17. AP view of the hip demonstrates an impacted fracture, shown as a white line.

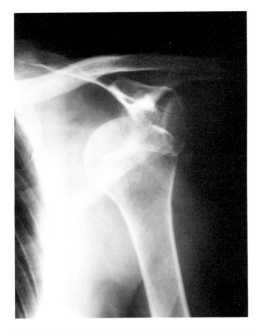

FIGURE 18. AP view of the shoulder demonstrates an antero-inferior dislocation of the head of humerus with a chip fracture of the posterolateral aspect of humeral head.

SUBLUXATIONS AND DISLOCATIONS

In some case of trauma, there is a disruption of the joint with or without a fracture. A complete separation of the articular surfaces is called a dislocation. If there is partial contact between the articular surfaces, it is called a subluxation. Dislocations most commonly occur in the shoulder. About 95% of shoulder dislocations are anterior, and 27% are associated with a compression fracture of the posterolateral aspect of the humeral head, or a fracture of the glenoid labrum that is known as a **Bankart's lesion** (Fig. 18). Repeated shoulder dislocation causes a hatchet-shaped deformity called the **Hill Sack's deformity**, which is best seen on the internal rotation view.

Posterior shoulder dislocations are rare but are commonly seen in patients with convulsions. The humeral head is in internal rotation. An anteroposterior film shows a lack of overlap of the head of humerus and glenoid causing a distortion of the normal elliptical radiodense area (Fig. 19). The space between the anterior rim of glenoid and the humeral head is less than 6 mm. The axillary view is diagnostic.

Lunate and perilunate dislocations are associated with fractures of wrist.[18] The clue is in the triangular shape of lunate on anteroposterior film in lunate dislocation (Figs. 15 and 20). The lateral film is diagnostic in both instances. In lunate dislocation it is dislocated dorsally. In perilunate dislocation only lunate is aligned with the distal radius, and the other carpal bones are dislocated dorsally (Fig. 21).

Acromioclavicular joint separation manifests as widening of the AC joint. An AP film with weightbearing will exaggerate the AC separation, making the diagnosis easy. It is customary to take films of both sides with and without weightbearing. Occasionally there is a **diastasis of symphysis pubis** along with other fractures involving the pelvis (Fig. 22). This type of injury is caused by either a fall

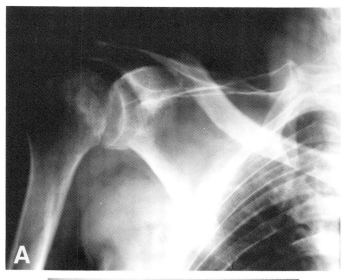

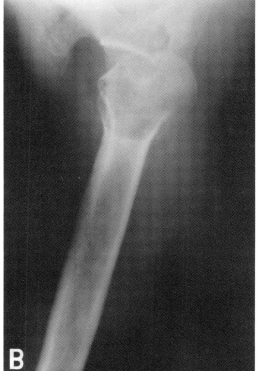

FIGURE 19. *A,* AP view of the shoulder. *B,* axillary view of the shoulder. AP view shows internal rotation of the humeral head and distortion of the elliptical dense area between the head of humerus and glenoid. Axillary view confirms the posterior dislocation.

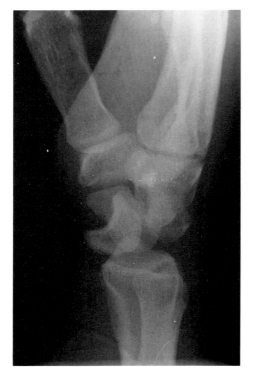

FIGURE 20. Lateral view of wrist shows a lunate dislocation. (AP view of this case is seen in Figure 15).

or an automobile accident.[2,24] There may be associated intra- or extraperitoneal rupture of the bladder and damage to adjacent neurovascular structures. A cystogram is the definitive study to use to diagnose a bladder rupture. Plain films may show soft tissue swelling or disruption of normal fat planes around the bladder.

When there is a fracture of one of the paired bones such as radius and ulna with an overlap of the fractured fragments, the other bone either breaks or there is an associated dislocation. In the case of a fracture of the radius, there is a dislocation of the inferior radio-ulnar joint at the wrist. This type of fracture dislocation is called **Galleazzi fracture** (*see* Fig. 1). A fracture of the ulna with dislocation of the proximal radio-ulnar joint at the elbow is called **Monteggia fracture**.[10]

RADIOLOGIC PROTOCOL FOR EVALUATION OF TRAUMA

Shoulder.   AP views are normally taken in internal and external rotation. They show fractures of humeral head and neck, clavicle, anterior dislocation of shoulder, and acromioclavicular dislocation.[22]

Extra views include the axillary view, which shows the posterior shoulder dislocation, and the transthoracic view if the axillary view is difficult to obtain due to pain. A stress view with weightbearing is done if acromioclavicular dislocation is suspected.

Elbow.   AP and lateral views are done routinely. The AP view shows fractures of distal humerus, medial, and lateral epicondyle, and valgus or varus deformity. The lateral film shows the fat pad sign, fractures of radial head and olecranon, and dislocation of radial head or the elbow.[19]

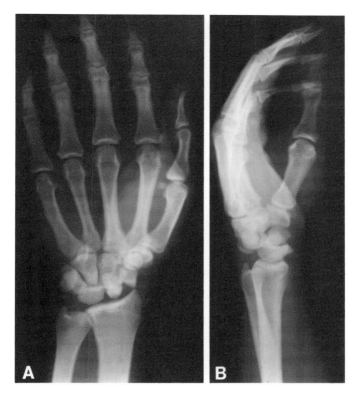

FIGURE 21. *A,* AP view of the wrist. *B,* lateral view of the wrist. AP and lateral views demonstrate a perilunate dislocation. Note that only lunate is in normal position and all the other carpal bones are dislocated dorsally.

External and internal oblique views may also be necessary. They show fractures of the lateral and medial epicondyle, radial head, and coronoid process.

Hand and Wrist. Posteroanterior (PA), lateral, and oblique views are done routinely. The PA film helps in fractures of the distal radius and ulna, carpal bones, metacarpals, and phalanges. The lateral film is useful in fractures of the triquetrum and hamate as well as lunate and perilunate dislocations. The oblique films are useful in fractures of metacarpals and phalanges.[17,26]

Pelvis and Hip. AP and lateral films are routine. The AP film shows fractures of the femoral head and neck, ischium, ilium, pubis, dislocation of the hip, and valgus or varus deformity of the hip. The lateral film, also known as the "frog leg" view, shows fractures of the femoral neck and greater or lesser trochanter. This view is helpful in subtle fractures. If the fracture is obvious on AP view, a lateral film is usually not performed, because it is too painful for the patient.

Knee. AP and lateral views are routine. The AP film shows fractures of the femoral and tibial condyles, tibial spine, proximal tibia and fibula, and osteochondritis dissecans. The lateral view may help in fractures of the patella and assessment of joint effusion.[21]

Additional views in the knee include a tunnel view and axial or "sunrise" view. The tunnel view shows fracture of the posterior aspect of femoral condyles,

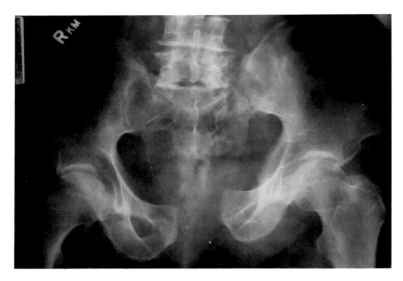

FIGURE 22.   AP view of the pelvis shows diastasis of symphysis pubis and fracture of the left side of sacrum.

the intercondylar notch, osteochondritis dissecans, and the presence of loose bodies. The sunrise view shows fractures of the patella.

Ankle and Foot.   As a routine, AP, lateral, and oblique views are performed. The AP views helps in fractures of distal tibia, fibula, both malleoli, talus, navicular, cuboid, cuneiforms, metatarsals and phalanges, and tarso-metatarsal dislocation. The lateral view is useful in fractures of the distal tibia, fibula, calcaneus, and cuboid. The oblique view may be of further help in patients with fractures of the medial and lateral malleoli, metatarsals, and phalanges.

A stress view in AP projection is useful when assessing the instability of the ankle joint.[20] This film is done with forcible inversion and eversion of the foot. There is increased space in the talo-tibial joint, indicating abnormal movement and possible damage to surrounding ligaments.

Cervical Spine.   Routinely AP, lateral, AP with open mouth, and both oblique views are done. The AP view shows fractures of third to seventh cervical vertebra. The open mouth view is helpful in fractures of lateral masses of the first cervical vertebra and odontoid process. The lateral film helps in fractures of first cervical vertebra, odontoid process, bodies of the second to the seventh cervical vertebra, the spinous processes, and atlanto-axial subluxation. The alignment of vertebral bodies is determined by the smooth curve of the anterior and posterior margins of the vertebral bodies. A sudden step indicates a subluxation. The prevertebral soft tissues measure only 4–5 mm up to the level of thyroid cartilage and, if increased, indicate a hematoma. The oblique views show the neural foramina.[4,11]

An extra "swimmer's view" of C7–T1 junction in lateral projection is done if the seventh cervical vertebra is not seen clearly on the regular lateral film. Lateral views in flexion and extension are useful in assessment of instability or loss of alignment of the cervical spine. In a patient with suspected cervical spine trauma, it is vital that he or she is not moved before assessing the atlanto-axial joint. A horizontal beam lateral film (a shoot through film with the patient supine) is first performed and checked before any more views are done.

Thoracic Spine. AP and lateral views are done. The AP film shows transverse processes and fractures of vertebral bodies. A penetrated AP film is useful in showing a paraspinal soft tissue bulge. The lateral film shows fractures of vertebral bodies, vertebral endplates, spinous processes, and loss of alignment.[17]

Lumbar Spine. Lateral and oblique views are performed routinely. A localized view of the lumbosacral junction is also done routinely. The AP and lateral views of the lumbar spine show findings similar to those in thoracic spine. The lateral lumbar spine may also show spondylolisthesis, meaning a forward slip of a vertebral body as compared to the one below. The oblique views show the facet joints and defect in pars interarticularis, indicating spondylolysis.[15]

COMPLICATIONS OF FRACTURE

Postreduction and serial films are done to evaluate the healing and diagnose any complications as early as possible. One should check alignment, callus formation, and the approximation of the fractured fragments. As the fracture heals, the fracture line becomes indistinct. The callus decreases in size and bridges the gap and finally becomes dense and sclerotic. Radiographic evidence of a bony union takes longer than clinical union.

Delayed Union. If a fracture does not unite within a reasonable length of time for that fracture, a diagnosis of delayed union is made. Delayed union is commonly seen in elderly patients, in pathologic fractures, and in cases with infection and inadequate immobilization. Radiographic findings of delayed union are a widening of the fracture line with ill-defined margins.[12]

Nonunion. With nonunion, there is little or no callus formation, and the fracture simply fails to unite. The two fragments are usually joined by dense scar tissue surrounded by sclerosis. Nonunion is common in fractures of the neck of the femur and scaphoid (Fig. 23). Nonunion is further divided into reactive or hypertrophic types, nonreactive or atrophic types, and infected types. In the reactive type of nonunion there is a large amount of callus and sclerosis of bone ends. A bone scan will show an increased uptake of radioisotope. The atrophic type of nonunion shows very little callus formation, and the bone scan shows little or no uptake of radioisotope. The infected type of nonunion may show periosteal reaction, sclerosis of bone and, rarely, sequestrum.[12]

Malunion. In a case of malunion, the fracture does unite but in an abnormal position. There is varus or valgus deformity. There may be shortening of the bone due to overlap of fragments.

Disuse Osteoporosis. Disuse osteoporosis is a fairly common condition. The films show patchy areas of decreased bone density, thinning of cortices, and coarsening of the trabecular pattern caused by disappearance of finer trabeculae.

Sudeck's Atrophy. Another type of complication, Sudeck's atrophy, is characterized by extensive spotty osteoporosis out of proportion to the original trauma. There is considerable soft tissue swelling, which may be difficult to visualize on the films.[16,25]

Volkmann's Ischemic Contractures. This complication is caused by vascular obstruction due to tight splints, bandages, or plaster. Volkmann's contractures most commonly occur in the wrist and hand after a supracondylar fracture of distal humerus.

Myositis Ossificans.   Myositis ossificans is caused by ossification of a soft tissue hematoma. Posttraumatic myositis ossificans develops relatively rapidly, in 4–6 weeks after trauma. The films show a radiolucent center with dense ossification on the outside. The mass of ossification is separated from the adjacent bone by a radiolucent band. A CT scan shows myossitis ossificans much earlier than plain films.

Avascular Necrosis.   Avascular necrosis (AVN) is caused by a lack of blood supply to a bone fragment. Common sites of AVN follow fractures of femoral head, proximal pole of scaphoid, and body of talus. The first radiographic finding is a radiolucent crescent in the head of femur. Surrounding sclerosis develops later. There is fragmentation and, later, collapse of the bone. MRI is much more sensitive in diagnosing early AVN and is the examination of choice with negative plain films. In the case of scaphoid fracture with AVN, there is sclerosis in the proximal fragment (Fig. 23).

Injury to Blood Vessels.   There may be injury to major blood vessels along with skeletal trauma (Fig. 24). Clinically there is a rapidly growing hematoma and decreased pulse distally. A CT scan may indicate trauma to blood vessels by demonstrating soft tissue swelling and hematoma. An emergency angiogram is the only definitive way to diagnose this condition.[6]

In summary, the treatment of skeletal trauma has been revolutionized by the discovery of x-rays. Generally, plain films are adequate in uncomplicated fractures. In cases with complex trauma, other imaging modalities play a complementary role in the diagnosis and treatment of fractures. Each case should be evaluated on its merit and appropriate studies ordered.

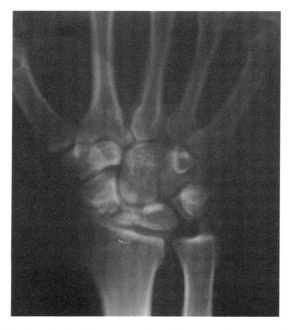

FIGURE 23.   AP view of wrist shows nonunion of fracture of the scaphoid with avascular necrosis shown as sclerosis of the proximal fragment.

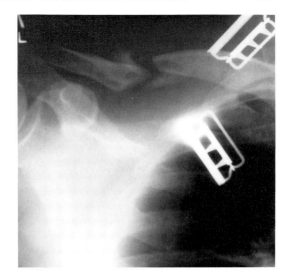

FIGURE 24. AP view of the clavicle shows a comminuted fracture of the clavicle with loose bony fragments compressing subclavian vessels.

ACKNOWLEDGMENTS

We would like to thank Reuben Garcia, RT, and Frederick Frias, RT, for their invaluable help.

REFERENCES

1. Blum GM, Crues J III, Sheehan W: MRI of occult bony trauma: The missing link. Appl Radiol 22:15–21, 1993.
2. Cohen MA, Sadller AH: Treatment of pelvic fractures and associated dislocations. Orthop Rev 15:142–153, 1986.
3. Daffner RH, Pavlov H: Stress fractures—current topics. AJR 159:245–252, 1992.
4. Daffner RH: Evaluation of cervical vertebral injuries. Semin Roentgen 27:239–253, 1992.
5. Dalinka MK, Boorstein JM, Zlatkin MB: Computed tomography of musculoskeletal trauma. Radiol Clin North Am 27:933–944, 1989.
6. Damron T, McBeath A: Diagnosis and management of vascular injuries associated with skeletal trauma. Orthop Rev 19:1063–1070, 1990.
7. Deutsch AL, Mink JH: Magnetic resonance imaging of musculoskeletal injuries. Radiol Clin North Am 27:983–1002, 1989.
8. Deutsch AL, Mink JH: Magnetic resonance imaging of injury to bone and articular cartilage: Emphasis on radiographically occult abnormalities. Orthop Rev 19:66–75, 1990.
9. Gelberman RH, Wolock BS, Siegel DB: Fractures and non union of carpal scaphoid. J Bone Joint Surg 71:1560–1565, 1989.
10. Greenspan A: Orthopedic Radiology. Philadelphia, JB Lippincott, 1988.
11. Harris JH Jr, et al: A practical classification of acute cervical spine injuries. Orthop Clin North Am 17:15–30, 1896.
12. Harris JH Jr: Musculoskeletal trauma; management and complications. Curr Opin Radiology 2:669–677, 1990.
13. Johnson EE: Intra-articular fractures of the calcaneus: Diagnosis and surgical management. Orthop 13:1091–1100, October 1990.
13a. Juhl JH, Crummy AB (eds): Paul and Juhl's Essentials of Radiographic Imaging. 6th ed. Philadelphia, JB Lippincott, 1993.
14. Karasick D, Burk DL Jr, Gross GW: Trauma to the elbow and forearm. Semin Roentgen 26:318–330, 1991.
15. Kricun ME, Kricun R: Fractures of the lumbar spine. Semin Roentgen 27:262–270, 1992.
16. Martinez CR, Di Pasquale TG, Helfet DR, et al: Evaluation of acetabular fractures with two and three dimensional CT. Radio Graphics 12:227–242, 1992.
17. Meyer S: Thoracic spine trauma. Semin Roentgen 27:254–261, 1992.

18. Meyer S: Radiographic evaluation of wrist trauma. Semin Roentgen 26:300–317, 1991.
19. Miller MD: Orthopedic trauma in elderly. Emerg Med Clin North Am 8:325–339, 1990.
20. Mitchell MJ, Ho C, Howard BA, et al: Diagnostic imaging of trauma of ankle and foot, I. Fractures about the ankle. J Foot Surg 28:174–179, 1989.
21. Mitchell MJ, Ho C, Resnick D, Sartoris DJ: Diagnostic imaging of lower extremity trauma. Radiol Clin North Am 27:909–928, 1989.
22. Neustadter LM, Weiss MJ: Trauma to the shoulder girdle. Semin Roentgen 26:331–343, 1991.
23. [Reference deleted.]
24. Pitt M, Ruth JT, Benjamin JB: Trauma to the pelvic ring and acetabulum. Semin Roentgen 27:299–218, 1992.
25. Resnick D, Niwayama G: Diagnosis of Bone and Joint Disorders. 2nd ed. Philadelphia, WB Saunders, 1988.
26. Wolfe SW, Dick HM: Articular fractures of the hand, Part I. Guidelines of assessment. Orthop Rev 20:27–32, 1991.

MARILYN STRONG, RN
CYNTHIA CATINDIG, RN
ANNA MARIE CHENEY, RN, MSN
MARLYN DELIM, RN

CARIDAD DIVINA, RNC, MSN
BARBARA FLYNN, RN
PAMELA SANTELLANO, RN

THE NURSE'S ROLE
IN FRACTURE REHABILITATION

From The Nursing Service
Veterans Health Administration
Medical Center
Sepulveda, California

The authors of this chapter approach patient care from a perspective that emphasizes the principles represented by Orem's self-care deficit theory of nursing.[28] Self-care refers to learned and deliberate actions that people perform in response to known needs. Nurses assess patients' self-care abilities and needs. If deficits exist, nurses design plans of care and designate who (nurse, patient, family) will carry out each part of the plan. Rehabilitation begins the moment patients are seen by the first health care provider and continues with every subsequent encounter. The goal is to increase patients' self-care abilities, decrease their needs, or both.

The major responsibilities of nurses in rehabilitation of fracture patients are promotion of self-care, provision of direct care, prevention of deformities and complications, and referral for continued services when needed.[58] Successful orthopedic nurses know anatomy and physiology and understand why and how to use multiple types of orthopedic equipment, including abduction pillows, cushions, sandbags, lumbar corsets, splints, braces, immobilizers, overhead slings, traction equipment, and continuous passive motion machines.

Physical limitations, however temporary, may have an impact on patients' psychological and emotional status. They may experience a series of emotional reactions, such as denial, depression, and helplessness. Sensitive nurses recognize these reactions and plan care accordingly. Nurses use their knowledge, skills, and caring attitudes to help patients gain confidence and adapt more readily.

This chapter aims to describe the role of nurses in fracture rehabilitation from the time of the fracture through healing and recovery. Nurses may encounter patients at any point along the continuum: at the site of the injury, in the emergency room, in the operating room, in a clinic, in the hospital, or at home.[14,16,18–20,29,55] In all settings, nurses aim to restore patients' capacity for self-care. Collaboration among members of the health care team—physicians, surgeons, nurses, physical therapists, social workers, occupational therapists, and dietitians—is crucial to the successful rehabilitation of fracture patients.[51,61] The major sections of this chapter address the nursing process, special nursing issues with fracture patients, complications, and discharge planning. Although discharge planning is separated for emphasis, readers should be aware that it is an integral part of the nursing process from the first encounter with patients. Issues particular to causes of fractures (trauma or disease), to location of fracture, and to age of patients are addressed throughout these sections.

THE NURSING PROCESS

Assessment

Assessment of fracture patients includes a history, physical exam, and psychosocial data. It may be necessary to involve "significant others" if patients are unable to give a complete accounting of the events surrounding the fracture or of the living situation.[22] The participation of significant others may be needed in discharge planning and in teaching the patient how to cope with the fracture, its treatment, and the aftermath of the treatment.

Health care providers involved with patients early in the fracture experience collect historical information that helps determine the cause and type of injury sustained. It is important to understand the cause of the fracture and whether it resulted from trauma alone or some other contributing reason. Other reasons to consider include diseases that weaken bones such as osteoporosis and cancer; conditions that make patients prone to fall such as neurologic deficits, Parkinson's disease, and cerebral vascular accident (stroke); environmental hazards such as highly polished floors, poor lighting, or obstructions; or drug-induced conditions such as drowsiness, lightheadedness, dizziness, or hypotension.[27] Knowledge of the factors involved provides guidance in developing rehabilitation plans.

A thorough history includes information regarding the type of force encountered, sounds heard, the position in which the patient was found, allergies, medications, concurrent medical conditions, and the patient's orientation to time, place, and person. Evers and Werpachowski admonish nurses to be alert to the possibility of physical abuse as a cause of the fracture.[22]

The physical assessment starts with attention to the head and works down toward the toes, focusing both on the site of injury and the unaffected areas. The unaffected and affected sides are compared to determine the effects of the fracture. Note should be taken of bruises, abrasions, skin color, temperature, and condition; edema and type (whether nonpitting or pitting); abduction, adduction, external rotation, and length of legs in comparison to one another. The patient should be asked about pain onset and character. The onset of pain may be gradual or immediate depending on the type of fracture.

Hip Fractures. Patients sustaining fractures of the hip have generally been subjected to trauma related to falls resulting in direct blows over the greater trochanter. The incidence of hip fracture is clearly related to osteoporosis. Cornell[17] reports that 5% of patients 65 and older occupying a hospital bed are recovering from a hip fracture. Nurses caring for fracture patients must be knowledgeable about age-related assessments and interventions.[4,11,12,15,17]

The two primary categories of hip fracture are the femoral neck fracture and the intertrochanteric fracture. Careful examination of the affected area and the entire extremity is essential. Common findings include discoloration/ecchymosis over the greater trochanter extending into the groin and surrounding tissue; swelling in hip and thigh region; shortening and external rotation of the limb; and complaints of pain increased with movement.

Upper/Lower Extremity Fractures. The nursing literature is surprisingly sparse with respect to upper and lower extremity fractures. This may be due to the fact that these patients primarily undergo ambulatory care or are hospitalized for short periods only. Kendrick's[35] description of her personal experience with a tibial fracture underscores the need for nurses to be sensitive to the needs of these patients.

Pelvic Fractures. Because pelvic fractures are most commonly associated with multiple injuries resulting from motor vehicle and industrial accidents,[32,52] emergency room and critical care nurses are likely to encounter patients with pelvic fractures. Johnson[32] warns that hemorrhage is a major cause of death in patients with pelvic fracture. Peter[52] describes assessment of instability of a fractured pelvis by applying alternating pressure on the iliac crests and noting asymmetry with complaint of pain. Genge[25] cites Iverson and Clawson, noting that pain, crepitus, or tenderness upon palpation over the symphysis pubis, anterior spines, iliac crests, sacrum, or coccyx are signs of a pelvic fracture. After the fracture is stabilized and the hypovolemia is being treated, one should assess the genitourinary tract for the possibility of associated injury.[43]

Spinal Fractures. Spinal fractures, including cervical spinal fractures, result from both trauma and disease, particularly osteoporosis.[2,15] Patients present with a history of trauma, acute pain that may be incapacitating, and tenderness at the site of the fracture.[15] Adelstein[2] recommends use of an assessment format for cervical fracture patients that rates pain, muscle spasm, limitation of range of motion, and numbness on a scale of absent, mild, moderate, and severe. Each factor is assessed for the muscles of the neck, the scapula border, the upper forearm, the forearm, the hands and the fingers. She also recommends a detailed assessment of motor and sensory function. McKenna and McCarthy[41] recommend spinal cord testing every hour for 4 hours postoperatively or until the results are stable and every 4 hours thereafter, and they include a documentation format for motor, sensory, and autonomic testing of spinal cord functioning.

Facial Fractures. Moncada and Black[44] outline nursing assessment concerns with patients with facial fractures as focused on airway patency, skin integrity, ability to eat and drink, ability to speak, vision, potential cerebrospinal fluid leak, self concept, and pain. Facial fractures are seldom life-threatening; however, nursing care is crucial because the effects of facial fractures can be disabling and/ or disfiguring.

For all types of fractures, neurovascular assessment is crucial to quality nursing care of fracture patients throughout the fracture episode. Table 1 summarizes the elements of neurovascular assessment to be considered.[24,37,45,46,48]

TABLE 1. Neurovascular Assessment

Factors to Assess	Assessment Techniques	Findings	Implications
Skin color	Visualize; compare to unaffected side.	Pale/white Bluish/mottled Red	Arterial insufficiency Inadequate venous return Impaired circulation
Skin temperature	Feel with back of hand; compare to unaffected side.	Cooler Warmer	Arterial insufficiency Inadequate venous return
Capillary refill	Count the number of seconds it takes for color to return to a toe or fingernail bed after blanching; if it is not possible to press on the toe nail due to calcification, deformity or pinning, press on the tip of the toe on the skin	Over 3 seconds	Suggests slowed peripheral perfusion
Pulses	Compare to contralateral pulse; if lower extremity check posterior tibial and pedal pulse (use pads of fingers, not thumb); in upper extremity check radial pulse. If unable to detect may use a Doppler.	Pulses: 4+ strong, bounding (normal) 3+ easily palpated 2+ difficult to palpate 1+ weak, thready 0 absent	If pulse on the affected side is diminished, suspect impaired circulation; if no pulse on affected side, notify MD immediately.
Sensation	Passive movement	Pain distal to injury that increases with movement, numb, tingling.	Suspect compartment syndrome, notify MD immediately.
	Pin pricks, light touch	Hypesthesia, anesthesia	Serious damage to a limb
Pain	Ask patient about: Location	Poorly localized	Associated with blood vessels, joints, fascia, or periosteum
		Chest, shoulder	Suspect pulmonary embolism
	Duration	Persistent at rest On passive movement and increasing on dorsiflexion	Suspect thrombophlebitis Muscle ischemia, compartment syndrome
	Quality/type	Throbbing Aching Burning under cast	Probably due to injury/ surgery. Suspect thrombophlebitis Possible skin irritation
Motion	Ask patient to dorsiflex and plantar flex lower extremities and move toes	Inability to flex or extend the toes	Suggests nerve compression on the peroneal nerve

The frequency of neurovascular assessment depends on the patient's condition. At the time of injury and postoperatively, assessments should be done every 15 minutes for an hour and then every hour until the patient's condition is stable. Subsequently, routine assessments are conducted every 4 hours unless the patient's condition changes.[41,45] Casts, skeletal traction, external fixator pins, and splints are assessed every shift for position, loosening, drainage around pins, pain, redness or tenderness, tightness or swelling.

Surveillance, defined by McCloskey and Bulechek as "purposeful and ongoing acquisition, interpretation and synthesis of patient data for clinical decision making,"[40] is an important component of the nurse's role. Much of the data gathered in physical assessment provides physicians with data crucial to effective medical treatment.[57] Three serious medical complications to which nurses must be alert are compartment syndrome, pulmonary embolism, and fat embolism. Early recognition of these complications is essential in preventing long-term disability or death.

Compartment Syndrome. Slye[60] quotes Matsen, Winquist, and Krugmire's definition of compartment syndrome, "a condition in which increased pressure in a limited space compromises the circulation and function of the tissues within that space." A compartment consists of blood vessels, bone, nerves, and muscles contained within inelastic boundaries composed of skin, epimysium, and fascia.[56] Compartment syndrome most commonly occurs in the lower leg and forearm. External pressure from casts, splints, or dressings and edema of the extremity or intracompartmental hemorrhage may cause compartment syndrome. Early detection and treatment are critical. The hallmark sign of impending compartment syndrome is pain on passive stretch.[58] Patients complain of severe pain that is not relieved by narcotics and increases when the affected part is elevated. Pressure over the involved part and passive movement of the distal extremities (fingers or toes) causes pain, indicating early ischemic changes.[56] Neurovascular assessment reveals altered or diminished sensation distal to the involved part; progressive weakness of the muscles results in diminished movement. Absent distal pulses, cool skin temperature, and pallor are late signs.[56]

Fat Embolism. Fat embolism is associated with severe trauma as seen in multiple fractures and crush injuries, especially those caused by high-energy forces such as motor vehicle and industrial accidents.[58,60] The most common fractures include those of the pelvis, femur, tibia, and ribs. Fat globules released from the marrow and local tissues surrounding the area of the trauma enter the pulmonary vasculature by way of the circulatory system and cause hypoxemia 24–48 hours after the trauma.[60] Vigilant nurses watch for signs and symptoms including dyspnea, restlessness or agitation, confusion, tachypnea, tachycardia, and high fever. Petechia, indicative of capillary fragility, form over the chest, axilla, and neck in slightly more than half of patients.[60]

Pulmonary Embolism. Pulmonary embolism, often associated with pelvic and hip fractures, results from deep vein thrombi that form in patients who are immobilized for long periods. The thrombus breaks loose, travels through the circulatory system, and lodges in the pulmonary vasculature, causing a partial or complete obstruction of the pulmonary artery or its subdivisions. Pulmonary emboli strike suddenly and can be deadly.[30] Signs and symptoms of pulmonary embolism include unexplained dyspnea, pleuritic chest pain, tachypnea, tachycardia, low grade fever, restlessness, and apprehension.

Psychosocial Data. Psychosocial data are an important part of the assessment. Patients and significant others are involved as much as possible, beginning with the asessment and throughout the nursing process. Their perceptions of the cause of the fracture, the meaning of the pain, and the care provided are very important to successful rehabilitation.[9,16,18–20] One must assess disturbances of sleep patterns, sensitivity to noises, anxiety related to the cause of the fracture, disruptions of interpersonal relationships and roles, frustrations related to impaired functioning, tolerance of and preference for activities,[35] mental status, knowledge, and ability to understand and carry out instructions.[12] Patients' living situations play a part in discharge planning and must be determined early in the process to allow effective planning.

Common Nursing Diagnoses

The National Association of Orthopaedic Nurses conducted a survey of its membership in 1990 to determine the most common nursing diagnoses used with orthopedic patients. The resulting list serves as the basis for the Guidelines for Orthopaedic Nursing[48] to be used in conjunction with the American Nurses Association Standards of Clinical Nursing Practice.[5] Table 2 lists and defines the 11 nursing diagnoses identified in the survey.

Nursing diagnoses are independent of medical diagnoses; however, a medical diagnosis and treatment can be expected to be similar to specific nursing diagnoses. They may vary depending on the patient's place on the continuum from fracture to recovery and rehabilitation.[59] Patients are assessed individually to determine which nursing diagnoses apply to them. Table 3 lists some additional nursing diagnoses consistent with the effects of a fracture and its treatment that are commonly used by the authors of this chapter.

Only a few of the nursing diagnoses identified in Tables 2 and 3 are explored in depth in this chapter. Pain, impaired physical mobility, and the specific self-care deficits are addressed beginning on page 237 under *Special Nursing Issues*. Impaired skin integrity and high risk for peripheral neurovascular dysfunction are discussed beginning on page 243 under *Complications*. High risk for injury and self-care deficit are discussed beginning on page 246 under *Discharge Planning*.

Intervention

Bulechek and McCloskey[10] define nursing intervention as "any direct care treatment that a nurse performs on behalf of a client. These treatments include nurse-initiated treatments resulting from nursing diagnoses, physician-initiated treatments resulting from medical diagnoses, and performance of the daily essential functions for the client who cannot do these." Interventions include

TABLE 2.   Common Nursing Diagnoses in Fracture Rehabilitation[48]

Diagnosis	Definition
Pain (acute)	State of severe discomfort or uncomfortable sensation
Pain (chronic, nonmalignant)	Pain that persists after tissue damage has healed or in the absence of evident tissue damage
Impaired physical mobility	Experience or risk of experiencing limitation of physical movement
Activity intolerance	Insufficient physiologic or psychologic energy to endure or complete required or desired activities
Impaired adjustment	Unable to modify lifestyle/behavior in a manner consistent with a change in health status
Impaired skin integrity	Experience or risk of experiencing damage to epidermal or dermal tissue
High risk for infection	At risk to be invaded by opportunistic or pathogenic agent
High risk for injury	At risk of harm because of physiologic deficit, lack of awareness or hazards, maturational age
High risk for disuse syndrome	At risk for the adverse effects of immobility, including impaired skin integrity, infection, injury, constipation, altered respiratory function, altered peripheral tissue perfusion, activity intolerance, sensory-perceptual alterations, powerlessness, body image disturbance
Post trauma response	Experiencing a sustained painful response to an overwhelming traumatic event
High risk for peripheral neurovascular dysfunction	At risk of experiencing a change in circulation, sensation, or motion (emphasis on compartment syndrome)

TABLE 3. Additional Nursing Diagnoses to Consider in Fracture Rehabilitation[13]

Self-care deficit:
  feeding
  bathing/hygiene
  dressing/grooming
  toileting
  instrumental self-care
	Impaired ability to perform or complete for oneself:
	  feeding
	  bathing/hygiene
	  dressing/grooming
	  toileting
	Impaired ability to perform activities/access services essential for managing a household

Diversional activity deficit	Experience or risk of experiencing decreased stimulation from leisure activity
Ineffective individual coping	Experience or risk of experiencing an inability to manage internal or environmental stressors adequately due to inadequate resources (physical, psychological, behavioral, and/or cognitive)
Potential complication: Fat embolism	At risk to experience obstruction of one or more pulmonary arteries from a fat embolus
Potential complication: Pulmonary embolism	Experience or risk of experiencing obstruction of one or more pulmonary arteries from a blood clot, air or fat embolism

activities carried out in collaboration with the patient and other members of the interdisciplinary health care team. The Iowa Intervention Project[10,40] is constructing a taxonomy of nursing interventions. The results of their work are expected to allow computerized care planning, determination of staffing requirements, and nursing research. Table 4 lists nursing interventions commonly used for fracture patients gleaned from the Nursing Interventions Classification (NIC). As the Iowa Intervention Project evolves, additional interventions will be identified and catalogued.

Physician-initiated treatments resulting from fractures, such as cast care, external fixation devices, and traction, are presented in this section. Nurse-initiated treatments are presented in the other three sections.

Fractures are immobilized to permit healing of the bone, to stabilize an unstable fracture, to relieve pain, and to assist in maintaining alignment.[47]

TABLE 4. Common Nursing Interventions[10,40]

Intervention	Associated Nursing (Medical) Diagnosis
Pain management	Pain
Analgesic administration	Pain
Positioning	Impaired physical mobility
Cast care: Wet	(Fracture)
Cast care: Maintenance	(Fracture)
Discharge planning	
Traction care	(Fracture)
Self-care assistance:	Self-care deficit:
bowel management	toileting
dry skin	bathing/hygiene
hygiene (includes moving)	bathing/hygiene
feeding	feeding
Limit setting	Ineffective individual coping; diversional activity deficit
Contracting	Ineffective individual coping; diversional activity deficit
Pressure management	Impaired physical mobility; impaired skin integrity
Pressure ulcer prevention	Impaired physical mobility; impaired skin integrity
Pressure ulcer care	Impaired skin integrity

Immobilization methods include casts, internal and external fixation devices, and traction. The use of traction is declining as the use of fixation devices increases. Fixation devices permit patients to become mobile much more quickly, thus decreasing the negative effects of immobility, such as pulmonary stasis, deep vein thrombosis, bone loss, and intolerance of activity.[21]

Cast Care. Nursing preparations and observations of the patient and the site to be encased are vital for the safety and comfort of the patient. Observations are made of the neurovascular status of the tissues, skin integrity, open areas, rash, bruises, edema, deformity, and dirt or foreign material.[47] Skin preparation over the part to be casted may include gently cleansing with soap and water and drying thoroughly.

Prior to cast application, one must explain to the patient the purpose of the cast, tell the patient to expect the sensation of heat during the drying process, and instruct the patient on the care of the cast. Generally, a firm mattress or a bed board underneath the mattress should be used to prevent sagging. It takes about 24–48 hours for a cast to dry thoroughly. A freshly applied cast should be exposed to air. A wet cast is gray and lusterless in appearance, dull to percussion, feels damp, and has a musty odor. A dry cast is white and shiny, resonant when percussed, firm and odorless.[37]

Several types of casting materials are used, with plaster of Paris being the most common. Plaster casts are easy to apply, durable, strong, and set rapidly even though they take time to dry thoroughly. Synthetic casts are made primarily of plastic or fiberglass. They have three advantages: (1) They harden and dry immediately, reaching maximum strength and being weightbearing in about 20 minutes; (2) they are water-resistant, and (3) they are lightweight.

It is important for the cast to be dried from inside out and not be dried too quickly or the inner portions of the cast may remain damp and become moldy. Rapid drying also may burn the skin beneath the cast or cause the cast to crack. While the cast is still drying, one should use only the palms of the hands to lift the cast because fingers cause indentations that can cause pressure and pressure ulcers when the cast dries. Initial cast care is important during drying to prevent changes in cast surfaces. The cast needs to dry on a smooth surface; constrictions of any sort must be avoided.[37]

The casted extremity must be kept elevated to prevent swelling, especially for the first 24–48 hours after casting. The cast should be placed on a soft pillow rather than a hard surface to avoid flattening of the cast. Elevation of the casted extremity may be done with pillows or slings attached to an overhead frame or IV stand. If a leg cast is applied, the leg is elevated above the level of the heart; if an arm cast is applied, each joint should be elevated higher than the preceding joint, i.e., elbow higher than the shoulder, hand higher than the elbow.

Taking meticulous care of the skin by washing and drying the skin thoroughly, massaging the skin gently with emollient lotion, periodically inspecting the skin, and turning the patient frequently are vital in the care of the patient with cast. When giving skin care, nurses should reach as far as possible under the cast with their fingers to remove plaster crumbs. The rough edges are padded by applying adhesive strips or "petals" around the edges or pulling the stockinette lining inside the case over the edge of the cast. During skin care one can also inspect the condition of the cast, its fit, and for any sign of cracking or softening, especially on the heel.

The cast should be kept clean and dry during rehabilitation. No sharp objects should be slipped under cast because of the danger of injuring the skin and causing an infection. All fingers and toes should be moved to prevent stiffness of joints and promote circulation to reduce swelling. If the cast gets wet, it can be dried with a portable hair dryer held at least 18 inches from the cast. Patients must be cautioned to avoid getting the cast hot with the hair dryer.

Written home care instructions or a cast care booklet should be given upon discharge to the patient or significant other. See page 246 under *Discharge Planning.*

External Fixation Devices. Internal and external fixation devices are being used increasingly frequently to stabilize fractures and allow for early mobilization of patients.

When external fixation devices are placed in an upper or lower extremity, the involved limb should be elevated above the level of the heart. This is usually done with pillows, but a stockinette and IV pole may be used for maximum elevation. Elevation is important during the first week to promote venous drainage and to decrease edema.[22] It is important when turning the patient not to hold the fixation device.[52]

Halo traction is a metal brace attached to the skull with four pins and attached to a plastic vest that affords patients more mobility. Patients in halo braces need assistance in positioning and sometimes use small pillows or wedges under their heads. This relieves pressure at the pin sites and provides reassurance that the pins are not hanging in mid air.[50]

Although the potential for infection at pin sites demands meticulous pin site care,[2] consensus about what constitutes a standard for pin care is lacking in the nursing literature.[26,32] Mandzuk[38] presents a thorough review of the literature and a survey of current practice in which practicing nurses reported using alcohol, hydrogen peroxide, povidone, normal saline, and soap and water. Frequency of pin site care varied from never to every other day. More recently, Jones-Walton[34] reports use of hydrogen peroxide by more than 91% of respondents. She further reports that two to three treatments using a clean rather than sterile technique was the norm. Jones-Walton[33] questions whether pin site care is necessary or effective based on comparing outcomes of patients who receive care and those for whom surgeons wrote specific orders for no pin site care. The choice of cleansing solution requires consideration of information that antiseptics, including hydrogen peroxide, destroy cell function and that normal saline is preferable.[3] Careful assessment of the site for signs of infection and loosening appears to be a minimal expectation.[2,25,50] Infection rates and the effects of various pin-site care protocols must be investigated further.[33,34]

Nurses have a responsibility to monitor patients carefully to identify early signs and symptoms of infection that might result from the presence of the pins. The most frequent signs and symptoms of infections and loosening are classified as either minor or major.[33] Minor reactions are characterized by redness, swelling, drainage, tenderness, or pain that improves spontaneously or after lancing. Major reactions are the same symptoms that do not improve after treatment. These symptoms are classified as reactions if they last longer than 72 hours, indicating a potential problem. Early detection of pin site infection may prevent the need to remove the pins, thus preserving the potential for effective traction and avoiding osteomyelitis.[28] Documentation by the nurse is important after pin care on every shift, until symptoms are resolved or need further attention. Bright red blood or purulent drainage around the pin sites is more severe and should be reported to the physician immediately. It is also important to check for tension and loosening of pins. Infected or loosened pins must be removed.[25]

Patients hospitalized for orthopedic problems now have shorter stays and go home with fixation devices.[16] Nurses should teach patients pin-site care as soon as it is feasible. They should stress cleaning and explain aseptic (clean) techniques in terms patients can understand. Nurses need to observe return demonstrations and document patients' or significant others' ability to carry out pin-site care. Patients also need to report any signs of infection, numbness, tingling, loss of sensation, or unrelieved pain. Patients with halo braces usually need someone else to do the pin-site care.[50] Nurses also must tell patients not to tamper with hardware, explaining that they could misalign the fracture and delay healing and that only the physician should adjust it.

Traction. Traction, the application of pulling forces, reduces a fracture, maintains alignment, and rests the body part. Types of traction most commonly used for fractures include skin and skeletal traction. Skin traction provides moderate pull (5–7 pounds of weight) for short periods and is often used as a temporary measure prior to open reduction or skeletal traction.[63] Skeletal traction is applied by means of surgically implanted pins, tongs, screws, or wires attached to a holder from which the traction force is hung. This type of traction allows for more force (15–30 pounds). These medical interventions require attention from nurses to ensure the integrity of traction; the nurses must inspect ropes for placement in pulleys and to verify the absence of knots, check the weights to be sure they are hanging freely and are consistent with the physicians' orders, and check the points of contact with patients. If skeletal traction is used, nurses must check the pin or wire sites daily for signs of infection and loosening, as with external fixation devices. If skin traction is used, nurses must check patients' skin for signs of irritation or inflammation. Neurovascular status is assessed hourly for the first 24 hours and then every 4 hours unless a change is noted.[31] The line of force is maintained continuously: Weights are neither removed nor lifted. Weights must be handled with extreme care to avoid muscle contractions and disruption of bone fragments. Patients remain supine with the head of the bed never elevated more than 20°.[63] An increase in pain may be a warning that the line of pull requires adjustment or that the peroneal nerve is compressed.

In addition to ensuring the integrity of the medical treatment, nurses face special issues and potential complications with traction patients, as they do with cast and external fixation patients. Special issues include pain management, impaired physical mobility, and self-care activities, and complications include impaired skin integrity and peripheral neurovascular dysfunction.

Electrical Stimulators. Barden and Sinkora[8] provide the primary source in the nursing literature for information about electrical stimulation for the treatment of nonunion of bone fractures. Their thorough review article summarizes the physiologic principles underlying the use of electrical stimulators and the primary methods of treatment, including direct current, inductive, and capacitive-coupled stimulation. Direct current stimulation is accomplished by means of a surgically implanted device; healing takes an average of 16 weeks for noninfected and 35 weeks for infected nonunited fractures. Inductive stimulation involves placement of a transducer or coil to the skin or cast from 3–10 hours daily for about 6 months. Capacitive-coupled stimulation uses electrodes in place 24 hours a day, and the average time to achieve successful union is 22.5 weeks. Barden and Sinkora report that the primary nursing management concerns are anxiety, potential for noncompliance, knowledge deficit, and impaired mobility. Since the treatment is used for nonunion of long bone fractures, patients have already been subject to many months of unsuccessful treatment of their fractures. They and their significant others are likely to be anxious both about the lack of successful union of the fracture and perhaps about the use of electricity. Because patient compliance is necessary for the success of inductive and capacitive-coupled stimulation, careful education of patients and their significant others is critical.

Evaluation

Three developments in health care delivery can be expected to affect the evaluation of patient care: critical pathways or care maps, emphasis on patient outcomes, and clinical practice guidelines.

Critical pathways and care maps are gaining momentum as methods to anticipate and evaluate the care of patients as pressure for managed care increases. Metcalf[42] reports a generalized orthopedic critical path developed by nurses, physicians, and others to identify key elements in the care of orthopedic patients. The critical path spells out aspects of care and the expected timeline for progress. The purpose is to improve the quality of care and to decrease the variations among providers. Metcalf reports on a generalized critical pathway focused primarily on inpatient care; however, as the momentum for managed care increases, the need for more specific critical pathways or care maps that span entire episodes of illness regardless of the site where care is provided will become increasingly acute.

Emphasis on patient outcomes is increasingly evident in the nursing research literature and in the Agenda for Change of the Joint Commission for the Accreditation of Health Care Organizations. Previously, evaluation schemes focused primarily on structure and process in the delivery of health care with little attention to patient outcomes. Recently, however, the emphasis has shifted and patient outcomes have assumed a more important position in evaluating care. This shift in emphasis currently is reported primarily in the nursing management and research literature; in the future, the clinical practice literature can be expected to attend more overtly to patient outcomes.

Clinical practice guidelines such as those published by the National Association of Orthopaedic Nurses[48] and the Agency for Health Care Policy and Research (AHCPR)[1,54] reflect the trend toward increasing accountability for care provided. Clinicians can expect the care they provide to be evaluated against both patient outcomes and standards of practice in the community reflected in published guidelines. These final two trends affect nurses in all specialties; nurses caring for fracture rehabilitation patients must be familiar with these trends and documents.

SPECIAL NURSING ISSUES

Important factors creating demand for nursing care are pain management, impaired physical mobility, self-care activities, limit setting, and contracting with patients.

Pain Management

Any state-of-the-art paper that discusses pain management must refer readers to the AHCPR's clinical practice guideline *Acute Pain Management: Operative or Medical Procedures and Trauma.*[1] Table 5 presents the summary recommendations.

TABLE 5. Acute Pain Management Clinical Practice Guidelines: Summary Recommendations[1]

1. Promise patients attentive analgesic care.
2. Chart and display assessment of pain relief.
3. Define pain and relief levels to trigger a review.
4. Survey patient satisfaction.
5. Analgesic drug treatment should comply with several basic principles: Unless contraindicated, every patient should receive an around-the-clock postoperative regimen of an NSAID; for patients unable to take medications by mouth, it may be necessary to use the parenteral or rectal route; analgesic orders should allow for the great variation in individual opioid requirements, including a regularly scheduled dose and "rescue" doses for instances in which the usual regimen is insufficient.
6. Specialized analgesic technologies ... should be governed by policies and standardized procedures that define the acceptable levels of patient monitoring and appropriate roles and limits of practice for all groups of health care providers involved. The policy should include definitions of physician and nurse accountability, physician and nurse responsibility to the patient, and the role of the pharmacy.
7. Nonpharmacologic interventions ... are intended to supplement, not replace, pharmacologic interventions. Staff should give patients information about these interventions and support patients in using them.
8. Monitor the efficacy of pain treatment.

According to these clinical practice guidelines, "the single most reliable indication of the existence and intensity of acute pain—and any resultant affective discomfort or distress—is the patient's self report."[1] Several years ago, the American Pain Society adopted Merskey's definition describing pain as "an unpleasant sensory and emotional experience associated with actual or potential tissue damage."[6] McCaffery defines pain as "whatever the experiencing person says it is, existing whenever the experiencing person says its does."[39]

The key to promoting effective rehabilitation begins with effective management of acute pain. Pain management offers a significant challenge for nurses caring for patients who have sustained most types of fractures. Following a fracture, pain is acute regardless of trauma or underlying disease. For nurses this requires careful and consistent assessment of pain as reported by patients. Neither behavior nor vital signs can substitute for self-report.[1]

Because of the varied personal and cultural beliefs held by nurses and patients concerning what constitutes pain, careful initial assessment of patients' experiences with pain is an important factor in managing pain. Determining how a particular patient responds to prior instances (pain history) helps to establish a guide for pain control. Patients need to take an active part in their own pain management to ensure its effectiveness.

The introduction and use of a pain scale is an increasingly accepted means of determining severity of pain. Patient education in the use of a pain scale improves its use. The AHCPR guidelines suggest several varieties of pain scales available for use in clinical practice.[1] Examples are shown in Figure 1.

Pharmacologic Management. The two major classes of analgesics used include central acting analgesics (opioids) and peripheral acting analgesics (nonsteroidal antiinflammatory drugs). Concurrent use of both of these classes of analgesics opioids and NSAIDs often provides more effective analgesia than either of the classes alone.[1]

Analgesics often are ordered *as required* by the physician in less than therapeutic doses. As a result, patients are undermedicated because nurses medicate only when patients request it and might make patients wait if their

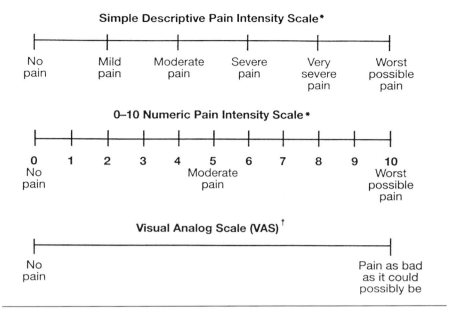

FIGURE 1. Pain Intensity Scales[1]

behavior fails to look sufficiently "painful."[46] This pattern of analgesic administration leads to ineffective pain management.

One of the most important aspects of pain management is to adopt a preventive approach. Around-the-clock dosing gives control to the patient. Patients are assured of medication for pain without having to ask. Orders for additional medication for breakthrough pain, which occurs when activities increase the use of the affected area, should be available to patients. Medication should be offered before procedures, physical therapy, or activities that increase the use of the affected area or cause additional pain.

Of the newer technologies in use, patient controlled analgesia (PCA) has been found to be an effective way to improve patient comfort and is used in many hospitals. PCA is administered intravenously or subcutaneously through the use of an infusion pump. The primary physician orders the dose of medication to be given. Central acting analgesics are the drugs of choice, morphine being the prototype.[46]

The effectiveness and success of PCA are determined primarily by careful selection of patients. Those with a history of chronic pulmonary disease, altered mental status, physical inability, allergic reactions to narcotics, and history of drug abuse are usually considered poor candidates for PCA.[58]

Nursing considerations when administering PCA are the same as when administering analgesics by conventional methods. Assessment and documentation are important to determine extent of patient comfort, and patients must be taught how infusion pumps work.

Another technique increasing both in popularity and use is epidural analgesia, which is used for acute postoperative pain and is effective for pelvic and lower extremity involvement. Central acting analgesics, primarily morphine, are the drugs of choice. Specific nursing considerations include close and consistent monitoring of patient status. Respiratory depression can be induced by the use of epidural analgesia usually within the first 2 hours of administration.[46]

Nonpharmacologic Methods. As the immediate and acute pain subsides, there are many treatment modalities for pain management that do not involve the use of medications and some of which are independent nursing interventions. It is important for nurses to become familiar with the techniques listed in Table 6 and implement them when caring for the patients.

Impaired Physical Mobility

Immobilizing a fracture is basic to medical treatment. Nurses' concerns include and extend beyond the immobilized fracture to the resulting impairment of physical mobility of the patient. For example, a cast immobilizes a leg and impairs the patient's ability to move. Balcombe, Davis, and Lim[7] state that moving, mobility, mobilizing, and activity are fundamental considerations in orthopedic nursing. They propose a model for orthopedic nursing with mobility as the core concept. Mobility-related nursing care considerations include self concept, diet, mental state, breathing, sleep, movement, pain, aspirations for health, behavior, and hygiene. Impaired physical mobility creates a cascade of concerns for nurses such as pressure management and prevention of secondary medical problems resulting from circulatory and pulmonary stasis such as pulmonary embolism and pneumonia.[25,41] Inactivity can also lead to further functional loss and bone loss, a particular problem with elderly patients.[11,15,17]

Positioning. Proper positioning is crucial to maintaining body alignment, relieving pressure, and promoting circulation and drainage. When patients are bedbound and unable to move without assistance, pull sheets are placed under them to facilitate log rolling or moving. Patients' positions should be changed every 2 hours.[40,54] Patients should be taught to assist with turning by grasping the bed rails for support, and if possible, they should be encouraged to turn themselves. Use of pillows and bolsters to support the back and buttocks enhances comfort, maintains alignment, and helps patients to maintain the position. Elevating affected limbs 20° or greater, above the level of the heart, improves venous return as appropriate.[40]

Pressure Management. McCloskey and Bulechek[40] identify pressure management as minimizing pressure to body parts. They include specific activities, such as padding rough cast edges and traction connections, and using toe pleats or bed cradles. The AHCPR clinical guidelines for the prediction and prevention of pressure sores in adults[54] summarize the best information available on pressure management. The guidelines, listed in Table 7, specifically address pressure management as part of a goal to protect against the adverse effects of external

TABLE 6.   Nonpharmacologic Interventions for Postoperative Pain[1]

Cognitive-Behavioral	Physical Agents
Education/instruction	Applications of heat or cold
Relaxation	Massage, exercise and immobilization
Imagery	Transcutaneous electrical nerve stimulaton
Music distraction	
Biofeedback	

TABLE 7. Pressure Ulcer Prediction and Prevention Algorithm Guidelines[54]

1. Activity or Mobility Deficit	Bed- or chair-bound individuals or those whose ability to reposition is impaired should be considered at risk for pressure ulcers. Identification of additional risk factors (immobility, moisture/incontinence, and nutritional deficit) should be undertaken to direct specific preventive treatment regimens.
2. Educational Program	Educational programs for the prevention of pressure ulcers should be structured, organized, and comprehensive and directed at all levels of health care providers, patients, and family or caregivers.
3. Reassessment	Active, mobile individuals should be periodically reassessed for changes in activity and mobility status. The frequency of reassessment depends on patient status and institutional policy.
4. Risk Assessment Tools	Clinicians are encouraged to select and use a method of risk assessment that ensures systematic evaluation of individual risk factors. Many risk assessment tools exist but only the Norton Scale and the Braden Scale have been tested extensively. Risk assessment tools include the following risk factors: mobility/activity impairment, moisture/incontinence, and impaired nutrition. Altered level of consciousness (or altered sensory perception) is also identified as a risk factor in most assessment tools. Identification of individual risk factors is helpful in directing care.
5. Mobility/Activity Deficit	*Mechanical Loading and Support Surface Guideline* For bed-bound individual: <ul><li>Reposition at least every 2 hours</li><li>Use pillows or foam wedges to keep bony prominences from direct contact.</li><li>Use devices that totally relieve pressure on the heels.</li><li>Avoid positioning directly on the trochanter.</li><li>Elevate the head of the bed as little and for as short a time as possible.</li><li>Use lifting devices to move rather than drag individuals during transfers and position changes.</li><li>Place at-risk individuals on a pressure-reducing mattress.</li></ul> **Do not use donut-type devices.** For chair-bound individuals: <ul><li>Reposition at least every hour.</li><li>Have patient shift weight every 15 minutes if able.</li><li>Use pressure-reducing devices for seating surfaces. **Do not use donut-type devices.**</li><li>Consider postural alignment, distribution of weight, balance and stability, and pressure relief when positioning individuals in chairs or wheelchairs.</li><li>Use a written plan.</li></ul> *Skin Care and Early Treatment Guideline* <ul><li>Inspect skin at least once a day.</li><li>Individualize bathing schedule. Avoid hot water. Use a mild cleansing agent.</li><li>Minimize environmental factors such as low humidity and cold air. Use moisturizers for dry skin.</li><li>Avoid massage over bony prominences.</li><li>Use proper positioning, transferring, and turning techniques.</li><li>Use lubricants to reduce friction injuries.</li><li>Institute a rehabilitation program.</li><li>Monitor and document interventions and outcomes.</li></ul>
6. Moisture/ Incontinence	<ul><li>Cleanse skin at time of soiling.</li><li>Minimize skin exposure to moisture. Assess and treat urinary incontinence. When moisture cannot be controlled, use underpads or briefs that are absorbent and present a quick-drying surface to the skin.</li></ul>
7. Nutritional deficit	<ul><li>Investigate factors that compromise an apparently well-nourished individual's dietary intake (especially protein or calories) and offer him or her support with eating.</li><li>Plan and implement a nutritional support and/or supplementation program for nutritionally compromised individuals.</li></ul>

mechanical forces: pressure, friction, and shear. The guidelines include specific recommendations for bed-bound and chair-bound patients, including frequency of position changes, use of devices/special surfaces to relieve pressure on bony prominences (especially the heels), avoiding placement on the trochanter, use of lifting devices, and use of a written plan for pressure management. Devices to keep weight off heels, ankles, and the sacrum while the patient is in bed should be used in immobile patients or those unable to recall or comply with preventive instructions while on bed rest.[23]

Preventing Complications of Inactivity. Inactivity leads to serious consequences related to pulmonary stasis, disuse of muscles, and circulatory stasis. Nursing responsibilities include teaching patients how to prevent complications. Bed-bound patients should be taught how to do deep breathing and coughing exercises, how to use incentive spirometry, and how to use pulmonary treatments such as hand-held nebulizers or an intermittent positive pressure breathing apparatus. Frequent position changes are important to prevent pulmonary and circulatory stasis and to relieve pressure.

Range of motion exercises prevent atrophy and stiffness. Exercises, which may vary in type depending upon patients' needs, may be active (motion is performed by the patient), passive (another person manipulates the patient's limbs), active-resistive (the patient actively performs as much of the motion as possible, with help as needed).[37] Active and passive exercises should be done at least three times daily either by a physical therapist or nurse. Patients should be reminded to exercise both the affected extremity and the unaffected extremity. For patients whose fractures allow, sit-ups or pull-ups strengthen the arms and shoulders to ease other movement. Quadriceps and gluteal sitting exercises strengthen the muscles needed to prepare patients for ambulating. Nurses collaborate with physical therapists to teach and encourage patients to use exercises to promote circulation and prevent the complications of inactivity.[31] Nurses play an important role in teaching the importance of and encouraging weightbearing activities as early as possible in a fracture episode, which helps to mitigate the loss of bone.

Circulatory stasis is alleviated by elevating affected parts, performing range of motion exercises, and using anti-embolism stockings. Patients should be advised to exercise the joints above and below the cast and to wiggle fingers or toes to stimulate circulation and increase venous return.

Self-care Activities

Nursing diagnoses specify five self-care deficits: feeding, bathing/hygiene, dressing/grooming, toileting, and instrumental self-care.[13] Patients in casts, with fixation devices, or in traction may be unable to accomplish one or another of these self-care activities temporarily or for an extended time. Nurses work with occupational therapists to teach patients to use adaptive devices or alternate ways to accomplish the tasks. The goal of care is to help patients regain self-care as soon as possible. Nurses assess patients' abilities and design interventions to maximize self-care and to increase patients' potential for independent function. Nurses encourage patients to increase activities as far as they are able to tolerate. Self-care activities should be flexible and modified according to patients' needs and lifestyle. Nurses facilitate self-care by ensuring accessibility of call bells, bed-side stands, trapezes, overbed tables, and assistive devices such as reachers, long-handled combs, or sock aids. Nurses support patients by giving justifiable praise for their efforts and accomplishments. Independence in self-care affords patients a sense of purpose and dignity.

Olson and Ustanko[50] report a study of the self-care needs of patients in the halo brace. The most commonly reported difficulties among their respondents were bathing, dressing, and finding clothing that fit over the brace. The majority of patients reported needing help with bathing and grooming.

Limit Setting

Patients with fractures may exhibit difficult or demanding behavior related to anxiety or grief concerning their injury. In addition to having acute pain, they may have a sense of having lost control of what happens to them. Their emotional and behavioral responses present a challenge for the nursing staff.

Patients who sustain injuries may have lifestyles that include activities such as fighting, driving under the influence of alcohol or drugs, and illegal activities. Alcohol and drug use are implicated in a high percentage of accidental orthopedic injuries. Problematic behavior and personality problems may be the cause rather than the effect of traumatic injuries.[36]

Patients whose fractures require long-term care in the hospital or rehabilitation unit may become quite familiar with the nursing staff, the layout of the hospital and hospital routines, and can become quite regimented and demanding, dictating their plans of care. Patients manifest problem behavior by demanding special considerations, using verbally abusive language, acting out, refusing to keep therapy appointments, and attempting to pit one staff member against another. These disruptive behaviors interfere with effective nursing interventions and impede progress toward self-care.

The single most effective measure in controlling behavior problems is the use of limit setting. Limit setting is an overall term used to describe interventions that decrease problematic behaviors. The basic strategy of limit setting is to give the patient structure by communicating expected behavior.[36,40] The use of direct statements focused on what is expected of patients rather than on what they should not be doing is an effective means of directing behavior. A key factor in limit setting is consistency. Nurses initiating plans of care need to include specific nursing interventions and make sure the information is communicated to all of the nursing staff providing the care. All personnel coming in contact with patients understand the limits and consistently apply them to patients.

Contracting with Patients

Another means of minimizing problematic behavior in patients is the use of a behavioral contract.[10,40] Behavioral contracts include patients in their design, delineate mutually agreed upon expected outcomes, and are in writing. Patients have copies to which they can refer to assess their own progress during hospitalization. Behavioral contracts are effective when used for slow progress and ongoing complaints of pain. As with limit setting, communication of plans to all personnel and consistent responses to patients are crucial to the success of this intervention.

COMPLICATIONS

Impaired Skin Integrity

Surveys indicate that the incidence of pressure sores in hospitals ranges from 2.7–29.5%.[55] Cummings[18] cites Versluysen's study of patients with a fractured neck of femur, which notes that 66% developed pressure sores. Another report states that up to 96% of pressure sores occur over bony prominences on the lower half of the body, including the calcaneus and the malleolus of the ankle.[62] Breakdown of the skin on the feet results in increased use of medical resources, added nursing time for dressing changes, and extended hospitalization.

Prevention of Pressure Sores.   In many, if not all instances, pressure sores can be avoided by meticulous skin care, relief of pressure over bony prominences, and nutritional support. Preventive measures are initiated by nurses; however, involving patients in the prevention of skin breakdown by extensive patient education should be a fundamental goal. The AHCPR's clinical practice guideline *Pressure Ulcers in Adults: Prediction and Prevention*[54] recommends a preferred management path as depicted in Figure 2 and further explicated in Table 7.

All bony prominences, back, buttocks, heels, and ears are potential pressure points. Back care should be carried out at least every 3–4 hours to increase circulation. Patients in traction are at high risk for skin breakdown over the heel. Inspecting the heel is the only way to evaluate heel status. The antiembolism hose must be removed at least twice daily to detect early impairment of skin integrity. Heel protectors should be applied[54] but should be removed for heel inspection.

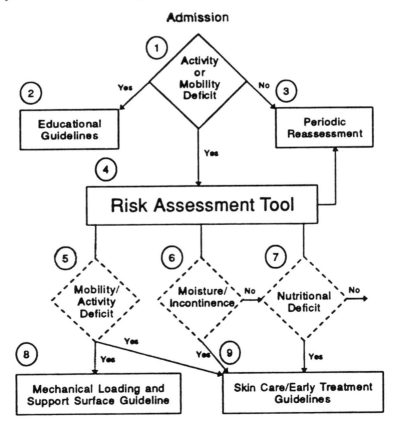

FIGURE 2.   Pressure Ulcer Prediction and Prevention Algorithm.[54]

It is imperative that patient education includes notifying the nurse if discomfort is felt in the heels. Heels can also be kept off the bed by placing a folded bath blanket under the calf. However, it is important to place the blanket so it does not put pressure on the popliteal space or the Achilles tendon.

With a trapeze, patients can lift themselves for some aspects of care and inspections, thereby relieving pressure on the sacral area and improving circulation. Patients should also be instructed to place their unaffected feet flat on the bed and push with the foot (not the heel) when raising themselves with the trapeze. Patients who are in traction frequently encounter skin impairment associated with tapes and wrapping bandages. Irritation from tape may come from various sources. When the stress of weight causes the adhesive tapes to slip, the skin is often pulled off. The skin needs to be checked carefully for drainage or odor whenever tape is placed for long periods. Patients also need to be questioned concerning skin discomfort.

Patients who have Steinmann pins in the tibia need to pull themselves up in bed frequently. Unfortunately, they often use their elbows rather than the trapeze, causing skin impairment. For this reason it is imperative that nurses provide patient education on the importance of position changes and the proper use of the trapeze.

Cervical Traction. Patients in cervical traction must have the occiput, chin, ears, and mandible inspected daily. Cornstarch helps keep the chin dry.[54] With a physician's order, patients with highly sensitive skin may be permitted to pull the chin piece down for a few seconds at frequent intervals to prevent skin irritation.

Pelvic Sling Traction. The iliac crest is very vulnerable to pressure. Special padding over the crests of thin patients helps relieve pressure. Elbows may become reddened as patients shift position. Elbow pads and lotion should be used as indicated.[54]

Buck's Traction. The patient generally is able to lift the top half of the body off the bed with the use of a trapeze. The patient may be turned 45° to either side with a pillow between the legs. The pillow maintains the line of pull in the affected leg. The affected heel must be kept off the mattress.

Russell's Traction. The skin at the edges of the sling needs to be inspected frequently for irritation. The foot plate may also be a source of irritation. Placing an abdominal (ABD) pad between the sole of the foot and the foot spreader provides some foot support. Heels should be kept off the mattress. The unaffected extremity and elbows also need close inspection.

Treatment of Pressure Sores. The emphasis in the literature currently is on prevention; however, Alterescu and Alterescu[3] address treatment of pressure sores if preventive measures fail. They enumerate four fundamental guidelines: (1) correct the underlying pathology; (2) debride necrotic tissue; (3) reduce bacteria/maintain host defenses; and (4) maintain a physiologic environment. They emphasize reducing pressure and increasing the frequency of changes of position. They evaluate multiple types of products designed to reduce sources of irritation, including friction, pressure, moisture, and shear. The items they evaluate range from gel cushions and pads to air-filled items, water-filled items, spot relief products, and specialized beds. They maintain that the choice of device is based on the assessment of what is best for an individual patient.

High Risk for Peripheral Neurovascular Dysfunction

The NAON Guidelines for Orthopaedic Nursing[48] identify high risks for peripheral neurovascular dysfunction among the most common nursing diagnoses seen in orthopedic patients. The expected outcomes of nursing and patient education interventions are the prevention or early detection of compartment syndrome. Patients are taught neurovascular assessment and to report uncontrolled pain, coolness, weakness, or diminished sensation immediately.[56] Immediate goals and independent nursing interventions are to decrease tissue pressure; restore local blood flow and minimize functional loss by lowering the extremity to the level of the heart and avoiding pressure on the affected area; and take precise neurovascular assessment and report accurate information to the physician promptly.[60] The physician may bivalve the cast or take the patient to surgery.

DISCHARGE PLANNING

Discharge planning is an essential component of rehabilitation nursing. It fosters continuity of care by ensuring that post-hospital nursing care needs are identified early prior to discharge and that plans are made to meet these needs. Planning discharge and rehabilitation of fracture patients begins on admission to the hospital.[11] The complexity of discharge planning depends on the needs of individual patients. The discharge planning assessment considers living arrangements, support systems, financial status, transportation, occupation, premorbid level of functioning, and comorbid conditions that affect patients' abilities to live safely and independently. Referrals to appropriate agencies for necessary support service are arranged.[16]

An interdisciplinary team approach assures comprehensive and coordinated care before and after discharge. The interdisciplinary team may include physicians, nurses, discharge planners, social workers, dietitians, physical therapists, and occupational therapists. Regular team meetings facilitate evaluations of patients' progress. The nurse who provides the greatest percentage of care for the patient brings to meetings the patient's level of self-care, pain management, skin assessment, and progress as viewed at the bedside. The nurse will usually be the one to identify psychosocial aspects such as helplessness, behavior problems, and family involvement. Collaboration among the disciplines is critical to attaining treatment goals.[51,61] Pittman, Morton, Edwards, and Holmes[53] emphasize the importance of careful documentation in multidisciplinary discharge planning.

The importance of good communication among the health disciplines and between the patient and family cannot be overemphasized. A cohesive group committed to meeting individual patient needs promotes effective planning best when the members involve patients and their families in the design and implementation of plans.

Instrumental Self-Care Deficit

Carpenito[13] defines instrumental self-care deficit as an impaired ability to perform activities or access services essential for managing a home. These activities and services include using a telephone, laundering, preparing meals, and shopping. Home health care referrals and requests for community services such as Meals-on-Wheels and day health care may need be arranged with patients or the consent of significant others to ensure a smooth transition from hospital to community. North, Meeusen, and Hollinsworth[49] recommend overnight passes as a way to identify needs that have been overlooked and to boost patients' confidence prior to discharge.

Patient/Family Education

Nurses initiate teaching on medication management, wound care, or any knowledge or skill deficit. Patients requiring hospitalization for orthopedic procedures now have shorter stays due to changes in orthopedic medical and nursing practice as a result of trends such as cost containment, advances in technology, and consumer activism.[16] For discharge to home, patients require clear and concise education concerning follow-up appointments, use of pain medications, any activity limits, use of equipment, signs and symptoms of potential complications, and what to do in the event of a complication. Patients and significant others should be taught neurovascular assessment skills and the signs and symptoms of infection. Both written materials and verbal instructions should be supplied. Patients should also be given the name of a person and/or phone number they can call for questions. Prepared discharge is one way of assuring patients are ready to manage their care at home.

Alywahby[4] recommends teaching strategies to enhance learning for older patients. She recommends well-organized teaching materials, time for patients to rehearse the information or skill, emphasis on relationships among items, and attention to the physical environment during the teaching-learning situation. Anxiety, overarousal, and interference from previously learned information may interfere with patients' ability to learn. Teaching strategies must take this into account and offer patients opportunities to decrease anxiety, clarify conflicting information, and achieve a sense of mastery.

Promote Healing.   Nutrition and hydration are essential to the healing process. Cornell[17] specifically addresses the importance of nutrition in elderly patients with fractures, pointing out that elderly patients are often malnourished and that nutritional replacement should be handled aggressively. Kendrick[35] suggests low-fat, high-fiber diets rich in calcium to promote healing, prevent constipation, and prevent weight gain.

Post Cast Care.   The sight and sound of an electric cast cutter can be frightening to patients. One must prepare patients for the sound and reassure them that the blade will not cut them. The skin under the casted area is commonly mottled and contains crusts of dead skin, oil, and exudate. Patients may experience increased tenderness, pain, stiffness, edema, and muscle weakness. Muscles may appear flabby and slightly atrophied. New aches and pains may appear with movements. Edema of the leg or foot frequently occurs after a long leg cast is removed. Patients should be instructed to elevate the affected limb and use antiembolism stockings to promote circulation. Increased activity, prescribed exercises, and improvement in muscle tone and circulation will lessen the edema.

High Risk for Injury.   The potential for injury must be considered in patients discharged with immobilization devices (casts, external fixation devices, traction) or after the devices are removed. Homes should be evaluated for safety hazards such as loose carpeting, highly waxed or slippery floors, electrical cords, scatter rugs, steps, pets, poor lighting, and uneven surfaces. Patients with fractures related to diseases such as osteoporosis may need rehabilitative assistance to restructure activities to reduce the possibility of future fractures.

The key to quality discharge planning is a comprehensive assessment of patients' individual needs and having a coordinated treatment care plan involving providers from various health care disciplines. From the initial assessment, identified areas of concern should be brought to the attention of the discharge planning team. Successful discharge planning is a centralized, coordinated multidisciplinary process that ensures that all patients are prepared adequately for discharge and have a plan for continuing care after they leave the hospital. According to Pittman et al., a discharge plan "must be based on a philosophy of patient care that each patient is an individual, taking into consideration the patient's emotional, social and economic history as well as specific needs for continuing care."[53]

ACKNOWLEDGMENT

The authors thank Hannah Dean, RN, PhD, for her consultation and editorial assistance in the preparation of this manuscript.

REFERENCES
1. Acute pain management: Operative or medical procedures and trauma. Washington, DC, US Dept of Health and Human Services, 1992, Agency for Health Care Policy and Research publication 92-0032.
2. Adelstein W: C_1-C_2 fractures and dislocations. J Neurosci Nurs 21:149–159, 1989.
3. Alterescu V, Alterescu KB: Pressure ulcers: Assessment and treatment. Orthop Nurs 11:37–49, 1992.
4. Alywahby NF: Principles of teaching for individual learning of older adults. Rehabil Nurs 14:330–333, 1989.
5. American Nurses Association: Standards of Clinical Nursing Practice. Kansas City, MO, American Nurses Association, 1991.
6. American Pain Society: Principles of Analgesic Use in the Treatment of Acute Pain and Chronic Cancer Pain: A Concise Guide to Medical Practice. 2nd ed. Skokie, IL, American Pain Society, 1989.
7. Balcombe K, Davis P, Lim E: A nursing model for orthopedics. Nurs Stand 5(49):26–28, 1991.
8. Barden RM, Sinkora GL: Bone stimulators for fusions and fractures. Nurs Clin North Am 26:89–103, 1991.
9. Blazek M: One diagnosis in 10 minutes, please! J Emerg Nurs 15:462, 1989.
10. Bulechek GM, McCloskey JC: Nursing Interventions: Essential Nursing Treatments. 2nd ed. Philadelphia, WB Saunders, 1992.
11. Butler M: Geriatric rehabilitation nursing. Rehabil Nurs 16:318–321, 1991.
12. Calvani DL, Douris KR: Functional assessment: A holistic approach to rehabilitation of the geriatric client. Rehabil Nurs 16:330–335, 1991.
13. Carpenito LJ: Nursing Diagnosis: Application to Practice. 4th ed. Philadelphia, JB Lippincott, 1992.
14. Cochran S: Action stat! Open fracture. Nursing87 17(5):33, 1987.
15. Cohen LD: Fractures of the osteoporotic spine. Orthop Clin North Am 21:143–150, 1990.
16. Connolly ML: Ambulatory surgery and prepared discharges: Effects on orthopedic patients and nursing practice. Nurs Clin North Am 26:105–112, 1991.
17. Cornell CN: Management of fractures in patients with osteoporosis. Orthop Clin North Am 21:125–141, 1990.
18. Cummings J: Managing the patient with fractured femur. Part I. Nurs Stand 5(25)(suppl):11–13, 1991.
19. Cummings J: Managing the patient with fractured femur. Part II. Nurs Stand 5(36)(suppl):11–13, 1991.
20. Cummings J: Managing the patient with fractured femur. Part III. Nurs Stand 5(50)(suppl):11–13, 1991.
21. Dunwoody CJ: Pelvic fracture patient care: Reflections on the past, implications for the future. Nurs Clin North Am 26:65–72, 1991.
22. Evers JA, Werpachowski D: Dealing with fractures. RN 47(11):53–55, 57, 1984.
23. Farrell J: Illustrated Guide to Orthopedic Nursing. 3rd ed. Philadelphia, JB Lippincott, 1986.
24. Farrell J: Orthopedic pain: What does it mean? Am J Nurs 84:466–469, 1984.
25. Genge ML: Orthopaedic trauma: Pelvic fractures. Orthop Nurs 5(1):11–19, 1986.
26. Goldberger DK, Kruse L, Stender R: A survey of external fixator pin care techniques. Clin Nurse Specialist 1:166–169, 1987.
27. Harper A: Initial assessement and management of femoral neck fractures in the elderly. Orthop Nurs 4:55–58, 1985.
28. Hartweg DL: Dorothea Orem: Self-care Deficit Theory. Newbury Park, CA, Sage, 1991.
29. Head JM: Multilevel spine fractures: Intraoperative nursing management. J Neurosci Nurs 22:370–374, 1990.
30. Holcomb S: Pulmonary embolism: Preventing a disaster. RN 54(9):52–58, 1991.

31. Ignatavicius DD, Bayne MV: Medical-Surgical Nursing: A Nursing Process Approach. Philadelphia, WB Saunders, 1991.
32. Johnson L: Operative management of unstable pelvic fractures. Orthop Nurs 8:21–25, 1989.
33. Jones-Walton P: Effects of pin care on pin reactions in adults with extremity fracture treated with skeletal traction and external fixation. Orthop Nurs 7:29–33, 1988.
34. Jones-Walton P: Clinical standards in skeletal traction pin site care. Orthop Nurs 10:12–16, 1991.
35. Kendrick DW: Now I stand up for my patients. RN 56(4):37–39, 1993.
36. Kestler V: Limitsetting: Dealing with difficult patients. Orthop Nurs 10(6):19–23, 1991.
37. Luckmann J, Sorenson KC: Medical-Surgical Nursing: A Psychophysiologic Approach. 3rd ed. Philadelphia, WB Saunders, 1987.
38. Mandzuk LL: External pinsite care: A review of the literature and nursing practice. CONA Journal 13(1):10–15, 1991.
39. McCaffrey M, Beebe A: Pain: Clinical Manual for Nursing Practice. St. Louis, Mosby, 1989.
40. McCloskey JC, Bulecheck GM: Iowa Intervention Project: Nursing Interventions Classification (NIC). St. Louis, Mosby-Year Book, 1992.
41. McKenna ME, McCarthy C: Nursing management of the patient with a spinal fracture. CONA Journal 10(3):4–9, 1988.
42. Metcalf EM: The orthopaedic critical path. Orthop Nurs 10(6):25–31, 1991.
43. Meyer PS: Urologic complications associated with pelvic fractures. Orthop Nurs 8(4):41–44, 48, 1989.
44. Moncada G, Black J: Facial fractures. Plastic Surgical Nursing 6:125–125, 1986.
45. Monk HL: Fractures are never simple. RN 56(4):30–35, 1993.
46. Mooney NE: Pain management in the orthopedic patient. Nurs Clin North Am 26:73–87, 1991.
47. Mourad LA: Orthopedic Disorders. St. Louis, Mosby, 1991.
48. National Association of Orthopaedic Nurses: Guidelines for Orthopaedic Nursing. Pitman, NJ, Anthony J. Janetti, 1992.
49. North M, Meeusen M, Hollinsworth P: Discharge planning: Increasing client and nurse satisfaction. Rehabil Nurs 16:327–329, 1991.
50. Olson B, Ustanko L: Self-care needs of patients in the halo brace. Orthop Nurs 9(1):27–33, 52, 1990.
51. Pachter S, Flics SS: Integrated care of patients with fractured hip by nursing and physical therapy. In Scherubel JC (ed): Patients and Purse Strings II. New York, National League for Nursing, 1988, pp 441–443.
52. Peter NK: Care of patients with traumatic pelvic fractures. Crit Care Nurse 8(3):62, 1988.
53. Pittman L, Morton W, Edwards L, Holmes D: Patient discharge planning documentation in an Australian multidisciplinary rehabilitation setting. Rehabil Nurs 17:327–331, 1992.
54. Pressure ulcers in adults: Prediction and prevention. Washington, DC, US Dept of Health and Human Services, 1992, Agency for Health Care Policy and Research publication 92-0047.
55. Redheffer GM, Bailey M: Assessing and splinting fractures. Nursing89 19(6):51–59, 1989.
56. Ross D: Acute compartment syndrome. Orthop Nurs 10(2):33–38, 1991.
57. Rubenstein LV, Chang BL, Keeler EB, Kahn KL: Measuring the quality of nursing surveillance activities for five diseases before and after implementation of the DRG-based prospective payment system. Proceedings of Patient Outcomes Research: Examining the Effectiveness of Nursing Practice, a conference sponsored by the National Center for Nursing Research. Bethesda, MD, publication 93-3411.
58. Salmond SW, Mooney NE, Verdisco LA: National Association of Orthopaedic Nurses: Core Curriculum for Orthopaedic Nursing. 2nd ed. Pitman, NJ, Anthony J. Janetti, 1991.
59. Sawin KJ, Heard L: Nursing diagnoses used most frequently in rehabiliation nursing. Rehabil Nurs 17:256–262, 1992.
60. Slye DA: Orthopedic complications: Compartment syndrome, fat embolism syndrome, and venous thromboembolism. Nurs Clin North Am 26:113–132, 1991.
61. Walsh CR: Collaborative practice: A coordinated approach to patient care. Orthop Nurs 10(5):52–60, 1991.
62. Yetzer EA, Sullivan RL: The foot at risk: Identification and prevention of skin breakdown. Rehabil Nurs 17:247–251, 1992.
63. Zimmer Traction Handbook: A Complete Reference Guide to the Basics of Traction. Zimmer, 1992.

PULIYODIL A. PHILIP, MD
EDWARD S. TRAISMAN, MD
MERSAMMA PHILIP, MD

MUSCULOSKELETAL INJURIES IN CHILD ABUSE

From the Northwestern University
  Medical School (PAP, EST, MP)
  and
Rehabilitation Institute of Chicago
  (PAP, EST)
  and
Children's Memorial Hospital
  (PAP, EST)
Chicago, Illinois

Reprint requests to:
Puliyodil A. Philip, MD
Rehabilitation Institute of
  Chicago
345 East Superior Street
Chicago, IL 60611

The term *battered child syndrome* was first defined in 1961 to make physicians aware of the manifestations of physical abuse of children.[48] Since then, child abuse has expanded to include sexual abuse, failure to thrive, neglect, poisoning, emotional abuse, burns, and Munchausen's syndrome by proxy.[16,56] Physical abuse is defined as nonaccidental injury caused by a caretaker. The injury causes tissue damage that can result in bruises, burns, fractures, head injury, lacerations, or organ damage. The use of an object to inflict injury on any body part is abuse.[25,48] Child abuse occurs in 16.3 per 1,000 children in the United States with 9.2 per 1,000 children suffering physical, emotional, or sexual abuse.[55] Child abuse affects 650,000–1 million children up to age 18 annually.[16,56] In 1992, 2.9 million children—45 out of every 1,000 children—were reported as abused nationwide. This is an increase of 8% from 1991 (Fig. 1). Most abused children are boys with an average age of 6–7.[8,16] Moderate injury occurred in 72% of reported cases, with 15% of children suffering serious injury. One in a thousand children die annually from abuse.[25,55] Fatality is highest from abuse in children younger than 1 year old.[6] Many cases do go unnoticed, and therefore, unfortunately, unreported. Physicians and other health care workers must be aware of this condition when dealing with childhood injury. Once child abuse has been established, appropriate legal action must be initiated and followed through.

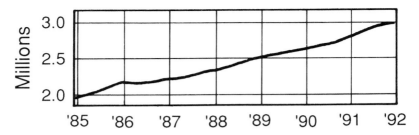

FIGURE 1. Estimated number of children abused nationwide. From the National Committee for Prevention of Child Abuse.

Poverty is a large factor contributing to abuse. Poor families have a much higher rate of abuse.[5,8,16] Exposure to violence and abuse within the family increases the risk of abuse[5,16] (30% of abused children abuse other children as adults).[5,8] Parents inflict abuse in a majority of cases, with poor, single mothers being the most common offenders.[5,16,25] These predisposing factors exist regardless of racial background.[8,37] It is important to remember that any person of any background can be guilty of child abuse. In pediatrics and other child care related programs, child abuse education exists to increase the awareness of this condition and help identify the abusers and their victims. Physicians, attorneys, nurses, coroners, dentists, psychologists, speech pathologists, teachers, and child care workers are mandated to report suspected cases of abuse. However, while all 50 states have child abuse legislation, the laws allow for a wide range of interpretation and, therefore, reports of abuse may vary.[25] Reporter interpretation of what constitutes discipline, accident, or abuse, along with monetary, legal or personal issues,[37,46] may influence the decision to file a case of abuse.

In pediatrics and physiatry, patients with injuries are a common occurrence. The medical evaluation of most injuries is straightforward; however, to differentiate accident from abuse can be difficult. Physicians must take into account ritual or cultural "norms" when considering between intentional or non-intentional injury. For example, corporal punishment was common in American families and schools well into the 20th century.[23] The avoidance of medical care in favor of religious healing could be viewed as neglect. In many states, obtaining court custody to render medical treatment (e.g., surgery, transfusions) is common practice. "Cupping" in Eastern Europe or rubbing heated coins or spoons along the skin in Southeast Asia[14] is an accepted practice and may cause burns. Physicians and immigrant families need to educate one another about their cultural differences with respect to medical treatment[24] to avoid false allegations of abuse.

In this chapter, we will review common types of musculoskeletal injuries and how physical abuse can be differentiated from accidental injury. A management plan for the treatment of abused children will be outlined. Other areas of abuse (sexual, neglect, failure to thrive, and Munchausen's by proxy) will not be discussed.

FRACTURES

In children, especially infants and toddlers, it is hard to differentiate between intentional or accidental fractures. More than half (58–66%) of abused children are younger than 3 but have 94% of all intentional fractures.[19,48] Half of all known abused children with fractures are younger than 1.[19,36] In consecutive studies of fractures in children, Leventhal et al. found that 39% of abused children with fractures are younger than 1 year old and that 8% of all fractures in children older than 2 is the result of abuse.[33] Accidental fractures can occur in infants and toddlers after minor (from a height of less than 4 feet) or significant (more than 4 feet) falls.[17,19,31,33] More significant injury occurs due to falls from greater heights.[35] With any fracture due to a "minor" fall that is associated with multiple injuries or internal injuries, abuse should be considered. Most accidental fractures occur in school-age children.[19]

The plausibility of an event resulting in a fracture can be determined by experience and medical knowledge. For example, the story of a 2-month-old rolling from a couch and suffering a skull fracture with an intracranial hemorrhage is unlikely in view of the severity of the injury, "minor" amount of trauma, and that, developmentally, a 2-month-old cannot roll over. To a trained physician this history would be alarming and raise concerns for abuse. Leventhal et al. found that of all cases resulting in fractures in their study, 60% of the children suffered a fall; 11% of all falls were the result of abuse, and 9% were equivocal in origin.[33]

Most children who suffer an accidental fracture are brought to medical attention within hours. These children are usually in pain and are crying, and the affected extremity is swollen or bruised.[19] A delay in seeking medical attention is seen in abuse cases.[47] Abused children with fractures may present with an unclear history of a swollen extremity, change in use of the affected limb, and minimal pain. This type of history is seen in half of abuse cases.[33]

The mechanism of skeletal injuries includes direct blows, twisting forces, shaking, and squeezing.[38] The diagnosis of the battered child syndrome depends on the discrepancy between alleged mechanisms of injury and the mechanisms that are actually responsible. Transverse or spiral (oblique) diaphyseal fractures are usually caused by direct blows. These fractures are common but not pathognomonic of the battered child syndrome. For example, a transverse fracture of a long bone in a 3-month-old baby is a much more suspicious injury than the same in a 6-year-old child. A direct blow to the clavicle results in a mid shaft fracture, which is common finding in the battered child syndrome. Direct blows to the scapula can also result in nonspecific linear or stellate fractures. These fractures are uncommon in infants and young children, and their presence should arouse suspicion. Direct blows to the face produce a variety of facial and mandibular fractures that frequently are associated with intracranial injury. Child abuse should be considered in these cases.

Twisting is another mechanism of skeletal injury in child abuse. Long-bone spiral (oblique) fractures are very specific for child abuse in preambulatory infants and generally a result of the application of twisting force to an extremity (Figs. 2 and 3). These types of fractures in older ambulatory children are not specific for child abuse. A toddler who accidentally falls and twists the lower extremity can sustain a spiral fracture of the tibia. This is commonly known as a toddler's fracture. Spiral fractures of the femur can also occur accidentally in toddlers, but they are frequently caused by child abuse and should be thoroughly evaluated.[54] Because the junction of epiphysis and metaphysis is one of the weakest parts of the long bones, twisting forces can produce epiphyseal-metaphyseal fractures and separation[27,51] (Fig. 4). Similar injuries also can result when the child is shaken violently and the extremities are allowed to dangle and lash back and forth (Fig. 5). Bleeding into the adjacent joint is commonly seen with these types

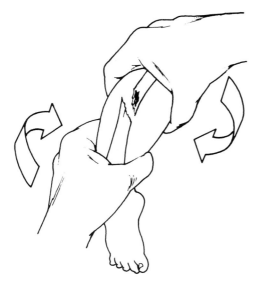

FIGURE 2. Spiral fractures in very young children are often due to abuse. The application of force in such a case is shown.

of fractures. Shaking injuries result when the infant is grasped around the torso and shaken violently back and forth or when one extremity is violently shaken. This mechanism produces epiphyseal-metaphyseal fractures[51] (Fig. 6). There can be associated frank dislocation of the spine, including compression fractures.

Squeezing injuries produce fractures at the points of maximal stress: posteriorly, laterally, and anteriorly at the costochondral junctions. They are often bilateral. Rib fractures in infants are very specific for child abuse. Cardiopulmonary resuscitation rarely causes fractures in infants. Multiple fractures at different stages of healing is a classic feature of the battered child syndrome.

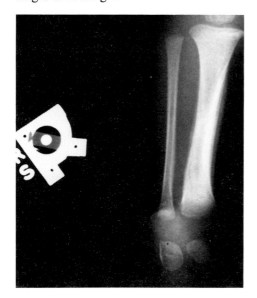

FIGURE 3. Spiral (oblique) fracture of tibia with diffuse callous formation.

FIGURE 4. Avulsion of metaphysis with epiphysis and separation of periosteum. (From Silverman FN: Radiology and other imaging procedures. In Helfer RE, Kempe RS (eds): The Battered Child. 4th ed. Chicago, University of Chicago Press, 1987, pp 214–246; with permission.)

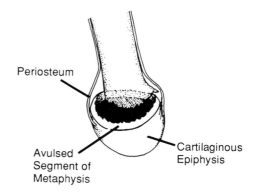

The mechanisms causing fractures in the battered child syndrome may also result in tendon avulsions, unusual muscle and tendon injuries, and periosteal avulsions (Fig. 7). In older children, multiple injuries to the small bones of the hands can occur. Any injury that can occur accidentally also may be the result of intentional trauma.

By dating a fracture radiographically, important historical discrepancies may be detected that will indicate abuse. It is relatively easy to date a fracture in its early stages, but it is more difficult later[57] (Table 1). In order to date a fracture, one should look for soft tissue changes, visibility of a fracture line, calcification of callus, and ossification of newly laid periosteal bone.

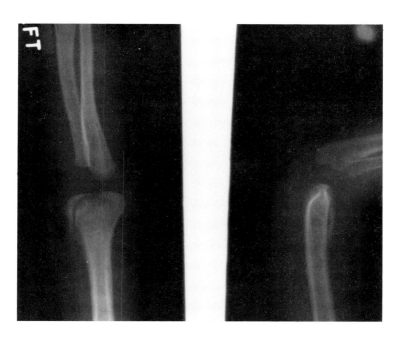

FIGURE 5. Epiphyseal metaphyseal fracture separation.

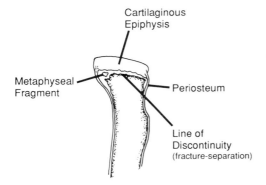

Cartilaginous
Epiphysis

Metaphyseal
Fragment

Periosteum

Line of
Discontinuity
(fracture-separation)

FIGURE 6.   Salter type 2 epiphyseal fracture. (From Silverman FN: Radiology and other imaging procedures. In Helfer RE, Kempe RS (eds): The Battered Child. 4th ed. Chicago, University of Chicago Press, 1987, pp 214–246; with permission.)

The types of skeletal lesions suggestive, if not diagnostic, of abuse include multiple, often symmetric fractures of the limbs, occult bone lesions, posterior rib fractures (Fig. 8), multiple fractures at different stages of healing indicating multiple injuries over time, bone injuries that appear out of proportion to the clinical history provided, and a combination of skeletal and nonskeletal injuries (cranial, cerebral, ophthalmologic, and cutaneous).

A skeletal survey should be considered in the following circumstances: (1) on any child younger than 2 who is suspected of being abused; (2) when the history or injury suggests physical abuse; (3) in older children with severe bruising, localized pain, limp, or reluctance to use arm or leg; (4) when a history of skeletal injury is present; and (5) in children dying in unusual or suspicious circumstances.[12]

The fractures seen with abuse are, in general, different than those seen with accidents. While not pathognomonic of abuse, the radiographic findings (Table 2) of fractures from abuse are very specific for nonaccidental injury.[19]

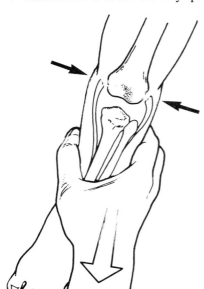

FIGURE 7.   A sudden jerk on the extremity produces tendon avulsions.

TABLE 1. Dating of Fractures

Age of Fracture	Radiologic Findings
0–10 days	Soft tissue swelling Fluid in joints Visible fracture lines Visible fracture fragments
10 days–8 weeks	Layered periosteal new bone Subtle and then heavy callus Bone resorption along fracture line Metaphyseal fragments
8 weeks and longer	Thicker maturing periosteal new bone Dense and smoother callus Metaphyseal fragments within callus Less visible fracture line Cortical deformities and bumps

Accidental fractures usually include[37] (1) clavicle fracture; (2) distal extremity fracture in a child older than 1; (3) supracondylar humerus fracture; and (4) femur fracture in a child older than 1 with a history of running and falling.[33] A negative skeletal survey or bone scan in association with the above fractures supports a nonintentional injury.

Other causes of fractures must be considered when differentiating abuse from accidental trauma. Osteogenesis imperfecta[1,43] (Table 3), Caffey's disease,[32] rickets of prematurity, osteoporosis, copper deficiency, osteomyelitis, and stress fractures are conditions that can account for fractures.[19] Behavior and chromosomal abnormalities must also be considered.[25]

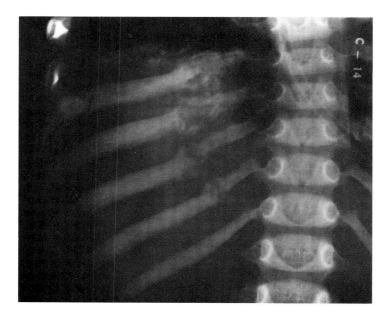

FIGURE 8. Multiple and bilateral rib fractures.

TABLE 2.   Radiologic Features of Child Abuse

Multiple fractures, posterior rib fractures
Multiple fractures showing different stages of healing
Scapular, acromial, or sternal fractures
Bucket handle and metaphyseal corner fractures
Unsuspected fractures without history of trauma
Visceral injuries such as duodenal or jejunal hematoma
Head injuries not compatible with mechanism of injury
Unexplained fractures with normal bone mineralization
Transverse, spiral, or oblique fractures in nonambulatory infants
Fracture separations of distal humeral/femoral epihysis

BURNS

Burns are potentially serious injuries and account for approximately 10% of all abuse injuries.[18,48] Burns resulting from abuse account for up to 25% of all burn hospitalizations in children.[21,44] It is therefore important to differentiate accidental from intentional burns.

Burns are caused in a variety of ways. The severity of the burn is determined by the method of burn, duration of exposure, temperature, and skin thickness.[21] Burns may occur under the following circumstances:

1. Scalds result from hot liquids, especially water, being poured, splashed, or dropped on the victim. They cause blistering, weeping, and peeling of the skin.

2. Contact with a hot object results in a well outlined injury in the shape of the object. The burn does not usually blister and is uniform in severity.

3. Flames cause charring of the victim.

4. Cigarette burns are circular if made by direct contact, and they are linear if the cigarette brushes against the skin.

5. Electric burns are deep and have entry and exit wounds.

6. Chemical burns discolor and scar the affected area.

7. Friction burns blister over bony areas, and the blisters may be open.

8. Radiant burns result from standing near a source of heat, such as a fire. They produce erythema and blistering of the skin.[21]

The duration of exposure and temperature resulting in the burn are important factors (Table 4). For example, water at 140° F will cause a first- or second-degree burn within 3 seconds of exposure[40] and a third-degree burn in 15 seconds.[25] However, a first- or second-degree burn will result from exposure to 120° F water

TABLE 3.   Findings Related to Child Abuse vs. Osteogenesis Imperfecta

Finding	Child Abuse	Osteogenesis Imperfecta
Family history	Common	Common
Incidence	Common	Rare
Short stature	Occasionally	Common
Hearing impairment	Uncommon	Common
Blue sclera	Rare	Common
Abnormal teeth	Rare	Common
Joint laxity	Rare	Common
Osteoporosis	Rare	Common
Fracture recurrence	Rare	Common
Abnormal fracture healing	Rare	Common

TABLE 4. Time Required to Develop First- or Second-Degree Burns on Human Skin

Time of Exposure in Seconds	Water temperature in °C (°F)
70	52 (126)
30	54 (129)
14	56 (133)
6	58 (136)
3	60 (140)
1.6	62 (144)
1	64 (147)

for 90 seconds or more. Also, thinner skin will suffer more damaging burns than thick skin.[21] Accidental burns usually result from carelessness (e.g., spills) or a lapse in supervision. Inflicted burns are the result of discipline, or they create sexual or sadistic pleasure in the abuser.[21,44] As in the evaluation of fractures, history, physical examination, and medical knowledge are important factors to use to distinguish accidental from intentional burns.

With inflicted burns, the history and burn pattern do not correlate.[21,44] For example, a well demarcated burn from being forced into a hot bathtub is not consistent with a history of falling into the tub, where the burn pattern would be irregular, demonstrating a splash effect. The developmental level of the child and siblings must also correlate with the history.[25,44,49,53] A child not old enough to climb into a bathtub should not have well delineated burns on his or her lower extremities, and abusive caretakers may say the sibling carried the victim and dropped him or her into the hot bath.[25] Delay in seeking treatment for a serious burn is common with inflicted burns.[44,49] Usually, a caretaker other than the one who inflicted the injury seeks treatment for the child.[44] The history will therefore be vague and raise the index of suspicion. Variability of history among caregivers is seen in abuse cases.[49,53] The abusive caretaker will deny the seriousness of the injury and commonly say the child "did not cry."[44] People who intentionally burn children are usually hostile to the medical staff, resist treatment, or blame the child for the event. The parents or caretakers who accidentally burn a child are guilty, defensive (resist the idea that the burn was intentional), and seek rapid medical attention in most cases. Abusive caregivers may be depressed or once abused themselves.[21]

The burn pattern and location are of paramount importance in differentiating abuse from accidental burns. Hot liquids or objects used to burn children[49] may leave characteristic markings.[25] However, because even accidental burns may be well demarcated, location must also be documented. Inflicted burns usually occur about the face, head, perineum, buttocks, and genitalia. The palmar and dorsal surface of the hand, soles of feet, and legs also are involved in abusive burns. Intentional burns usually spare flexion areas because a child will withdraw from hot liquids, and the burn is well delineated—for instance, at the waist if the child is dipped in water.[21,25]

Accidental burns usually occur in older infants and toddlers over the face, head, upper body, and shoulders, because most of these burns result from pulling hot substances onto themselves. The burn is typically a splash burn with irregular borders. If a child is accidently burned by a hot object, the burn is usually superficial and not serious because the child will withdraw from pain.[21] Obviously, burns also occur from playing with matches, from housefires, fireworks, or explosives.

With accidental burns, poor parental or guardian supervision may have occurred.[44] Counseling the family on safety issues is warranted.

The treatment of burns is the same regardless of whether they are intentional or accidental; however, clinical management of the family situation and long-term follow-up will vary. This will be discussed later in this chapter.

HEAD INJURY

Head trauma is very common in physical medicine and rehabilitation practice, but it accounts for less than 10% of all physical abuse injuries in children.[4,25] However, a large percentage of abuse-related deaths in children younger than 2 result from head injury.[4,50] The types of head injury most commonly seen are skull fracture and intracranial hemorrhage that is isolated or associated with skull fracture.

Skull fractures do not take on characteristic findings that will significantly differentiate abuse from accidental injury. In studies by Meservy et al. and Leventhal et al., linear skull fractures of the parietal bone occurred in about 90% of intentional and accidental skull fractures in children younger than 2 years old.[33,39] Hobbs found the same percentage for accidental injury; however, in abused children younger than 2, 79% of patients suffered multiple, depressed, widening, or growing fractures [20] (Fig. 9). Leventhal et al. and Mesery et al. agree on the higher incidence of complicated skull fractures in abused children.[25,39] Skull fractures associated with intracranial hemorrhage (subarachnoid, subdural, or intracerebral) are more prevalent with child abuse.[45]

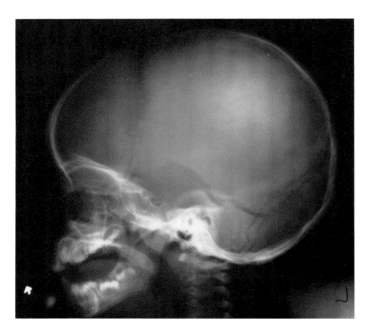

FIGURE 9. Spread sutures indicating increased intracranial pressure. This was secondary to a subdural hematoma.

As with differentiation of fractures and burns, a detailed history and physical examination are important. A consistent, plausible history in conjunction with physical findings may help delineate abuse from accidental injury. Skull fractures with other associated injuries (burns, bruising, fractures) are highly suggestive of abuse. Falls account for a majority of all fractures in children. When obtaining the history, it is necessary to know the distance of the fall. In children younger than 5, falls of less than 90 cm (3 feet) usually do not result in a skull fracture; however, when fracture does occur, it is linear and uncomplicated.[2,17,20,31] Leventhal et al. report that falls of even as little as 60 cm (2 feet) can result in skull fractures.[33] Complicated fractures occur with falls further than 120 cm (4 feet).

Shaken impact (or shaken baby) syndrome is another major cause of head injury in abused children younger than 3.[4] This results in subdural hematoma, subarachnoid hemorrhage, and/or cerebral edema (Fig. 10). Anoxia and possible hematoma also may occur.[4] Apnea and cardiopulmonary arrest can result from associated cervical medullary injury. The child usually presents with an altered state of consciousness (lethargy to coma), seizures, or posturing, or dies.[4] A history that is not compatible with the clinical findings, in addition to other signs of abuse, is consistent with shaken impact syndrome. Anoxia, infection, toxins, or metabolic disease may also present with changes in level of consciousness or death and should be considered in the differential diagnosis.

Accidents can result in a similar clinical picture; however, the event, such as a motor vehicle accident, is usually witnessed. A careful history and physical examination is crucial for proper identification of abuse cases. Retinal hemorrhages are almost pathognomonic ($> 80\%$)[34] for shaken impact syndrome because of the forces generated to cause them. Coagulopathies, vasculitis, and hypertension also can cause retinal hemorrhages. These disease entities can be confirmed by examination and laboratory findings.[34]

The mechanism by which head injury occurs in shaken impact syndrome is acceleration-deceleration forces. When these forces are applied to a child, the brain

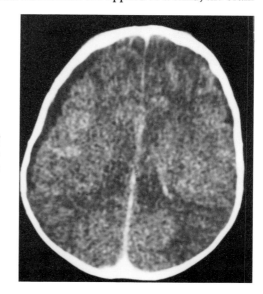

FIGURE 10. CT scan of the brain of a child with shaken baby syndrome showing subdural hematoma and brain edema.

moves in the opposite direction as the skull. Shearing of cerebral meningeal vessels and brain contusion or laceration cause intracranial injury.[28] Simple shaking does not generate forces sufficient to cause injury;[19] however, if the child is thrown after shaking, markedly greater acceleration forces occur that will result in the above-mentioned intracranial injuries.[10]

Spinal cord injury can result from shaken impact syndrome or trauma to the spine[4,19] and can lead to dislocation, subluxation, or vertebral column fracture.

BRUISES AND SKIN INJURIES

Bruises and skin injuries are very prevalent in both intentional and accidental injuries. Skin manifestations may be isolated or associated with other injuries. The history and careful examination of the patient's skin findings may delineate abuse from accidental trauma.

The physician must be able to date the bruise (Table 5). Bruises of various ages are suggestive of abuse. Location is also important. Bruising about the face, neck, trunk, genitals, buttocks, and thighs are suggestive of abuse.[11] With accidental trauma, bruising usually is to the forehead and lower legs and arms. Accidental bruises may be associated with lacerations.[42] Abused children often have bruising over the back and forearms as they try to defend themselves from the beating.[30] Inflicted bruises also may be isolated, whereas accidental bruises can be generalized. For example, a fall down steps will cause bruising over various parts of the body rather than just the back, as occurs with an intentional beating. Skin markings characteristic of an object are indicative of abuse. In most cases, hand marks about the face or neck and human bite marks are highly suggestive of abuse.[30]

Laboratory data such as prothrombin time, partial thromboplastin time, bleeding time, and platelets to rule out coagulopathy are important to determine the cause of bruising.[41] Other disease processes, such as meningococcal sepsis, osteogenesis imperfecta,[1] Ehler-Danlos syndrome, and vasculitis (especially Schönlein-Henoch purpura[30]), may cause diffuse ecchymotic lesions. Poisonings with coumadin or salicylates can result in bruising. Mongolian spots may be falsely identified as bruises or allergic shiners. Children with psychological (autism) or genetic abnormalities (Lesch-Nyhan syndrome) may have self-inflicted bruising.[25] It must be realized that any child, despite underlying disease that may mimic abuse, can be abused.

IDENTIFICATION OF CHILD ABUSE

Despite an abundance of statistical information, differentiation of accidental from intentional injury is dependent on history, physical examination, laboratory data, and level of suspicion.

TABLE 5.   Dating of Bruises

Age of Bruise	Findings
0–2 days	Tender and swollen; Red, blue
0–5 days	Blue, purple
5–7 days	Green
7–10 days	Yellow
10–14 days	Brown
2–4 weeks	Resolved

History

The history provides the single most important source of information. An adequate history, or the lack of it, is critical in identifying abuse in children. A careful history must be obtained from the parents and caregivers. The history may reveal stress within the family that needs attention. A pattern of frequent injuries should raise suspicion. Attempts should be made to obtain information regarding the child's past medical history, and contacts must be made with previous health care providers.[5,56] If a child requires admission to the hospital for assessment and treatment, the parents must be told why, and their reactions may be an important clue and should be noted in the medical records. Parents should be informed of the physician's and health care worker's legal responsibility to report suspected child abuse.

All attempts must be made to interview the child, and the interview must be conducted as privately as possible. Clear, short, and open-ended questions should be directed to the child. A child's statements may be influenced by an adult. However, these statements should never be discounted.

In obtaining a history, factors important to discern are plausibility of event or injury, accuracy of the story among witnesses and/or caretakers, discrepancies of the event between caretakers or parents, and the reason for seeking medical care when the involved parties are questioned individually. Accoridng to Leventhal et al., 40% of abused children present with a false history. Falls from a bed, couch, or changing table, while frequently used as an explanation for injuries, are unlikely to result in serious injury. When there is delay in seeking medical care after a significant injury, careful evaluations must be made because of the high risk of abuse. Discrepancies or contradictions in the histories obtained from the parents, child, witnesses, or other caregivers raise suspicion of abuse. Conflicting stories sometimes merely reflect the lack of first-hand information. The history should be dated and the time it is obtained documented. The history giver and time and place of the alleged abuse should be named. The alleged instigator of the abuse should also be named. Past history of medical, social, or abuse problems must be documented.

Examination

The evaluation should be conducted by a team including, but not limited to, physician, nurse, and social worker. Other health care professionals should also be included, as needed. The assessment in suspected child abuse requires careful attention to detail and documentation.[22] The team must consider whether the history is consistent with the injury the child has suffered. A thorough physical examination must be performed, and the details of the findings must be carefully documented. Diagrams and physical descriptions including size, shape, color, and location of the injuries must be documented.

Dating of Injuries

The timing of injury will play an important role in the assessment of the abused child. The time of injury can be narrowed down by noting the color of the resultant bruise or the stage of healing of burn injuries. Chronic or acute fractures and subdural hematomas can be estimated using x-rays and other imaging techniques.

Photographs

All injuries should be photographed, if possible, by a medical photographer.[25] The photos should be dated and timed. Instant photographs should be supplemented with higher quality pictures for a more permanent record.

Imaging Techniques

Computed tomography (CT), magnetic resonance imaging (MRI), scintigraphy, and radiographs are valuable methods of evaluation to determine chronic or acute injury to the skeletal system and other organ systems.[29] Skeletal surveys are useful in children who are young, but they are infrequently indicated in school-age children.[12] Radionuclide bone scans are more sensitive than conventional radiography in detecting acute trauma even hours after injury[29] (Fig. 11). Bone scans do not replace skeletal surveys and other radiographs. CT scans are useful in detecting subtle intracranial injuries, especially intracerebral ones, as well as intraabdominal injuries.

Laboratory Studies

Hematologic evaluations including prothrombin time, partial thromboplastin time, fibrinogen, platelet aggregation, bleeding time, factor VIII, factor VIII-related antigens, factor IX, and other laboratory studies will help to document conditions such as hemophilia, von Willebrand disease, or other bleeding disorders.[41] If the hematologic evaluation is normal, a collagen vascular disorder should also be investigated. A child with a medical condition including hematologic disorders can also be abused, and the diagnosis of such conditions does not exclude the possibility of child abuse.

Role of Physicians, Health Care Workers, and Other Professionals

Physicians, medical professionals, law enforcement officers, teachers, and child care providers are responsible for reporting, assessing, treating, and investigating abused children and their families.[15] Hospital personnel often see injured or ill children who have been abused or neglected. Studies have documented that many physicians have limited knowledge about different aspects of child abuse, in part due to the deficiency of formal instruction in residency programs and medical schools.[7] Physicians have the legal and ethical responsibility to report all cases of

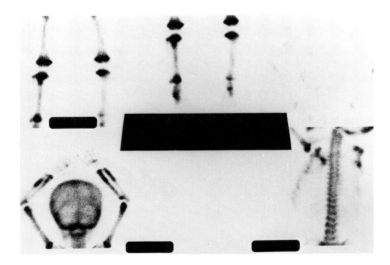

FIGURE 11.   Scintigram showing increased uptake due to trauma at multiple sites.

suspected child abuse.[3] All differential diagnoses evaluated with appropriate tests must be performed. It is not the physician's responsibility to prove that abuse occurred.

The identification of child abuse, as in other areas of medicine, is based on a thorough history, a complete physical examination, and appropriate use of laboratory tests. All risk factors must be identified, but a diagnosis cannot be reached based on the presence of risk factors alone. The ability to identify abuse is dependent on the belief that it can occur and that anyone can potentially abuse a child.

Management

Once the examination is completed, the child should be told that the evaluation is completed and whatever has happened was not his or her fault. Emergency medical care must be rendered to the child in the appropriate manner. The child must be kept as comfortable as possible, with fractures and other injuries treated with utmost care. The child should be put at ease at all times, and every step of the management should be explained to him or her. Long-term treatment, including rehabilitation, should be planned early.

The emotional trauma of the child due to abuse should receive careful attention.[13] The child may feel isolated, rejected, and terrorized. To avoid more permanent and serious behavioral, cognitive, emotional, or mental disorders in an abused child, it is necessary to provide intervention by child protective services as well as medical personnel. The child and parents or caregivers should receive appropriate evaluation and treatment. The plans regarding future child care, medical and rehabilitative care, and ways to avoid future abuse must be laid out carefully and explained to the child and parents/caregivers. Appropriate government agencies and community services must be involved to deal with the acute situation, provide ongoing care, protect the child, and to determine child custody issues. Psychological intervention needs to be instituted in most cases to meet the psychological, emotional, and behavioral needs of the child and the caregiver.

After documentation has occurred, the physician should inform the parents or caregiver of suspected abuse. An immediate report to the state protective service agency should be made by telephone. In most cases, the child needs to be hospitalized for protection and medical care. The hospital's protective service team consisting of a physician, nurse, social worker, protective service agency worker, and psychologist should be involved in such cases. The child's siblings must also be brought to medical attention to be evaluated for abuse and involved in the state protective agency for their protection.[12] It is important to follow the case from initial contact to its conclusion, including disposition or trial.[38,54] Medical follow-up for the abused child should be made available.

ABUSE OF THE DISABLED CHILD AND PREVENTION

Several studies have indicated a correlation between disabilities and child abuse. Many professionals believe that disabled children do constitute a high risk group for abuse. According to the report in the Central Registry for Child Abuse and Neglect published by the Utah's Department of Social Services, Division of Family Services, 623 of 5,127 children (12.15%) were identified as having "special characteristics."[52] Of the 623 abused children, 14% had mental retardation, 10% were physically handicapped, 5% had chronic illness, 3% were premature babies, and 68% were identified as emotionally disturbed. Disabled children are abused and neglected in as many different ways as are nondisabled children. Disabled children are often perceived as being "different," and this tends to be a factor for abuse. Physical abuse of these children can result in orthopedic, emotional, behavioral, neurologic, or any number of interrelated problems. A study by Kempe et al. found that 85 of 302 (28%) abused children in 71 hospitals had suffered neurologic damage and that 33 of the children died as a result of their injuries.[26] A handicapped baby born to parents who have the potential to abuse is clearly at risk for abuse.

The primary focus for prevention of child abuse is increasing public awareness and to inform parents of the stresses involved in child care and the resources that may be available to them.[9] Some prevention programs have been implemented through school systems. Although the awareness of child abuse has increased, it is not clear whether these programs actually prevent abuse. The secondary aspect of prevention targets populations at high risk for child abuse such as disadvantaged and single-parent families and teenage mothers. Family support, home visitation, and use of community and social support systems have resulted in a decrease in the incidence of maltreatment. The third measure attempts to treat families in which abuse has occurred in order to prevent recurrent abuse. Many services, including peer support, parenting education, skill development, and the measures to manage the effects of abuse on children, family, and society, appear to be valuable in preventing further abuse. As many as 58% of parents who undergo treatment fail to show a reduced potential for abuse, and many children continue to be abused even while their parents are being treated.

Sources for prevention and treatment have simply not kept pace with advances in diagnostic skills. More child protection workers and other professionals must be made available to deal with abused children and their families. Multidisciplinary efforts from the federal level to the neighborhood level must be emphasized and coordinated.

CONCLUSION

Child abuse afflicts hundreds of thousands of children each year and has long-term sequelae. Physicians and health care providers must understand and recognize this health and social problem. In this chapter we have discussed accidental and intentional trauma and how to differentiate between them. As with any disease, statistical information aids in the diagnosis but should not eliminate a diagnosis. Child abuse must be suspected when a child is evaluated for injury, especially when there are discrepancies in the history, physical findings, and the types of injuries. As more children are identified and appropriate treatment and preventative measures applied, it is hoped that fewer children will suffer and that children can be allowed to be children.

ACKNOWLEDGMENT

The authors wish to thank Constance Blade, MD, and Suzanne P. Kawaguchi for their assistance in review and preparation of this manuscript.

REFERENCES

1. Ablin DS, Greenspan A, Reinhart M, Grix A: Differentiation of child abuse from osteogenesis imperfecta. Am J Roentgenol 154:1035–1046, 1990.
2. Billmore ME, Myers PA: Serious head injury in infants: Accident or abuse? Pediatrics 75:340–342, 1985.

3. Brown RH, Truitt RB: Medical legal aspects of child abuse: The physicians' responsibilities. J Med Pract Manag 4:130–135, 1988.
4. Bruce DA: Neurosurgical aspects of child abuse. In Ludwig S, Kornberg AE (ed): Child Abuse: A Medical Reference. 2nd ed. New York, Churchill Livingstone, 1992.
5. Christian CW: Etiology and prevention of abuse: Family and individual factors. In Ludwig S, Kornberg AE (ed): Child Abuse: A Medical Reference. 2nd ed. New York, Churchill Livingstone, 1992.
6. Christoffel KK: Child abuse fatalities. In Ludwig S, Kornberg AE (ed): Child Abuse: A Medical Reference. 2nd ed. New York, Churchill Livingstone, 1992.
7. Dubowitz H: Child abuse programs and pediatric residency training. Pediatrics 82(suppl):477–480, 1988.
8. Dubowitz H: Pediatrician's role in preventing child maltreatment. Pediatr Clin North Am 37:989–1002, 1990.
9. Dubowitz H: Prevention of child maltreatment: What is known? Pediatrics 83:570–577, 1989.
10. Duhaime AC, Gennarelli TA, Thibault LE, et al: The shaken baby syndrome: A clinical pathological and biomechanical study. J Neurosurg 66:409–415, 1987.
11. Ellerstein NS: The cutaneous manifestations of child abuse and neglect. Am J Dis Child 133:906–909, 1979.
12. Ellerstein NS, Norris KJ: Value of radiologic skeletal survey in assessment of abused children. Pediatrics 74:1075–1079, 1984.
13. Garbarino J: The psychologically battered child: Toward a definition. Pediatr Ann 18:502–504, 1989.
14. Gelles S, Feingold M, Cao GIO: Pseudobattering in Vietnamese Children. Am J Dis Child130:857–858, 1976.
15. Hampton R, Newberges E: Child abuse incidence and reporting by hospitals: Significance of severity, class and race. Am J Public Health 75:56–60, 1985.
16. Helfer RE: The developmental cases of child abuse and neglect: An epidemiological approach. In Helfer RE, Kempe RS (eds): The Battered Child. 4th ed. Chicago, University of Chicago Press, 1987.
17. Helfer RE, Slovis TL, Black M: Injuries resulting when small children fall out of bed. Pediatrics 60:533–535, 1977.
18. Hight DW, Bakalar HR, Lloyd JR: Inflicted burns in children. JAMA 242:517–520, 1979.
19. Hobbs CJ: ABC of child abuse: Fractures. BMJ 298:1015–1018, 1989.
20. Hobbs CJ: Skull fracture and the diagnosis of abuse. Arch Dis Child 59:246–252, 1984.
21. Hobbs CJ: ABC of child abuse: Burns and scalds. BMJ 298:1302–1305, 1989.
22. Holter JC, Friedman SB: Child abuse: Early case findings in the emergency department. Pediatrics 42:128–138, 1968.
23. Hyman IA, Wise JH: Corporal Punishment in American Education. Philadelphia, Temple University Press, 1979.
24. Johnson CF, Coury DL: Child neglect: General concepts and medical neglect. In Ludwig S, Kornberg AE (ed): Child Abuse: A Medical Reference. 2nd ed. New York, Churchill Livingstone, 1992.
25. Johnson CF: Inflicted injury versus accidental injury. Pediatr Clin North Am 37:791–814, 1979.
26. Kempe CH, Silverman F, Steele BF, et al: The battered child syndrome. JAMA 181:17–24, 1962.
27. King J, Diefendorf D, Apthorp J: Analysis of 429 fractures in 189 battered children. J Pediatr Orthop 8:585–589, 1988.
28. Klein DM: Central nervous system injuries. In Ellerstein NS (ed): Child Abuse and Neglect: A Medical Reference. New York, Churchill Livingstone, 1981.
29. Kleinman PK (ed): Diagnostic Imaging of Child Abuse. Baltimore, Williams & Wilkins, 1987.
30. Kornberg AE: Skin and soft tissue injuries. In Ludwig S, Kornberg AE (eds): Child Abuse: A Medical Reference. 2nd ed. New York, Churchill Livingstone, 1992.
31. Kravitz H, Driessen G, Gomberg R, Korach A: Accidental falls from elevated surfaces in infants from birth to one year of age. Pediatrics 44(suppl):869–876, 1969.
32. Lamont AC, Young ID, Shannon RS: Diagnosis with unexplained injuries in children. BMJ 302–305, 1991.
33. Leventhal JM, Thomas SA, Rosenfield NS, Markowitz RI: Fractures in young children distinguishing child abuse from unintentional injuries. Am J Dis Child 147:87–92, 1992.
34. Levin AV: Ophthalmologic manifestations. In Ludwig S, Kornberg AE (eds): Child Abuse and Neglect: A Medical reference. 2nd ed. New York, Churchill Livingstone, 1992, pp 191–212.
35. Lyons TJ, Oates RK: Falling out of bed: A relatively benign outcome. Pediatrics 92:125–127, 1993.

36. McClelland CQ, Kingsbury GH: Fractures in the first year of life: A diagnostic dilemma. Am J Dis Child 136:26–29, 1982.
37. McDonald AE, Reece RM: Child abuse: Problems of reporting. Pediatr Clin North Am 26:785–791, 1979.
38. Merten DF, Radkowski MA, Leonidas JC: The abused child: A radiological reappraisal. Radiology 146:377–381, 1983.
39. Meservy CJ, Towbin R, McLaurin RL, et al: Radiographic characteristics of skull fractures resulting from child abuse. Am J Roentgenol 149:173–175, 1987.
40. Moritz AR, Henriques FC: Studies of thermal injury: Pathology and pathogenesis of cutaneous burn experimental study. Am J Pathol 23:915–941, 1947.
41. O'Hare AE, Eden OB: Bleeding disorders and non-accidental injury. Arch Dis Child 59:960–964, 1984.
42. Pascoe JM, Hildebrandy MH, Tarrier A, et al: Patterns of skin injury in non-accidental and accidental injury. Pediatrics 64:245–247, 1979.
43. Paterson CR, McAllion SJ: Osteogenesis imperfecta in the differential diagnosis of child abuse. BMJ 299:1451–1454, 1989.
44. Prescott PR: Hair dryer burns in children. Pediatrics 86:692–697, 1990.
45. Radkowski MA, Meten DF, Leonidas JC: The abused child: Criteria for the radiologic diagnosis. Radiographics 3:262–297, 1983.
46. Salsbury FT, Campbell RE: Evaluation of child abuse reporting by physicians. Am J Dis Child 193:393, 1985.
47. Schmitt BD: The child with non-accidental trauma. In Helfer RE, Kempe RS (eds): The Battered Child. 4th ed. Chicago, University of Chicago Press, 1987.
48. Schmitt BD, Kempe CH: Abuse and neglect of children. In Vaughan VC III, McKay RJ, Behrman RE, Nelson WE (eds): Nelson Textbook of Pediatrics. 11th ed. Philadelphia, WB Saunders, 1979.
49. Showers J, Garrison KM: Burn abuse: A four year study. J Trauma 28:1581–1583, 1988.
50. Showers J, Apolo J, Thomas J, et al: Fatal child abuse: A two decade review. Pediatr Emerg Care 1:66–70, 1985.
51. Silverman FN: Radiology and other imaging procedures. In Helfer RE, Kempe RS (eds): The Battered Child. 4th ed. Chicago, University of Chicago Press, 1987, pp 214–246.
52. State of Utah Department of Social Services, Division of Family Services: Central Registry for Child Abuse and Neglect, Annual Report for CY 1986, Salt Lake City, 1986.
53. Stone NA, Rinaldo L, Humphrey CT, Brown RH: Child abuse by burning. Surg Clin North Am 50:1919–1924, 1970.
54. Thomas SA, Rosefield NS, Leventhal JM, Markowitz RI: Long bone fractures in young children: Distinguishing accidental injuries from child abuse. Pediatrics 88:471–476, 1991.
55. US Department of Health and Human Services: Study Findings: Study of National Incidence and Prevalence of Child Abuse and Neglect. Washington, DC, Children's Bureau, National Center for Child Abuse, 1988.
56. US Department of Health and Human Services: Executive Summary: National Study of the Incidence and Severity of Child Abuse and Neglect. Washington, DC, National Center for Child Abuse and Neglect, 1984, publication OHDS 81-30329.
57. Warlock P, Stower M, Barbor P: Patterns of fractures in accidental and non-accidental injury in children: A comparative study. BMJ 293:100–102, 1986.

EDWARD G. McFARLAND, MD
MARK A. YOUNG, MD

BIOMECHANICAL PRINCIPLES IN REHABILITATION OF FRACTURES

From the Section of Sports
   Medicine and Shoulder Surgery
Department of Orthopaedic
   Surgery (EGM)
   and
Department of Physical Medicine
   and Rehabilitation (MAY)
Johns Hopkins University
Baltimore, Maryland

Reprint requests to:
Edward G. McFarland, MD
3901 Greenspring Ave.
Suite 301
Baltimore, MD 21211

Fracture treatment and rehabilitation is a challenge requiring a cooperative effort from the orthopedist and the rehabilitation specialist. Although bone is a living tissue, its composition dictates its response to forces and treatment according to biomechanical principles. These principles influence the fracture pattern, the specific orthopedic intervention and the timing, and intensity and type of rehabilitation. This chapter will briefly review these principles as they relate to fracture management and rehabilitative aftercare, discuss the influence of internal fixation devices on rehabilitation, and review illustrative examples that demonstrate these concepts. This review will discuss these principles as they relate primarily to the appendicular skeleton, or long bones, although the same principles also apply to spine fractures.

BONE BIOMECHANICS AND FRACTURES

Bone is the most rigid form of connective tissue. There are two types of bone, cortical and cancellous, which have different structural and mechanical properties. Cortical bone forms the outer surface of the bones and the cancellous, or spongy, bone is located within the compact bone. Cortical bone is stiffer than cancellous bone and can absorb large amounts of energy before it fails. However, cortical bone generally tolerates only small changes in length, less than 2%, before it fails. Cancellous bone can withstand length changes of up to 7% but cannot absorb as much energy as cortical bone prior to failure.

The relative amounts of cortical and cancellous bone in a given location significantly influence the biomechanics of that particular bone. The geometry and relative ratios of type of bone will influence how a particular bone will fracture and heal.[2,3,4,5] These factors also have important implications for rehabilitation.[6]

The material properties of bone determine its biomechanical behavior. Unlike a block of metal, bone is nonhomogeneous. Consequently, bone is also anisotropic, which means that it responds differently to a force applied to it depending on the direction from which the force is applied. Forces applied to the same bone from different directions tend to produce different fracture patterns (Fig. 1). Cortical bone is weaker in tension than in compression. Bone is also viscoelastic, which means that its material properties vary according to the rate at which the load is applied. At high rates of load, the bone absorbs more energy; when it fractures, the increased energy may lead to comminution and more soft tissue damage.

Bones experience a variety of forces from gravity, muscles, and externally applied sources. The applied load to the bone may produce classic or stereotypic fracture patterns (*see* Fig. 1). However, most fractures are the result of combined applied loads and show more complex patterns. When loaded in compression, long bones tend to fail in a line oblique to the long axis of the bone. When loaded in tension, the bone tends to fail perpendicularly to the long axis. When a bone bends, there tends to be a transverse fracture, but commonly the compression on one side of the bone with tension on the other side of the bone produces a short oblique fracture or a butterfly fragment. A butterfly fragment indicates a more complex failure mode, and the comminution may indicate absorption of high

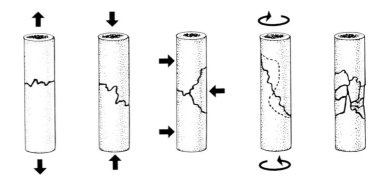

Fracture Pattern	Transverse	Oblique	Transverse with Oblique (Butterfly)	Spiral	Comminuted
Loading Mode	Tension	Compression	3 point bending	Tension	Combined
Energy	Moderate	Moderate	Moderate	Low	High

FIGURE 1. Bone's reaction to stress applied from different directions. The direction and amount of force determine the fracture pattern and, ultimately, the treatment and rehabilitation.

energy. Torsional loads tend to produce spiral fractures that course all the way around the bone.

Fractures that enter joints provide other biomechanical and treatment considerations. Incongruity of the articular cartilage surface can lead to cartilage breakdown and arthritis over time if it is uncorrected. The amount of incongruity acceptable varies from joint to joint and from weightbearing to nonweightbearing joints. Incongruity of the joint may also alter the joint's mechanics by shifting the center of axis or by altering relative ligament tension. This may result in loss of motion and increased stress concentration in localized areas of the articular surface. Joint surface incongruity can lead to degenerative arthritis, dysfunctional gait patterns, and impairment of activities of daily living. Joints tend to see significant translational and torsional loads, which can influence fracture and injury patterns.[3-5]

BIOMECHANICS OF FRACTURE MANAGEMENT

The goal of fracture treatment is to provide a structurally stable bone that allows full functional recovery of the extremity. Many factors influence the choice of treatment and the recovery of the injured extremity and the patient. The overall health of the patient influences wound and fracture healing. Systemic diseases such as hypothyroidism or cancer can influence the type of fracture fixation chosen and the length of healing. Polytrauma patients with multiple fractures and injuries are often treated more aggressively with internal fixation than patients with isolated extremity fractures. Open fractures, with lacerations to the surface, are contaminated to a varying degree, and the risk of infection can significantly affect the treatment choices. Surrounding soft tissue injury with damage to surrounding muscles, tendons, ligaments, or neurovascular structures also influences the treatment and the patient's recovery.

As bone heals, its biomechanical properties change.[2] A fractured bone basically has no structural integrity, and applied stress will cause motion, pain, and collapse of the affected part. Biologically, the healing bone attempts to restore its architecture and biomechanical stability. Once healing is complete, the bone can withstand functional stresses without refracture. Although a detailed review of bone healing can be obtained from other sources,[2,7,8,10] a few pertinent features will be reviewed here.

When a bone breaks, all of its component parts are disrupted. The blood supply to the involved fragments is compromised, and osteocyte death occurs proportionately. After a series of biochemical events, macrophages and osteoclasts begin to remove dead tissue and bone. Fibroblasts begin to produce collagen and fibrocartilage, which begins to stabilize the fracture site. This early callus is eventually invaded by blood vessels, and mineralization occurs. As the mineralized tissue and fibrocartilage is broken down by osteoclasts and macrophages, osteoblasts follow and produce bone. This callus is called secondary bone repair and can form within the bone canal (internal callus) or on the periosteal surface (external callus). Both types depend on an adequate blood supply and are consequently affected by surgical procedures that interrupt medullary or cortical blood supply.[8,9] Motion at the fracture site tends to increase this type of secondary callus formation. Continued motion or excessive motion can cause the callus to form insufficiently, leading to a nonunion. This underscores the importance of maintaining immobility in some fractures during the rehabilitative process. Bone that heals in an abnormal position or excessively angulated is called a malunion.

Bone also can heal in certain circumstances by direct bone healing without going through a fibrocartilage or mineralized connective tissue stage. Direct bone healing, or gap healing, can occur when bone ends are within 0.5–1.0 mm of each other. This type of healing is called primary bone healing and involves direct deposition of bone by osteoblasts into the gap. However, this type of healing does not tolerate motion and occurs primarily in very stable, nondisplaced fractures or in fractures rigidly fixed with surgical devices, especially plate and screw fixation.[2,9]

The choice of treatment for a fracture depends primarily on its location and configuration. Each treatment option has different effects on the type of bone healing and, consequently, on the biomechanics of the recovery. The treatment should restore normal alignment to the bone as closely as possible in all planes, depending on the bone. For example, humerus fractures can heal with significant angulation (e.g., 20°) in any plane and not affect upper extremity function. However, a tibia fracture with 15° of angulation can have significant effects at the knee and the ankle. Rotational deformity must be treated since most limbs do not tolerate the resulting abnormal stresses produced at proximal and distal joints.

Cast immobilization continues to be an acceptable and often preferred treatment of many fractures and is often encountered in the rehabilitation setting. Casts must be applied to resist deformation produced at the fracture site by gravity or by muscular pull on the fragments. To resist muscular deforming forces, immobilization of the joint both proximally and distally to the fracture must be achieved. The cast should be molded to provide three-point bending in fractures with an intact periosteum on one side of the fracture (Fig. 2). Unfortunately, the periosteum of adults is thin, and the fracture is frequently too unstable to be

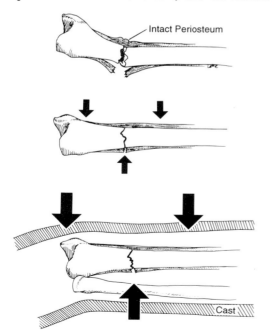

FIGURE 2. For fractures with an intact periosteum, the cast can be applied with three-point bending to stabilize the fracture.

controlled with a cast. Casts and fracture braces are essentially splints and have limited ability to control unstable fractures. This allows motion at the fracture site in unstable fractures, which in turn promotes the formation of external callus to varying degrees.

Long-term cast immobilization can also lead to what is called *cast disease.* Osteopenia of the immobilized extremity, loss of muscle mass, contracture of immobilized joints, and compensatory changes at other joints are a consequence of prolonged immobilization. Early mobilization and rehabilitation of patients with fractures have become recognized as important goals, especially in patients with polytrauma or spinal cord injuries. Although treatment of fractures with traction may be indicated in certain situations, such as when the patient is too sick for surgery or when immediate operative fixation is not available, the deleterious local effects on the extremity and systemic effects on the patient are significant and prolonged.

Rigid fixation of fractures has the potential advantage of minimizing the problems of prolonged immobilization. The goal is to provide rigid fixation that allows accurate reduction of the fracture and that allows early range of motion of the affected extremity and earlier mobilization of the patient. Types of fixation include external fixation and internal fixation. Internal fixation can be subdivided into extramedullary (plates and screws) and intramedullary (rods). Each type of fixation has biomechanical advantages and disadvantages that dictate when and where they are used. The biologic healing response is likewise affected by the biomechanical properties of the device, the amount of dissection necessary to implant the device, and the resultant disruption of the blood supply to the fracture site. Other factors, such as quality of the bone, will influence which type of fixation is used and how successfully it is applied.

Plate and screw fixation of fractures provides many advantages over cast fixation. Direct visualization of the fracture fragments at the time of surgery allows anatomic reduction of the fracture. The plate serves to reduce the fragments but also functions as a load-sharing device. How successfully load is transferred to the plate from the bone depends on many factors, such as location of the plate, the plate thickness, the status of the bone, and the security of the purchase of the screws. When a gap exists in the plate beneath the bone, the unsupported length between the implant and the proximal and distal segments of the bone represents the "working length" of the implant. This unsupported area creates large bending stress on the plate and can be quite large in some fractures, especially in comminuted fractures (Fig. 3). In these cases, the loads may be supported entirely by the plate. Fixation with screws alone must be supplemented by a cast or brace until healing is complete. In weightbearing joints, screw fixation alone must be used with caution and weightbearing protected until bony union occurs.

For any of these fixation devices, there is a race between bone healing and failure of the device. Initially, the loads across the fractures are relieved/shared by the device, but as the fracture heals the device experiences less stress until it becomes superfluous. However, if the fracture does *not* heal, the device continues to undergo stresses above its mechanical properties to survive. Consequently, the device fails and the extremity is impaired as the fracture recurs (Fig. 4).

Some plates act merely as buttresses and are not designed to be load-sharing. In these circumstances, range of motion of the extremity may be allowed but not the high stresses of weightbearing or functional loading (Fig. 5). Some plates can apply compression across the fracture to allow direct bone healing. Due to their rigidity, most plates do *not* allow motion at the fracture site, and, consequently,

Bending Open

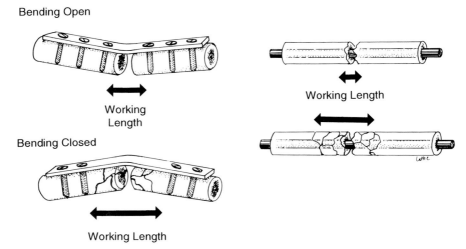

Working
Length

Working Length

Bending Closed

Working Length

FIGURE 3. The "working distance" of a plate or rod is the unsupported area. As this increases, the device must bear more stress.

little external callus is seen radiographically.[9] Generally, screw fixation alone without plates is inferior fixation, since the screws alone will not function as a load-sharing device.

Intramedullary rods are essentially internal splints and are currently the treatment of choice for fractures of the shafts of long weightbearing bones such as the femur and tibia. Intramedullary rods are placed from one end of the bone down the canal of the fragments and allow excellent restoration of anatomic alignment (Fig. 6). Even though the rods disrupt the endosteal blood supply to the fracture, they are not as rigid as plates, and the bone heals primarily with secondary callus.

A variety of rods are commercially available. Their strength varies according to diameter, cross-sectional shape (some are circular, others clover-leaf shaped), type of material composing the rod, and the presence of a slot in the rod down its entire length. Rods resist compressive loads well but are weakest in torsion. To prevent torsional slippage, many rods can now be locked at either end with screws. Initially, it was believed that these screws had to be removed to prevent stress shielding of the bone shaft, but currently these interlocking screws are left in place unless other circumstances arise.[2,5]

External fixation devices are available in a variety of patterns and configurations. They are currently used primarily for the treatment of open fractures or fractures with large defects (Fig. 7). The stability of the fixator is determined by its configuration and its interaction with the device-bone interface at the pins where they meet the bone. Stability is increased by using more pins, increasing the pin diameter, placing the pins closer to the fracture site, placing the side bar closer to the limb, placing the pins closer together, and placing compression at the fracture site with the device. When there is no bony contact at the fracture site, the external fixator must support the entire load of the bone. External fixators consequently can be subjected to high axial, distraction, torsional, and bending loads (*see* Fig. 3). Unfortunately, this can lead to stress at the pin-bone interface, which results in pin loosening and pin-tract infections. External fixators also tend

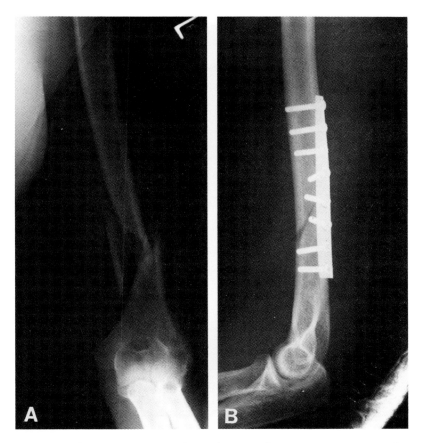

FIGURE 4 A and B. *A,* anteroposterior radiograph of a comminuted humerus fracture in a 40-year-old woman. *B,* because the fracture could not be held in a cast, it was treated with plate and screw fixation. *(Continued on following page)*

to bind down muscles and fascia with resulting loss of proximal or distal joint range of motion.[1,2,5]

BIOMECHANICS OF FRACTURE REHABILITATION

The rehabilitation process in patients with fractures necessitates a basic understanding of fracture biology and biomechanics. Most often, rehabilitation of fractures is directed by the orthopedic surgeon, but there has been increasing involvement of physiatrists and other health professionals in the process. A team approach has been shown to be beneficial in dealing with the impact of fractures upon the patient as a whole.[5,6] This is especially important in elderly patients with complex management problems or in polytrauma victims who need prolonged recovery and rehabilitation. Open communication among the members of the treating team is essential to optimize treatment of the patient.

The goals of rehabilitation of the fracture are to provide, first, full range of motion; second, restoration of strength; and last, full function of the extremity.

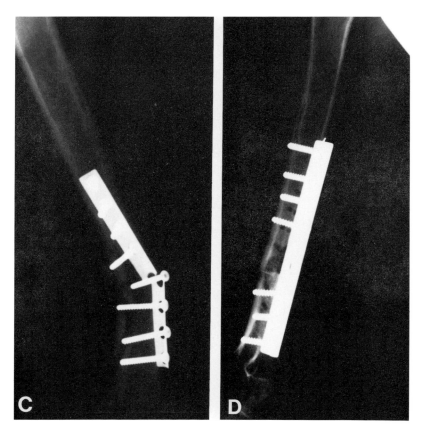

FIGURE 4 C and D. *C,* fixation failure occurred before the fracture healed. *D,* the nonunion was successfully treated by revision with a larger plate, bone grafting, and protected motion in a brace.

Full function implies different goals according to the particular patient. Full, pain-free range of motion may have more importance to a professional athlete than nonambulatory patients, depending on the circumstances. Judgments about how fast to progress in a rehabilitation program for fractures depend on many factors; each patient and each fracture must be considered individually. Fracture location, configuration, type of fixation, security of the fixation, and condition of the soft tissues are the primary factors to be considered in fracture rehabilitation.

For the physical medicine physician, the initial evaluation of the patient should include an understanding of the biomechanical and surgical issues discussed above. The orthopedist should provide ongoing information and direction about the relative stability of the fracture. The status of associated soft tissue or neurovascular symptoms should be ascertained. Associated injuries or medical conditions may influence the rehabilitation process and need to be evaluated.

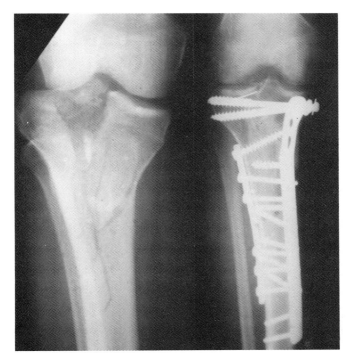

FIGURE 5. A displaced and comminuted tibial plateau fracture enters the joint and requires accurate reduction. The plates here function as a buttress and will not withstand high weightbearing loads.

The initial physical examination should establish the neurovascular status of the extremity. Atrophy or swelling should be noted. Active and passive range of motion should be measured if the fracture is not casted or splinted. Drainage from the incision or wound after surgery for fractures is not normal and should be brought to the attention of the surgeon. Swelling may indicate deep venous thrombosis, dependent edema, or infection. Crepitus at the fracture site, especially with pain, suggests a nonunion or fixation failure. Pin sites should be clean and not draining.

Range of motion and mobilization of the joints proximally and distally will depend on the extent to which the bone has healed and rigidity of the fixation. Generally, fractures treated with internal fixation can begin early range of motion, but clearance should be obtained from the orthopedist. Often, the extremity benefits from elevation and splinting when not performing motion exercises. Weightbearing should be allowed as dictated by the surgeon. Typically, lower extremity fractures are protected from full weightbearing until some degree of bony union is obtained. This is usually a clinical judgment since radiographs often lag behind in demonstrating bony union.[1,2,5,10] The presence or absence of callus on radiographs will depend on the type of fixation and may not be a reliable measure of healing.[1,2] Weightbearing is usually begun earlier with intramedullary rods than with plates, but many factors prevent providing

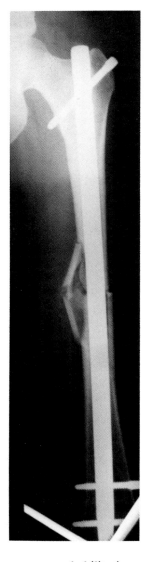

FIGURE 6.   An intramedullary rod in a fractured femur, with interlocking screws proximally and distally.

concrete rehabilitation guidelines. Each fracture and patient must be treated individually.

CASE STUDIES

Case 1

A 70-year-old hypertensive woman who lived alone fell and sustained a comminuted fracture of her hip (Fig. 8). She was otherwise in good health. She gave no history of syncope or palpitations prior to her fall. She was taken to surgery and, under epidural anesthesia, an open reduction and internal fixation

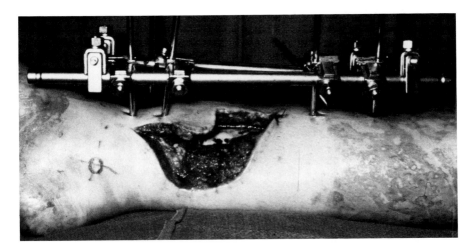

FIGURE 7.   An external fixator is applied to a comminuted, open tibial fracture. Screw holes are visible from a failed, infected plate that had been removed.

using a hip compression screw was performed. It was noted at the time of surgery that her bone was soft and that she had medial comminution in the area of the lesser trochanter. As a result of these findings, a longer side plate was used that allowed more stable shaft fixation of the device. This allowed a more rigid construct, capable of withstanding the stresses in the proximal femur. The patient was allowed to sit up in bed on the first postoperative day. On the second postoperative day, she was allowed to sit in a chair and was sent to therapy, where partial weightbearing was allowed (toe-touch progressing as tolerated). Gentle range of motion of the hip and knee was begun as tolerated several days after surgery. After 1 week in the hospital, she was transferred to an intermediate care nursing facility for 6 weeks. Quadriceps sets were begun as tolerated at 10 days. Out of concern for her bone quality, she used a walker for 6 weeks and was converted to using a cane prior to discharge to home.

This case demonstrates many of the principles of fracture management and care.[5,6] The forces acting on the intertrochanteric area are compression, shear bending, and torsion (Fig. 9). Comminution in this area and the patient's poor bone quality increase the stress on the fixation device. Studies have demonstrated that during ambulation the force acting on the femoral head is three to four times body weight.[3] Instrumented fracture fixation devices have demonstrated that forces acting on the implant during activities of daily living were nearly as high as those encountered during walking with external supports.[3] These studies were done with a nail plate, and it is unknown if the findings are applicable to other devices. Since most activities such as rolling over in bed or transferring cause high loads on these devices, most surgeons allow protected weightbearing until healing is demonstrated.

Case 2

A 50-year-old man tripped on his stairs, sustaining a fracture-dislocation of his left ankle (Fig. 10). His injury was closed with no lacerations. He was

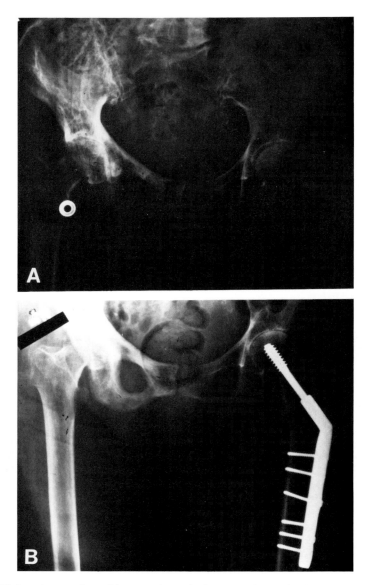

FIGURE 8. *A,* comminuted intertrochanteric fracture of the left hip. *B,* treatment with ORIF using a compression hip screw.

neurovascularly intact and had no other medical problems. A closed reduction of his talus was performed in the emergency room, and he later underwent open reduction–internal fixation of the fibula and tibia in the operating room. At the time of surgery, he was felt to have good bone, but his fibula was comminuted. To protect his fibular plate, he was kept nonweightbearing for 4 weeks after surgery.

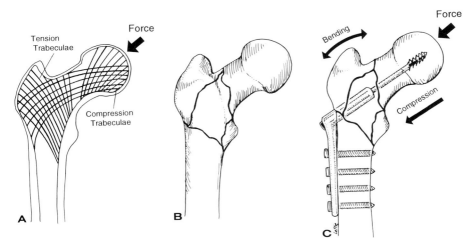

FIGURE 9.   *A,* the forces on the normal hip. *B,* intertrochanteric fractures frequently disrupt the medial side, where high compressive forces exist. *C,* ORIF attempts to restore this medial buttress and allows the fragments to collapse to a more stable position.

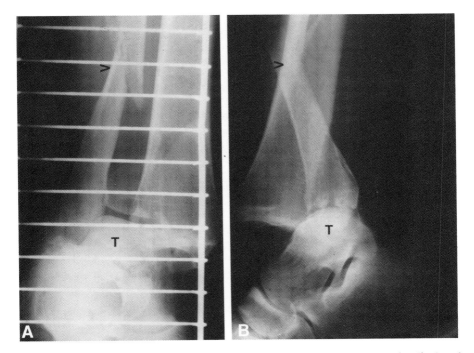

FIGURE 10 A and B.   Anteroposterior *(A)* and lateral *(B)* radiographs of a displaced ankle fracture with the broken fibula (open arrow) and dislocated talus (T).   *(Continued on following page)*

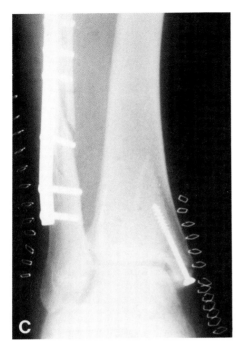

FIGURE 10 C. ORIF with plate and screws on the fibula and a screw in the medial malleolus.

Since the fixation was secure enough, range of motion exercises were begun 1 week after surgery, and he regained full function of the ankle.

This case demonstrates that even in the face of adequate fixation, comminution and lack of bone support can cause the postoperative care to be altered. A long "working distance" allows the plate to see more stress and biomechanically should be protected until some bony union has occurred. In ankle fractures where bone stock and fixation are adequate, weightbearing can often be begun within 2 weeks after surgery.

SUMMARY

Treatment and rehabilitation of fractures require an understanding of the biomechanical and biologic characteristics of bone fracture and healing. Interventions by the physician will be dictated by the fracture pattern and myriad other factors. Different types of fixation deal with the biomechanical forces differently. Successful rehabilitation requires that motion, strengthening, and weightbearing be begun at the right time to prevent failure of fixation. The race between fracture healing and failure of fixation requires knowledge of the biomechanical aspects of fracture treatment and rehabilitation.

ACKNOWLEDGMENTS

We would like to thank Dr. Ed Chao, Director of Biomechanics at Johns Hopkins University, for his review of this manuscript, and to Ms. Kris Hetman for her invaluable assistance.

REFERENCES

1. Aro HT, Wahner HT, Chao EYS: Healing patterns of transverse and oblique osteotomies in the canine tibia under external fixation. J Orthop Trauma 5:351–364, 1991.
2. Chao EYS, Aro HT: Biomechanics of fracture fixation. In Mow VC, Hayes WC (eds): Basic Orthopaedic Biomechanics. New York, Raven, 1991, pp 293–336.
3. Frankel VH, Nordin M: Basic Biomechanics of the Skeletal System. Philadelphia, Lea & Febiger, 1980.
4. Gonza ER, Harrington IJ: Biomechanics of Musculoskeletal Injury. Baltimore, Williams & Wilkins, 1989.
5. Hipp JJ, Cheal EJ, Hayes WC: Biomechanics of fractures. In Browner BD, Jupiter JJ, Levine AM, Trafton PG (eds): Skeletal Trauma. Philadelphia, WB Saunders, 1992, pp 95–126.
6. Lewis C, Knortz K (eds): Orthopedic Assessment and Treatment of the Geriatric Patient. St. Louis, Mosby, 1993.
7. Markel MD, Wikenheiser MA, Chao EYS: Formation of bone in tibial defects in a canine model. J Bone Joint Surg 73A:914–923, 1981.
8. McKibbin B: The biology of fracture healing in long bones. J Bone Joint Surg 60B:150–162, 1978.
9. Rand JA, An KN, Chao EYS, Kelly PJ: A comparison of the effect of open intramedullary nailing and compression-plate fixation on fracture-site blood flow and fracture healing. J Bone Joint Surg 63A:427–442, 1981.
10. Schenk RK: Biology of fracture repair. In Browner BD, Jupiter JJ, Levine AM, Trafton PG (eds): Skeletal Trauma. Philadelphia, WB Saunders, 1992, pp 31–76.

INDEX

Entries in **boldface type** signify complete articles.